Canine and Feline Respiratory Medicine: An Update

Editor

LYNELLE R. JOHNSON

VETERINARY CLINICS OF NORTH AMERICA: SMALL ANIMAL PRACTICE

www.vetsmall.theclinics.com

March 2020 • Volume 50 • Number 2

ELSEVIER

1600 John F. Kennedy Boulevard ● Suite 1800 ● Philadelphia, Pennsylvania, 19103-2899

http://www.vetsmall.theclinics.com

VETERINARY CLINICS OF NORTH AMERICA: SMALL ANIMAL PRACTICE Volume 50, Number 2
March 2020 ISSN 0195-5616, ISBN-13: 978-0-323-71173-9

Editor: Colleen Dietzler

Developmental Editor: Nicole Congleton

Veterinary Clinics of North America: Small Animal Practice (ISSN 0195-5616) is published bimonthly by Elsevier Inc., 360 Park Avenue South, New York, NY 10010-1710. Months of issue are January, March, May, July, September, and November. Business and Editorial Offices: 1600 John F. Kennedy Blvd., Ste. 1800, Philadelphia, PA 19103-2899. Customer Service Office: 3251 Riverport Lane, Maryland Heights, MO 63043. Periodicals postage paid at New York, NY and additional mailing offices. Subscription prices are $348.00 per year (domestic individuals), $705.00 per year (domestic institutions), $100.00 per year (domestic students/residents), $451.00 per year (Canadian individuals), $876.00 per year (Canadian institutions), $488.00 per year (international individuals), $876.00 per year (international institutions), $100.00 per year (Canadian students/residents), and $220.00 per year (international students/residents). To receive student/resident rate, orders must be accompanied by name of affiliated institution, date of term, and the *signature* of program/residency coordinator on institution letterhead. Orders will be billed at individual rate until proof of status is received. Foreign air speed delivery is included in all *Clinics* subscription prices. All prices are subject to change without notice. **POSTMASTER:** Send address changes to *Veterinary Clinics of North America: Small Animal Practice*, Elsevier Health Sciences Division, Subscription Customer Service, 3251 Riverport Lane, Maryland Heights, MO 63043. Customer Service (orders, claims, online, change of address): Elsevier Periodicals Customer Service, Elsevier Health Sciences Division Subscription **Customer Service 3251 Riverport Lane Maryland Heights, MO 63043. Tel: 1-800-654-2452 (U.S. and Canada); 314-447-8871 (outside U.S. and Canada). Fax: 314-447-8029. E-mail: journalscustomerservice-usa@elsevier.com (for print support); journalsonlinesupport-usa@elsevier.com (for online support).**

Reprints. For copies of 100 or more of articles in this publication, please contact the Commercial Reprints Department, Elsevier Inc., 360 Park Avenue South, New York, NY 10010-1710. Tel.: 212-633-3874; Fax: 212-633-3820; E-mail: reprints@elsevier.com.

Veterinary Clinics of North America: Small Animal Practice is also published in Japanese by Inter Zoo Publishing Co., Ltd., Aoyama Crystal-Bldg 5F, 3-5-12 Kitaaoyama, Minato-ku, Tokyo 107-0061, Japan.

Veterinary Clinics of North America: Small Animal Practice is covered in *Current Contents/Agriculture, Biology and Environmental Sciences, Science Citation Index, ASCA, MEDLINE/PubMed (Index Medicus), Excerpta Medica,* and *BIOSIS.*

Contributors

EDITOR

LYNELLE R. JOHNSON, DVM, MS, PhD
Diplomate, American College of Veterinary Internal Medicine (Small Animal Internal Medicine); Professor, Department of Medicine and Epidemiology, University of California, Davis, Veterinary Medicine: Medicine and Epidemiology, Davis, California, USA

AUTHORS

ANUSHA BALAKRISHNAN, BVSc
Diplomate, American College of Veterinary Emergency and Critical Care; Staff Criticalist, Cornell University Veterinary Specialists, Stamford, Connecticut, USA; Adjunct Assistant Clinical Professor, Emergency and Critical Care, Cornell University College of Veterinary Medicine, Ithaca, New York, USA

INGRID M. BALSA, DVM
Diplomate, American College of Veterinary Surgeons - Small Animal; Assistant Professor of Clinical Small Animal Surgery, Department of Veterinary Surgical and Radiological Sciences, School of Veterinary Medicine, University of California, Davis, Davis, California, USA

VANESSA R. BARRS, BVSc (Hons), PhD, MVetClinStud, FANZCVSc (Feline Medicine), GradCertEd (Higher Ed)
Chair Professor of Companion Animal Health, City University of Hong Kong, Department of Public Health & Infectious Diseases, Jockey Club College of Veterinary Medicine and Life Sciences, Kowloon, Hong Kong, SAR, China

LEAH A. COHN, DVM, PhD
Diplomate, American College of Veterinary Internal Medicine (Small Animal Internal Medicine); Professor, Department of Veterinary Medicine and Surgery, University of Missouri, Columbia, Missouri, USA

JONATHAN D. DEAR, MAS, DVM
Diplomate, American College of Veterinary Internal Medicine (Small Animal Internal Medicine); Assistant Professor of Clinical Internal Medicine, Department of Medicine and Epidemiology, University of California, Davis, Davis, California, USA

ANN DELLA MAGGIORE, DVM
Diplomate, American College of Veterinary Internal Medicine (Small Animal Internal Medicine); MarQueen Pet Emergency and Specialty Group, Roseville, California, USA

STEVEN E. EPSTEIN, DVM
Diplomate, American College of Veterinary Emergency and Critical Care; Associate Professor of Clinical Small Animal Emergency and Critical Care, Department of Veterinary Surgical and Radiological Sciences, School of Veterinary Medicine, University of California, Davis, Davis, California, USA

HENNA P. LAURILA, DVM, PhD
Clinical Teacher, Discipline of Small Animal Internal Medicine, Department of Equine and Small Animal Medicine, Faculty of Veterinary Medicine, University of Helsinki, Helsinki, Finland

CATRIONA M. MacPHAIL, DVM, PhD
Diplomate, American College of Veterinary Surgeons; ACVS Founding Fellow, Surgical Oncology; Professor, Small Animal Surgery, Department of Clinical Sciences, Colorado State University, Fort Collins, Colorado, USA

MINNA M. RAJAMÄKI, DVM, PhD
Adjunct Professor, Discipline of Small Animal Internal Medicine, Department of Equine and Small Animal Medicine, Faculty of Veterinary Medicine, University of Helsinki, Helsinki, Finland

KRYSTLE L. REAGAN, DVM, PhD
Infectious Disease Fellow, Veterinary Medical Teaching Hospital, University of California, Davis, Davis, California, USA

NICKI REED, BVM&S, Cert VR, MRCVS
Diploma in Small Animal Medicine (Feline), Diplomate, European College of Veterinary Internal Medicine Specialists - Companion Animals; Internal Medicine Specialist, Veterinary Specialists, Livingston, West Lothian, Scotland, United Kingdom

ELIZABETH ROZANSKI, DVM
Diplomate, American College of Veterinary Emergency and Critical Care, Diplomate, American College of Small Animal Internal Medicine (Small Animal Medicine); Section of Critical Care, Cummings School of Veterinary Medicine, North Grafton, Massachusetts, USA

JANE E. SYKES, BVSc (Hons), PhD
Professor of Small Animal Internal Medicine, Chief Veterinary Medical Officer and Associate Dean for Veterinary Medical Center Operations, Veterinary Medical Teaching Hospital, University of California, Davis, Davis, California, USA

JESSICA J. TALBOT, BVSc (Hons), BSc (Vet), PhD
University of Sydney, Faculty of Science, Sydney School of Veterinary Science, Camperdown, New South Wales, Australia

CARISSA W. TONG, BVM&S
Member of Royal College of Veterinary Surgeons, Resident, Emergency and Critical Care, Cornell University Veterinary Specialists, Stamford, Connecticut, USA

JULIE E. TRZIL, DVM, MS
Diplomate, American College of Veterinary Internal Medicine (Small Animal Internal Medicine); Internist, IndyVet Emergency and Specialty Hospital, Indianapolis, Indiana, USA

Contents

Preface: Respiratory Diseases in Dogs and Cats　　　　　　　　　ix

Lynelle R. Johnson

Clinical Application of Pulmonary Function Testing in Small Animals　　273

Anusha Balakrishnan and Carissa W. Tong

Pulmonary function tests (PFTs) are important diagnostic tools that have wide clinical applications in human and veterinary medicine. Widespread use of PFTs in measuring lung volumes in veterinary medicine was historically limited by the need for specialized equipment to accurately perform and interpret these tests, and by lack of patient cooperation. However, recent advances and modifications have allowed PFTs to be safely performed in conscious veterinary patients with minimal stress. This article focuses on the most commonly used tests of pulmonary function including tests of pulmonary mechanics and of gas exchange in the lungs.

Laryngeal Disease in Dogs and Cats: An Update　　　　　　　　　295

Catriona M. MacPhail

 Video content accompanies this article at http://www.vetsmall. theclinics.com

Laryngeal diseases are manifested by obstructive breathing patterns reflecting functional or mechanical upper airway obstruction. Laryngeal paralysis is the most common disease of the larynx. Diagnosis requires close attention to anesthetic plane and coordination of respiratory effort with laryngeal motion. Surgical arytenoid lateralization improves clinical signs and quality of life in dogs; however, aspiration pneumonia is a recognized complication, and generalized neuropathy can progress. Laryngeal collapse can result from any cause of chronic upper airway obstruction but is most often associated with brachycephalic obstructive airway syndrome. Although uncommon, laryngeal neoplasia has a guarded to grave prognosis regardless of treatment.

Chronic Rhinitis in the Cat: An Update　　　　　　　　　　　　311

Nicki Reed

The etiology of feline chronic rhinitis is incompletely understood and often is a diagnosis of exclusion. History, clinical signs, and investigations performed to reach this diagnosis are discussed. Several treatment options are provided, although cure of this frustrating disease is rarely achieved.

Fungal Rhinosinusitis and Disseminated Invasive Aspergillosis in Cats　　331

Vanessa R. Barrs and Jessica J. Talbot

Fungal rhinosinusitis, including sinonasal aspergillosis (SNA) and sinoorbital aspergillosis (SOA), is the most common type of aspergillosis encountered in cats. Other focal forms of aspergillosis including disseminated invasive aspergillosis occur less frequently. SOA is an invasive mycosis that is increasingly recognized and is most commonly caused by Aspergillus felis, a close relative of Aspergillus fumigatus. SNA can be invasive or noninvasive and is most commonly caused by A fumigatus and Aspergillus niger. Molecular methods are required to correctly identify the fungi that cause SNA and SOA. SNA has a favorable prognosis with treatment, whereas the prognosis for SOA remains poor.

Canine Nasal Disease: An Update   359

Leah A. Cohn

Nasal disease in dogs is common and is often accompanied by chronic nasal discharge with or without other clinical signs. A thorough history and physical examination often guide the most appropriate choice of diagnostic testing to provide the best chance of attaining a diagnosis as to cause, and therefore, the most appropriate treatment. The purpose of this article is to guide the practitioner through a logical approach to the evaluation of dogs that are presented with signs of nasal disease.

Feline Asthma: Diagnostic and Treatment Update   375

Julie E. Trzil

Asthma is an important allergic lower-airway disease in cats affecting approximately 1% to 5% of the pet cat population. New diagnostics are being developed to help better differentiate asthma from other lower-airway diseases and improve monitoring. In addition, new treatments are being developed to help in refractory cases or in those cases in which traditional therapeutics are contraindicated. This article discusses potential pitfalls in the diagnosis of asthma. In addition, current literature investigating new diagnostic tests and therapies for feline asthma is reviewed.

Canine Chronic Bronchitis: An Update   393

Elizabeth Rozanski

Chronic bronchitis is a syndrome defined by cough on most days for at least 2 months for which no specific cause can be identified. Older small breed dogs are most commonly affected, but bronchitis can also be documented in midsized and larger breed dogs. Diagnostic testing includes physical examination, laboratory testing, radiography, and airway evaluation via bronchoscopy, cytology, and culture. Treatment is directed at reducing exposure to irritants, reducing airway inflammation, and controlling cough.

Canine Infectious Respiratory Disease   405

Krystle L. Reagan and Jane E. Sykes

Canine infectious respiratory disease complex (CIRDC) refers to a syndrome of diseases that can be caused by several different bacterial and viral pathogens. These pathogens are often highly contagious, and coinfections are common. Clinical signs are frequently mild and self-limiting; however, some individual cases progress to severe disease. Clinical diagnosis of CIRDC is often based on history of exposure and physical examination findings; however, determining the etiologic agent requires application of specific diagnostic tests, and results can be difficult to interpret because of widespread subclinical infections.

An Update on Tracheal and Airway Collapse in Dogs   419

Ann Della Maggiore

Tracheal and airway collapse (bronchomalacia) are common causes of chronic cough in middle-aged to older dogs in which weakening of cartilage within the respiratory system leads to narrowing of airways, irritation, inflammation, partial to complete airway obstruction, and other secondary effects. Tracheomalacia occurs in small-breed dogs, whereas bronchomalacia can occur in any size dog. Successful treatment involves correct identification of the problem, recognition of concurrent disease processes, and appropriate medical therapy. Surgical intervention and intraluminal stenting are readily available so it is important to understand indications for such procedures.

Update on Canine Idiopathic Pulmonary Fibrosis in West Highland White Terriers   431

Henna P. Laurila and Minna M. Rajamäki

Canine idiopathic pulmonary fibrosis (CIPF) is a chronic, progressive, interstitial lung disease (ILD) affecting older West Highland white terriers (WHWTs). According to one classification, CIPF is a familial fibrotic ILD in the group of idiopathic interstitial pneumonias. Etiology is unknown but likely arises from interplay between genetic and environmental factors. CIPF shares features with human idiopathic pulmonary fibrosis and human nonspecific interstitial pneumonia. This article describes clinical signs, findings in physical examination, arterial oxygenation, diagnostic imaging, bronchoscopy, bronchoalveolar lavage, histopathology, disease course, and outcome of WHWTs with CIPF; compares canine and human diseases; summarizes biomarker research; and gives an overview of potential treatment.

Bacterial Pneumonia in Dogs and Cats: An Update   447

Jonathan D. Dear

Bacterial pneumonia is a common clinical diagnosis in dogs but seems to occur less often in cats. Underlying causes include viral infection, aspiration injury, foreign body inhalation, and defects in clearance of respiratory secretions. Identification of the specific organisms involved in disease, appropriate use of antibiotics and adjunct therapy, and control of risk factors for pneumonia improve management.

Canine and Feline Exudative Pleural Diseases   467

Steven E. Epstein and Ingrid M. Balsa

Exudative pleural diseases are a common cause of respiratory distress and systemic illness in dogs and cats. This article covers the pathophysiology, development, and classification of exudative pleural effusions. The most current diagnostic strategies, causes, imaging findings, and medical or surgical treatment options for select diseases are reviewed in detail.

VETERINARY CLINICS OF NORTH AMERICA: SMALL ANIMAL PRACTICE

FORTHCOMING ISSUES

May 2020
Small Animal Euthanasia: Updates on Clinical Practice
Beth Marchitelli, Tami Shearer, *Editors*

July 2020
Feline Practice: Integrating Medicine and Well-Being: Part I
Margie Scherk, *Editor*

September 2020
Feline Practice: Integrating Medicine and Well-Being: Part II
Margie Scherk, *Editor*

RECENT ISSUES

January 2020
Minimally Invasive Fracture Repair
Karl C. Maritato and
Matthew D. Barnhart, *Editors*

November 2019
Alternatives to Opioid Analgesia in Small Animal Anesthesia
Ciara Barr and Giacomo Gianotti, *Editors*

September 2019
Cancer in Companion Animals
Philip J. Bergman and Craig Clifford, *Editors*

SERIES OF RELATED INTEREST

Veterinary Clinics of North America: Exotic Animal Practice
https://www.vetexotic.theclinics.com/

THE CLINICS ARE NOW AVAILABLE ONLINE!
Access your subscription at:
www.theclinics.com

Preface

Respiratory Diseases in Dogs and Cats

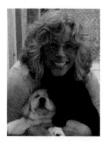

Lynelle R. Johnson, DVM, MS, PhD
Editor

Respiratory medicine remains a field rich in discovery through research as well as through clinical practice. This issue of *Veterinary Clinics of North America: Small Animal Practice* brings together a group of talented, practicing veterinarians from academic institutions and specialty hospitals that has extensive clinical experience managing cases involving the respiratory tract. Authors share their knowledge with the reader and provide a review of the literature on common diseases, including feline asthma, laryngeal paralysis, pneumonia, and bronchomalacia. Each author offers the reader insight gained from their experiences in clinical medicine and shares well-written and nicely illustrated articles. Each article appropriately references the current literature, allowing the reader to pursue further investigations as needed.

I am grateful to the authors for their devotion to the task set forth and am certain that readers will greatly appreciate their diagnostic and treatment recommendations. We hope that this issue of *Veterinary Clinics of North America: Small Animal Practice* will serve as a resource in the years to come. Patients and clients alike will benefit from the expertise offered by these brilliant and thoughtful clinicians.

Lynelle R. Johnson, DVM, MS, PhD
Department of Medicine and Epidemiology
University of California, Davis
2108 Tupper Hall
Davis, CA 95616, USA

E-mail address:
lrjohnson@ucdavis.edu

Vet Clin Small Anim 50 (2020) ix
https://doi.org/10.1016/j.cvsm.2019.11.005
0195-5616/20/© 2019 Published by Elsevier Inc.

vetsmall.theclinics.com

Clinical Application of Pulmonary Function Testing in Small Animals

Anusha Balakrishnan, BVSc[a,b],*, Carissa W. Tong, BVM&S, MRCVS[a]

KEYWORDS

- Pulmonary function testing • Spirometry • Tidal flow volume breathing loops
- Plethysmography • Arterial blood gas • Capnography • Pulse oximetry

KEY POINTS

- The most widely available tool for assessment of pulmonary function is pulse oximetry; however, it provides only a crude assessment of oxygenation.
- Lung function tests are divided broadly into those that measure lung mechanics and those that measure gas exchange capabilities.
- Pulmonary function tests (PFTs) do not identify specific diagnoses but instead are used to quantify the severity of respiratory system dysfunction.
- In some cases, these tests are used to determine the anatomic location of disease in the respiratory tract (eg, upper vs lower airway disease).

PULMONARY FUNCTION TESTING

Pulmonary function tests (PFTs) are widely used in human patients in respiratory medicine, sports medicine, and occupational health to provide an objective assessment of lung function. They provide information regarding the large and small airways and the pulmonary parenchyma, including the capillary bed. In human and veterinary medicine, PFTs are used to evaluate patients with known or suspected respiratory disease either as preanesthetic evaluation or to aid diagnosis, and monitoring the efficacy of therapeutic interventions to guide further treatments.

PFTs are generally benign, but specific contraindications exist. PFTs are dependent on patient effort; therefore, any concurrent thoracic or abdominal pain can inhibit obtaining optimal test results. Important contraindications include the following[1]:

[a] Emergency and Critical Care, Cornell University Veterinary Specialists, 880 Canal Street, Stamford, CT 06902, USA; [b] Emergency and Critical Care, Cornell University College of Veterinary Medicine, Ithaca, NY, USA
* Corresponding author. Cornell University Veterinary Specialists, 880 Canal Street, Stamford, CT 06902.
E-mail address: abalakrishnan@cuvs.org

Vet Clin Small Anim 50 (2020) 273–294
https://doi.org/10.1016/j.cvsm.2019.10.004
0195-5616/20/© 2019 Elsevier Inc. All rights reserved.

1. Pneumothorax
2. Hemoptysis of unknown origin
3. Hemodynamic instability, specifically pulmonary thromboembolism
4. Recent thoracoabdominal surgery
5. Recent ophthalmic surgery
6. Infectious respiratory disease

It is important to remember that PFTs do not identify specific diagnoses. Instead, they are used to quantify the severity of respiratory system dysfunction, and in some cases to determine the anatomic location of the disease in the respiratory tract. Widespread use of PFTs in measuring lung volumes in veterinary medicine was historically limited by the need for specialized equipment to accurately perform and interpret these tests, and by lack of patient cooperation. However, recent advances and modifications have allowed PFTs to be safely performed in conscious veterinary patients with minimal stress. Instruments, such as blood gas analyzers and pulse oximeters, are also readily available in most practices, and this type of PFT can easily be applied to small animal patients.

Tests of pulmonary function are broadly divided into two major categories: tests of lung mechanics and tests of pulmonary gas exchange.

TESTS OF LUNG MECHANICS

Lung mechanics reflect the physical properties of the lungs and evaluate the relationship between airway pressure, air flow, and lung volumes.

Spirometry

Spirometry is one of the most basic PFTs. It measures the volume of air or rate of airflow in and out of the respiratory system. It is the accepted standard for diagnosis of obstructive respiratory disease in human medicine[2–4] and is used to diagnose upper or lower airway obstructions in veterinary patients with such conditions as tracheal collapse, brachycephalic airway disease, and feline lower airway diseases. Spirometry can also be used to evaluate ventilatory function in patients with neuromuscular disease or postanesthesia. **Table 1** lists normal values for dogs and cats.

Table 1
Normal reported values for respiratory parameters in dogs and cats

Parameter	Unit	Dog	Cat
Tidal volume	mL	10–20 mL/kg	10–20 mL/kg
Minute ventilation	mL/min	150–250 mL/kg	150–250 mL/kg
Respiratory rate	bpm	32 ± 10	43 ± 7
Inspiratory time	ms	920 ± 350	716.6 ± 139.5
Expiratory time	ms	1170 ± 480	703.7 ± 133.0
Peak inspiratory flow	mL/s	740 ± 240	110.0 ± 26.6
Peak expiratory flow	mL/s	780 ± 230	113.7 ± 29.1
Dynamic compliance	mL/cm H_2O	117 ± 46	19.8
Static compliance	mL/cm H_2O	42.25 ± 32	NA
Lung resistance	cm H_2O/L/s	0.8–4.2	28.9

NA, not applicable.
Adapted from Rozanski EL, Hoffman AM. Pulmonary function testing in small animals. *Clin Tech Small Anim Prac* 1999;14(4):237-241; with permission.

Spirometry is performed using a handheld spirometer or a pneumotachograph, which is connected to an endotracheal tube in an anesthetized patient or attached to a tight face mask fitted over the snout of an awake patient. The pneumotachograph is used to measure flow rates and duration of the various segments of a given breath, including inspiratory time (TI), expiratory time (TE), tidal volume (VT), and peak inspiratory flow (PIF) and peak expiratory flow (PEF) rates.[2] Human patients undergoing spirometry are instructed to take a full inspiration and then exhale forcefully for as long as possible, thereby measuring the forced vital capacity. Because this is challenging in veterinary patients, the use of spirometry in veterinary medicine is confined to tests of spontaneous VTs in awake or anesthetized patients.

Tidal Breathing Flow-Volume Loops

Flow-volume loops are graphical representations of the relationship between dynamic parameters of airflow and volume during various stages of inspiration and expiration, allowing identification of airway obstruction. Adult human patients that are able to cooperate can complete the forced/maximum expiratory and/or inspiratory maneuvers that are needed to obtain maximum expiratory and inspiratory flow volumes. However, infants and critically ill patients and veterinary patients are not cooperative; therefore, tidal breathing flow-volume loops (TBFVLs) were introduced and subsequently used in veterinary medicine. In small animal patients, airway function is evaluated during tidal breathing by analyzing airflow patterns and waveforms using a face mask. Evaluation of awake patients is preferred to that of anesthetized patients, because their upper airway is not bypassed by endotracheal intubation.

To record TBFVL, patients should be calm and unsedated, standing and breathing room air in a nonstressful environment. A tight-fitting face mask of an appropriate size is placed over the mouth, including the lip commissures, and attached to a pneumotachograph. The patient should be allowed to adapt for 2 to 3 minutes before starting measurements. The pneumotachograph, along with an X-Y recorder to plot a graph, is used to document the relationship among air flow, volume, and time. In a spontaneous breath, the inspiratory arm of the loop is negative, and the expiratory arm is positive. Loops are analyzed to evaluate qualitative and quantitative parameters (**Fig. 1**). Qualitative parameters refer to the overall shape of the loop. Quantitative parameters include

- VT
- Respiratory rate (RR)
- PIF and PEF
- Midtidal inspiratory and expiratory flow rates (IF_{50}, EF_{50})
- Inspiratory and expiratory flow at end-expiratory volume plus 25% of VT
- TI and TE

TBFVL are useful in detecting changes in airflow in animals with fixed and dynamic upper airway obstructions.[5,6] Fixed upper airway obstructions, such as a laryngeal mass or end-stage collapse, cause limitations in airflow (flattening) in the inspiratory and expiratory portions of the loops (**Fig. 2**). Dynamic airflow obstructions cause more marked changes in one phase of the loop over the other, depending on the location of the obstruction (see **Fig. 2**A; **Fig. 3**). Dynamic upper airway obstruction, such as tracheal collapse or early laryngeal paralysis, causes flattening of the inspiratory phase, whereas dynamic lower airway obstruction, such as chronic bronchitis, causes concavity or flattening of the late expiratory phase of the loop (**Fig. 4**).[5,6]

TBFVL have been evaluated in healthy dogs and cats, and cats with lower airway disease and dogs with tracheal masses and tracheal collapse.[7–10] Cats with bronchial

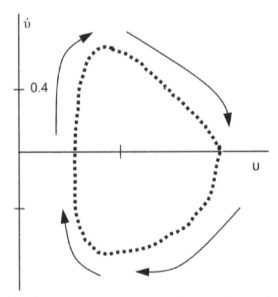

Fig. 1. Tidal breathing flow-volume loop from a conscious, healthy dog. Inspiratory gas flow increases gradually, reaching plateau at 40% inspiratory VT, which then returns to zero. Expiratory flow rises rapidly at the beginning of expiration, then ceases gradually to zero without any plateau. (*From* Adamama-Moraitou KK, Pardali D, Menexes G, Athanasiou LV, Kazakos G, Rallis TS. Tidal breathing flow volume loop analysis of 21 healthy, unsedated, young adult male Beagle dogs. Australian Veterinary Journal. 2013;91(6):226-232; with permission.)

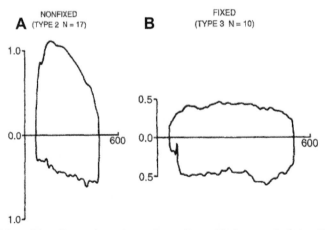

Fig. 2. Tidal breathing flow-volume loops from dogs with laryngeal obstruction. (*A*) Dog with a dynamic laryngeal obstruction; note the early decrease in peak inspiratory flow. (*B*) Dog with a fixed laryngeal obstruction where the inspiratory and expiratory portions of the loops are blunted. (*From* Amis TC, Kupershoek C. Tidal breathing flow-volume loop analysis for clinical assessment of airway obstruction in dogs. *Am J Vet Res* 1986;47:1002-1006; with permission.)

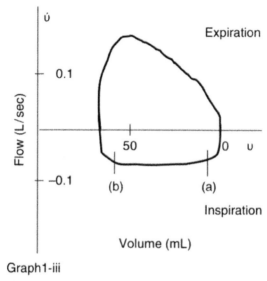

Graph1-iii

Fig. 3. Tidal breathing flow-volume loops in a dog with tracheal collapse. (a) Beginning of inspiratory plateau. (b) End of inspiratory plateau. (*From* Pardali D, Adamama-Moraitou KK, Rallis TS, Raptopoulos D, Gioulekas D. Tidal Breathing Flow-Volume Loop Analysis for the Diagnosis and Staging of Tracheal Collapse in Dogs. *Journal of Veterinary Internal Medicine.* 2010;24(4):832-842; with permission.)

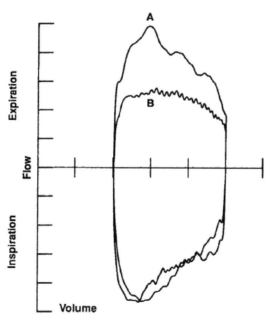

Fig. 4. Tidal breathing flow-volume loops of healthy and bronchitic cats. Note the similar inspiratory flow but marked difference in expiratory flow between normal (A) and bronchitic (B) cats. (*From* McKiernan BC, Dye JA, Rozanski EL. Tidal breathing flow-volume loops in healthy and bronchitic cats. *J Vet Intern Med* 1993;7:388-393; with permission.)

disease have an increased ratio of TE to TI, lower expiratory flow rates, decreased area under total and peak expiratory flow curves, and decreased tidal breathing expiratory volumes (see **Fig. 4**).[10–12] In dogs, the TE/TI, TI/total tidal volume (TTOT), and EF_{75}/IF_{75} can be used to differentiate healthy dogs from dogs clinically affected by tracheal collapse.[7] Because TBFVL has shown good agreement with tracheoscopy, it is used as a quick, noninvasive test for diagnosis of tracheal collapse.[7] Lack of available equipment and trained personnel has limited use of this technique in clinical practice.

Lung Compliance

Compliance, expressed in L/cm H_2O, is a measure of the distensibility of elastic lung tissue, and is described as the change in lung volume for a given change in airway pressure.[13,14] Compliance is routinely monitored during positive pressure ventilation in veterinary patients and the reported values reflect compliance of the lungs and the thoracic wall. Lung compliance is typically measured in intubated patients, with esophageal pressure measured as an approximation of intrapleural pressure to calculate transpulmonary pressure. A pneumotachometer that records respiratory volumes and a pressure transducer attached to the end of the endotracheal tube are required. At points of zero gas flow, pressures measured at the airway are equal to alveolar pressures. Compliance is highly dependent on the size of the patient; lung volumes developed by a given airway pressure are much larger in the lungs of a Great Dane compared with a Chihuahua.

Compliance is either static or dynamic. Static compliance is defined as the change in volume for a given change in transpulmonary pressure with zero gas flow.[15] To calculate static compliance, airway pressures and volumes are measured during a brief inspiratory hold (plateau). The inspiratory plateau allows redistribution of air throughout small airways that have variable time constants and are slower to open at the end of inspiration:

Static compliance = ΔV/(Plateau pressure – PEEP)

where ΔV = change in volume, and PEEP = positive end-expiratory pressure.

Dynamic compliance is defined as the change in volume for a given change in transpulmonary pressure during active gas flow, such as during inspiration and expiration in animals on positive pressure ventilation. Dynamic compliance is therefore the slope of the line between the two points of zero airflow at the end of exhalation and at the end of inspiration (**Fig. 5**)[15]:

Dynamic compliance = ΔV/(PIP-PEEP)

where ΔV = change in volume, PIP = peak inspiratory pressure, and PEEP = positive end-expiratory pressure.

In disease conditions where lung compliance is reduced, higher airway pressures are required to deliver a normal VT. Such diseases include[14]

- Acute respiratory distress syndrome (ARDS)
- Pneumonia
- Pulmonary fibrosis
- Pulmonary edema (cardiogenic and noncardiogenic)

Lung Resistance

Resistance, expressed as cm H_2O/L/s, is a measure of the amount of pressure required to deliver a given gas flow.[13] Lung resistance is a function of the

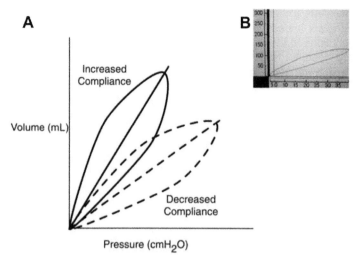

Fig. 5. (*A, B*) Illustration of pressure-volume loops and dynamic compliance. Note the markedly decreased dynamic compliance documented in the photograph (*B*) of a patient on a ventilator. (*From* Corona TM, Aumann M. Ventilator waveform interpretation in mechanically ventilated small animals. *J Vet Emerg Crit Care* 2011;21(5):496-514; with permission.)

nondistensible components of the respiratory system (the airways). It is a test of the patency of small bronchi that are deep within the lung. Lung resistance is measured using the same equipment as compliance.

In the normal lung, airway resistance is low, allowing for easy flow of air during either spontaneous or positive pressure breaths. Like compliance, resistance is dependent on body weight: larger flow rates are expected in bigger animals for a given change in airway pressure. Pathologic conditions that increase airway resistance include those that impede airflow in the small bronchi, such as canine chronic bronchitis and feline lower airway disease (bronchitis or feline asthma).

Whole-Body Plethysmography

Plethysmography measures the absolute lung volume and airway resistance and is considered the gold standard test for determining lung volumes in cases of airway obstruction.[16–18] It measures the total lung capacity, functional residual capacity, and residual volume of the lung. Plethysmography can occasionally overestimate lung volumes in patients that are panting or hyperventilating, with some human studies finding differences of 1 L when lung volumes are measured via plethysmography compared with helium dilution techniques.

Traditional plethysmography in human medicine involves placing the patient inside a sealed chamber with a single mouthpiece. At the end of normal expiration, the mouthpiece is closed, and the patient is then asked to make an inspiratory effort. As the patient inhales against the closed mouthpiece, the chest cavity and lungs expand, decreasing pressure within the lungs. The increase in thoracic volume increases pressure within the closed system of the box, and the volume of the box decreases to accommodate the new volume of the patient's body. The volume within the lungs is then calculated using Boyle's law. This is a useful way of evaluating a patient for objective evidence of lung disease.[16]

Traditional plethysmography in small animals is challenging because the increase in resistance to flow imposed on the animal during inspiration is usually not tolerated well. Modifications to the traditional methods have been made to allow ease of use in veterinary patients. Head out whole-body plethysmography was developed for use in dogs to overcome the tendency of canine patients to pant when in an enclosed box. In this technique, dogs are placed in an airtight glass box that has a fixed volume, with their heads protruding out of box. A pneumotachograph and face mask are then fitted over the nose and mouth and flow measurements are obtained.[17–19]

Barometric whole-body plethysmography (BWBP) has recently been introduced as a noninvasive PFT alternative. The animal is placed into a sealed chamber with preset bias flow. Bias flow refers to the amount of air that is applied via the inlet and outlet to prevent CO_2 buildup in the chamber. In this technique, respiration (nasal flow and thoracic movement) causes barometric pressure oscillations proportional to VT. Exhaled air, which is humidified and warmed, creates a larger pressure change than inspired air even though the flow rates are identical. Because the signals are not a direct measurement of airflow at the nasal opening (as in people), they are referred to as pseudoflow and pseudovolume estimates. A pneumotachograph of known resistance is mounted on the wall of the chamber in which the animal is placed, and a pressure transducer is connected to the recording device. The animal moves around the chamber freely and signals produced by inhaled and exhaled air are recorded. BWBP parameters under tidal breathing, including RR, pseudoflow (PIF, PEF), pseudovolume, and time-related variables (TI, TE, and relaxation time [RT]) can be recorded (**Fig. 6**).[20,21] Airway resistance is approximated using enhanced pause

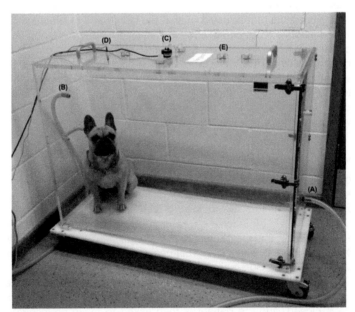

Fig. 6. Chamber used for barometric whole-body plethysmography in a French Bulldog. A pole of the chamber pressure differential transducer is opened to the top of the chamber (C). Two inlets (A, B) are connected to the front and back of the chamber to ventilate with bias air flow. An audio sensor is located at the top of the chamber (D) together with pneumotachograph screens (E). (*From* Liu N-C, Sargan DR, Adams VJ, Ladlow JF. Characterisation of Brachycephalic Obstructive Airway Syndrome in French Bulldogs Using Whole-Body Barometric Plethysmography. *PLOS ONE.* 2015;10(6):e0130741.)

(Penh) as a surrogate. Penh is a unitless index of airflow limitation or bronchoconstriction, and is calculated using the formula: Penh = PEF/PIF × (TE-RT)/RT.[20,22] BWBP has been evaluated in healthy, obese cats and cats with lower airway disease[20,22,23] and in healthy dogs and dogs with brachycephalic obstructive airway syndrome.[21,24–26] In cats, it has been shown that BWBP flow tracings are affected by artifactual waveforms caused by nonbreath movements or vocalizations; therefore, simultaneous visual monitoring is recommended.[27]

BWBP also has been extensively studied in brachycephalic breeds and Liu and colleagues[21,25] have established BWBP as a clinical tool to determine the severity of brachycephalic obstructive airway syndrome (BOAS) noninvasively and objectively (**Fig. 7**). Compared with a nonbrachycephalic dog, the flow tracing from a brachycephalic breed with clinical BOAS showed a flattened inspiratory phase with bursts of high-frequency flow oscillations during inspiration and occasionally during expiration (see **Fig. 7**). BWBP is a new tool for clinicians to diagnose BOAS, monitor disease progression, and for evaluating surgical outcomes without need for sedation or anesthesia, which carry a degree of risk in brachycephalic breeds.

Forced Oscillation Technique

The forced oscillation technique (FOT) is used in people to measure respiratory impedance and its two components: respiratory system resistance and reactance. Unlike spirometry, it requires passive cooperation and no forced expiratory maneuvers. It provides information on mechanical characteristics of the respiratory system that are complementary to spirometry. FOT measures lung function by using sinusoidal sound waves of single frequencies that are generated by a loudspeaker and passed into the lungs during tidal breathing. Higher frequencies (<20 Hz) travel shorter distance and are reflective of larger airways, whereas lower frequencies (<15 Hz) travel deep into the lungs and are reflective of small airways and the pulmonary parenchyma. The main limitation of FOT is that it does not distinguish between restrictive and obstructive lung disease.[28–30] To the authors' knowledge, this technique has not been explored in veterinary medicine.

TESTS OF PULMONARY GAS EXCHANGE
Diffusion Capacity of Carbon Monoxide

Diffusion capacity of carbon monoxide (DLCO) studies the diffusion of CO across the alveolar-capillary membrane. The test is based on the principle of hemoglobin having an increased affinity to preferentially bind carbon monoxide, as compared with oxygen. It is interpreted in conjunction with spirometry and lung volumes. When lung volumes and spirometry are normal but DLCO is lower than the predicted range, it indicates reduced diffusion. It is mainly used in people for the diagnosis of pulmonary arterial hypertension and systemic sclerosis, with or without concurrent interstitial lung disease. DLCO cannot definitively diagnose the previously mentioned conditions, but its value predicts mortality in a variety of diseases including neoplasia, interstitial lung disease, and severe pulmonary hypertension.[31,32] To the authors' knowledge, this technique has only been evaluated in large animal medicine.

Arterial Blood Gas Analysis

Arterial blood gas analysis is considered the gold standard test for evaluating oxygenation and ventilation.[33] Samples in small animal patients are drawn from various locations including the dorsal metatarsal, coccygeal, sublingual, femoral, or

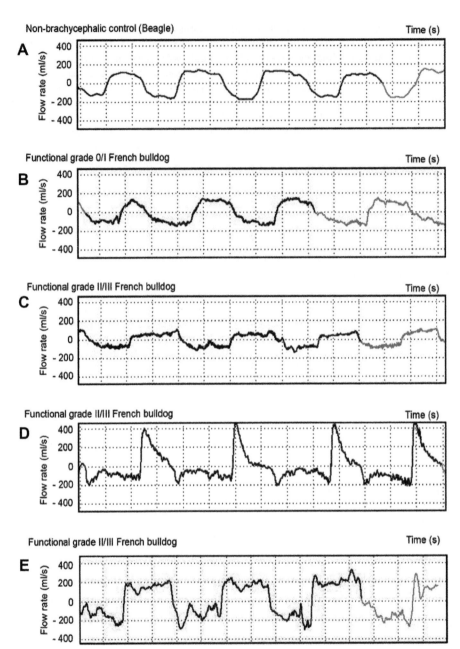

Fig. 7. Respiratory flow trace samples from barometric whole body plethysmography. (*A*) Flow traces of a nonbrachycephalic control. (*B*) Flow traces of a Function grade 0/1 French bulldog. (*C*) French Bulldog with grade I/III BOAS. (*D* and *E*) French Bulldog with grade III/III BOAS. (*From* Liu N-C, Sargan DR, Adams VJ, et al. Characterisation of Brachycephalic Obstructive Airway Syndrome in French Bulldogs Using Whole-Body Barometric Plethysmography. PLOS ONE 2015;10(6):e0130741; with permission.)

aural arteries. In animals requiring repeated sampling, arterial catheters are placed for easy access. Samples should be collected into preheparinized arterial blood gas syringes. All air bubbles should be removed to render the sample anaerobic, and the syringe capped and processed immediately. Samples can also be collected in regular 1- to 2-mL syringes that have been preheparinized by drawing up heparin and then squirting it out immediately. Samples not run within 5 to 10 minutes should be capped to avoid gas diffusion and equilibration with atmospheric oxygen and carbon dioxide and are refrigerated or placed on ice to prevent cell metabolism, which would distort the results.

A typical arterial blood gas measures the following values (reference ranges for dogs and cats are listed in **Table 2**):

- Pao_2
- $Paco_2$
- Arterial pH
- Other acid-base parameters are calculated rather than directly measured, including bicarbonate and base excess

Only arterial samples are used to evaluate oxygenation. Oxygenation is the process by which oxygen diffuses passively from the alveolus into the blood. Reduced oxygenation is termed hypoxemia. Hypoxemia is defined as a reduced arterial oxygen tension (Pao_2) lower than 80 mm Hg. For proper interpretation of an arterial blood gas analysis, an understanding of the major physiologic causes of hypoxemia is necessary. The main causes of hypoxemia include

- Decreased fraction of inspired oxygen (Fio_2)
- Ventilation-perfusion (V/Q) mismatch
- Anatomic shunts
- Diffusion impairment
- Hypoventilation

It is also prudent not to confuse hypoxemia with hypoxia. Hypoxia refers to reduced oxygen supply at the tissue level, which is not measured by a laboratory value. The four main causes of hypoxia include

1. Hypoxic hypoxia: reduced arterial oxygen tension (ie, decreased Pao_2)
2. Circulatory/stagnant hypoxia: reduced oxygen delivery secondary to reduced blood flow (eg, circulatory shock in sepsis, congestive heart failure)
3. Anemic hypoxia: reduced oxygen carrying capacity (eg, anemia, carbon monoxide poisoning)

Table 2		
Normal arterial blood gas values in dogs and cats		
Value	**Dog**	**Cat**
pH	7.31–7.46	7.21–7.41
Pao_2	92 mm Hg (80–105)	105 mm Hg (95–115)
$Paco_2$	37 mm Hg (32–43)	31 mm Hg (26–36)
Sao_2	>95%	>95%

Abbreviations: Sao_2, arterial oxygen saturation; Spo_2, oxygen saturation as measured by pulse oximetry.

From Balakrishnan A, King LG. Updates on pulmonary function testing in small animals. Vet Clin North Am Small Anim Pract. 2014;44(1):1-18; with permission.

4. Histotoxic hypoxia: inability to use oxygen even in the absence of hypoxemia (eg, cyanide poisoning)

Venous samples are not useful to evaluate oxygenation. Instead, serial measurement of venous oxygen concentrations is used to infer the ability of tissue to extract oxygen. Poor tissue perfusion can lead to high values for venous oxygen caused by reduced extraction.

Ventilation is the ability of the animal to move air in and out of the lungs. CO_2 is produced in tissues as a normal by-product of metabolism and eliminated through the airways. Elimination of CO_2 is dependent on minute ventilation, the volume of air moving through the airways in a given period of time (VT × RR), usually expressed as L/min. Because carbon dioxide is about 20 times more soluble than oxygen, there is a linear relationship between $Paco_2$ and minute ventilation. Disease processes that result in abnormal ventilation and are detected by changes in the $Paco_2$ are listed in **Table 3**.

If an arterial sample cannot be obtained, a venous sample is used to assess ventilation. Central venous samples obtained from a central vein, such as the jugular vein or caudal vena, or a mixed venous sample is obtained from a pulmonary artery catheter to evaluate $PcvCO_2$, which serves as a surrogate for alveolar ventilation. If these are not available, a peripheral venous sample is used to evaluate $PvCO_2$. However, caution is advised in regard to interpretation of $PvCO_2$, because peripheral venous samples reflect CO_2 production in the extremity sampled, rather than the whole body. In a normal animal, $PvCO_2$ is usually 5 mm Hg higher than $Paco_2$. This venous-arterial gradient occurs as CO_2 is removed from tissue and transported in venous blood back to the lungs as dissolved CO_2 in plasma (10%), and buffered within red blood cells as bicarbonate (90%). However, this gradient can dramatically increase in states of compromised perfusion or poor cardiac output.

Approach to assessment of an arterial blood gas sample is outlined in **Table 4**.

Oxygen-Tension-Based Indices

Alveolar to arterial oxygen gradient

Oxygenation of blood occurs following diffusion of air across the alveolar-capillary membrane. However, diffusion in normal animals does not occur to a perfect degree because a small amount of blood is shunted to bronchial and pleural vessels, to the coronary venous circulation, and to some areas of dead space ventilation. This normal physiologic difference in the resulting partial pressure of oxygen in the alveoli (PAO_2)

Table 3 Ventilatory abnormalities	
Hypoventilation: A Decrease in VT or in RR Can Lead to an Increase in $Paco_2$ (>35 mm Hg)	Hyperventilation: An Increase in VT or RR Leads to a Decrease $Paco_2$
Upper airway obstruction Respiratory center depression by anesthetic agents, especially opioids Respiratory center depression secondary to central nervous system disease Cervical myelopathy Diffuse neuromuscular disease Chest wall disease	Pain Anxiety Severe hypoxia

From Balakrishnan A, King LG. Updates on pulmonary function testing in small animals. Vet Clin North Am Small Anim Pract. 2014;44(1):1-18; with permission.

Table 4
Assessment of an arterial blood gas sample involves the following steps

1. Evaluation of acid-base status

Acidemic (pH <7.35)	Normal (pH 7.35–7.45)	Alkalemic (pH >7.45)
• Metabolic acidosis? • Respiratory acidosis? • Both?	• No acid base disorder? • Mixed acid-base disorder?	• Metabolic alkalosis? • Respiratory alkalosis? • Both?

2. Examination of alveolar ventilation ($Paco_2$)

Increased $Paco_2$ (>45 mm Hg)	Decreased $Paco_2$ (<35 mm Hg)
• Primary respiratory acidosis caused by hypoventilation • Compensatory response to a metabolic alkalosis	• Primary respiratory alkalosis • Compensatory response to a metabolic acidosis

3. Examination of HCO_3^- and BE

HCO_3^- increased (>24 mmol/L) or BE positive	HCO_3^- decreased (<18 mmol/L) or BE <-4
• Primary metabolic alkalosis • Compensatory response to a chronic respiratory acidosis	• Primary metabolic acidosis

Remember that the body never overcompensates. The primary process can usually be determined by evaluating the direction in which the pH is trending from 7.4. If the pH is <7.4, then the acidosis is the primary process. If the pH is >7.4, then the alkalosis is the primary process.

4. Evaluation of oxygenation (Pao_2)

- In healthy animals, Pao_2 should be about 4–5 times the Fio_2. When breathing room air (Fio_2 = 0.21), Pao_2 should be close to 100 mm Hg. In patients breathing 100% oxygen, Pao_2 should be approximately 500 mm Hg.
- When Fio_2 changes, equilibration to a new Fio_2 occurs within minutes. Therefore, representative samples can be obtained approximately 5 or more minutes after changing to a new Fio_2.
- When breathing room air, a Pao_2 of 75–90 mm Hg indicates mild hypoxemia, whereas a Pao_2 <60 mm Hg indicates severe hypoxemia.

Abbreviations: BE, base excess; HCO_3^-, bicarbonate.
From Balakrishnan A, King LG. Updates on pulmonary function testing in small animals. Vet Clin North Am Small Anim Pract. 2014;44(1):1-18; with permission.

and the arterial blood (Pao_2), that is, the alveolar to arterial (A-a) gradient, is about 5 to 10 mm Hg in an animal breathing room air (reference range <15 mm Hg).

The P_{AO_2} is derived from the alveolar gas equation:

$$P_{AO_2} = [(P_B - P_{H2O}) \times Fio_2] - [Paco_2/RQ]$$

where P_B = barometric pressure (mm Hg), P_{H2O} = water vapor pressure (mm Hg), RQ = respiratory quotient (ratio of CO_2 production to O_2 consumption), and $Paco_2$ = partial pressure of CO_2 in the arterial blood (mm Hg), which is used as an approximation of alveolar CO_2.

Using an atmospheric pressure of 760 mm Hg, water vapor pressure at 37°C of 47 mm Hg, an Fio_2 on room air of 0.21 (21%), and a typical RQ of a dog of 0.8, the equation is simplified as:

$$P(A-a)O_2 = 150 - Paco_2/0.8$$

The alveolar gas equation and A-a gradient provide a clinically useful method to evaluate the degree of pulmonary parenchymal disease, especially in situations where the $Paco_2$ is abnormal or variable when serial blood gases are being compared. Because $Paco_2$ is taken into consideration in the equation, hypoventilation or hyperventilation is excluded as a potential cause of hypoxemia. However, V/Q mismatch, shunting, and diffusion barriers all cause an increased A-a gradient.

"The 120 rule"

Assuming the alveolar barometric pressure and partial pressure of oxygen and water vapor do not change, the sum of $Paco_2$ and Pao_2 provides the clinician an idea of V/Q mismatch. Normal $Paco_2$ is approximately 40 mm Hg and Pao_2 is approximately 80 mm Hg, which adds up to 120 mm Hg. In general, an added value less than 120 mm Hg is an indication of V/Q mismatch. The lower the added value is, the greater the degree of V/Q mismatch.

Pao_2/Fio_2 ratio

The Pao_2/Fio_2 (PF) ratio is another clinically useful indicator of oxygenation status. It is particularly helpful for comparison of Pao_2 values between serial blood gases obtained when a patient is breathing varying concentrations of inspired oxygen. In a normal animal breathing room air with an Fio_2 of 0.21, Pao_2 is between 85 and 100 mm Hg, which results in a PF ratio of 400 to 500.

Abnormalities in the PF ratio can occur with any type of severe pulmonary dysfunction and are not diagnostic for a specific disease. However, this ratio has been used to characterize the severity of lung disease in animals with acute lung injury (ALI) and ARDS. Historically, a PF ratio less than 300 was considered consistent with VetALI, whereas a PF ratio less than 200 was indicative of VetARDS.[34] More recently, the Berlin definition proposed using varying degrees of ARDS in place of the term ALI[35]:

- Mild ARDS: PF ratio 200 to 300 with positive end-expiratory pressure >5 cm H_2O
- Moderate ARDS: PF ratio 100 to 200 with positive end-expiratory pressure >5 cm H_2O
- Severe ARDS: PF ratio less than 100 with positive end-expiratory pressure >5 cm H_2O

Pulse Oximetry

Pulse oximetry is a widely available, noninvasive indirect method for assessing oxygenation. It is extensively used in veterinary medicine, particularly during anesthesia and in the intensive care unit. Pulse oximetry is used for measurement of oxygenation at specified time-points; as a continuous real-time monitor during stressful procedures; or for immediate assessment of the need for interventions, such as oxygen supplementation.

Pulse oximeters report the oxygen saturation as measured by pulse oximetry (Spo_2), rather than the arterial oxygen saturation. Pulse oximeters use spectrophotometric technology, which measures oxygen saturation of hemoglobin by illuminating the skin and measuring the changes in light absorption of oxygenated blood (oxyhemoglobin) and deoxygenated blood (reduced hemoglobin) using two light wavelengths, 660 nm (red) and 940 nm (infrared). The pulsatile nature of blood flow is detected by the sensor and fluctuations in light absorption cause a rhythmic variation that is then translated into a ratio of oxyhemoglobin to reduced hemoglobin. The oxygen saturation of hemoglobin is calculated from this ratio.[33,36,37] Traditionally, pulse oximetry uses transmission sensors, that is, clips, where the light emitter and detector are on opposing surfaces of the tissue bed. Common clip probe placement sites in small animals include the tongue, lips, ear pinna, preputial or vulvar folds, or across digits. Recently, reflectance technology has been developed. Reflectance probes have the light emitter and detector on the same surface, adjacent to each other, so oxygen saturation is estimated from the back-scattered light rather than transmitted light. Common reflectance probe placement sites in small animals include ventral tail base, axillary, and inguinal regions.[37]

Hemoglobin carries most oxygen in the blood. The relationship between saturation of hemoglobin with oxygen and Pao_2 is not linear and is demonstrated by the oxyhemoglobin dissociation curve (**Fig. 8**). Each hemoglobin molecule carries four oxygen molecules when fully saturated. Binding of the first oxygen molecule causes a change in conformation of the hemoglobin molecule that allows more rapid binding of the other three molecules, thereby contributing to the shape of the curve. This curve is shifted to the right or left by several factors, such as temperature, pH, and Pco_2, thus altering the ease with which oxygen is loaded or unloaded onto or off hemoglobin.

A pulse oximetry reading of 100% correlates with a Pao_2 of about 120 mm Hg,[33] and a pulse oximeter reading greater than 95% is considered normal for most animals, resulting in a Pao_2 between 80 and 120 mm Hg. Mild to moderate hypoxemia is evidenced by values between 90% and 94%. A pulse oximeter reading of 90% indicates a Pao_2 of about 60 mm Hg. Severe, potentially life-threatening hypoxemia results in Spo_2 readings lower than 90%.

Recently, studies have been published in pediatrics and adults demonstrating the utility of the Spo_2/Fio_2 ratio (SF) as a surrogate for the PF ratio. In adults with ARDS, an SF ratio of 235 predicted a PF ratio of 200 with a sensitivity of 85% and

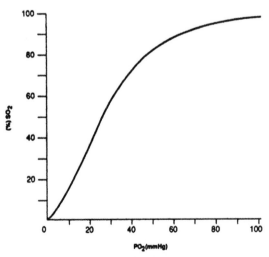

Fig. 8. Oxyhemoglobin dissociation curve. Note that hemoglobin is almost completely saturated with oxygen once the Po_2 is greater than about 70 mm Hg. This creates a safety margin for the patient as hypoxemia develops with lung disease. However, once the Po_2 drops lower than 60 mm Hg (which might occur as a result of high oxygen demands associated with stress of handling or transport), severe desaturation and hypoxemia are likely. (*Modified from* Balakrishnan A, King LG. Updates on pulmonary function testing in small animals. Vet Clin North Am Small Anim Pract. 2014;44(1):1-18; with permission.)

specificity of 85%. It was also useful in evaluating illness severity and predicting outcome in people with ARDS[38] and was a reliable, noninvasive surrogate of PF ratio to identify children with ALI or ARDS.[39] A pilot study in veterinary medicine showed good correlation between the SF and PF ratios in healthy dogs spontaneously breathing room air.[40] A prospective study is needed to confirm the relationship between SF and PF ratio in veterinary patients, although it seems to be a promising alternative by replacing invasive arterial blood sampling with noninvasive pulse oximetry.

Although standard pulse oximetry is inexpensive and easy to use and interpret, there are several inherent limitations to use of this technique. Because only two wavelengths are emitted, the device is unable to detect the dyshemoglobins, such as carboxyhemoglobin and methemoglobin. This becomes important in the clinical setting in the case of dyshemoglobinemias caused by carbon monoxide toxicity and conditions that cause methemoglobinemia, such as acetaminophen toxicity. Newer pulse oximeters have been developed that emit four or more different wavelengths and thus are able to detect additional hemoglobin species that may be present in the blood, known as pulse CO-oximeters. They measure what is known as fractional saturation, that is, oxyHb/(oxyHb + reduced hemoglobin + carboxyhemoglobin + methemoglobin).[29] Inaccurate readings have been reported when intravenous dyes (eg, methylene blue) have been used for diagnostics purposes, with excessive fluorescent light, in the presence of severe anemia, and with a hypoperfused state (eg, reduced cardiac output, peripheral vasoconstriction).[37] External motion can also cause excessive artifact and signal disruption. In critically ill animals that are anemic, decreased hemoglobin concentration results in markedly decreased total oxygen content of blood. The use of pulse oximetry in these patients can be misleading. Although oxygen saturation might be close to 100%, the total amount of hemoglobin is reduced, and the animal can still have dramatically low tissue oxygen delivery.[41,42] Pulse oximetry should be interpreted with caution in these animals.

End-Tidal Capnography

Measurement of the partial pressure of carbon dioxide in inhaled and exhaled gases during phasic breathing is known as capnography. This is a noninvasive tool that provides real-time information about ventilatory status, which is valuable for monitoring animals under general anesthesia and for critically ill animals that are intubated and/ or being mechanically ventilated.

Commercially available capnometers rely on infrared spectroscopy to detect exhaled CO_2 as it flows through a sensor device attached to the endotracheal tube. The amount of CO_2 is estimated by detecting variations in the absorption of light at a specific wavelength (4.26 μm).[43,44] There are two main types of capnometers:

- Mainstream capnometers: The CO_2 sensor is interposed between the endotracheal tube and the breathing circuit. CO_2 measurement is across the airway.
- Sidestream capnometers: The respiratory gases are continuously aspirated via an adaptor, which passes through a length of microtubing to a remote sensor where the CO_2 is measured. The transport of gas to the infrared measuring device results in a 1- to 4-second delay in CO_2 measurement and display on the capnogram. The use of sidestream capnometers attached to a nasal catheter has been evaluated in awake, spontaneously breathing dogs and their exhaled CO_2 content correlated well with the $Paco_2$. Animals with underlying respiratory pathology likely have elevated end-tidal CO_2 ($Etco_2$) and $Paco_2$ levels that would support hypoventilation.[44,45] However, a

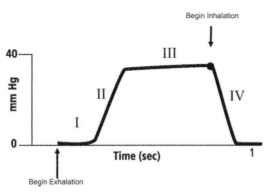

Fig. 9. Normal capnogram. (*From* Krauss B, Hess DR. Capnography for procedural sedation and analgesia in the emergency department. *Ann Emerg Med* 2007;50(2):176–7; with permission. See text for discussion of the four phases of the capnogram.)

falsely normal or low reading can occur in some animals despite the presence of hypoventilation.

A typical capnogram consists of four distinct phases (**Fig. 9**)[45]:

1. Beginning of exhalation: Zero baseline as CO_2-poor atmospheric air from anatomic dead space is eliminated.
2. Exhalation: As CO_2-rich air from the lower airways begins to mix with dead space air, there is a gradual increase in exhaled CO_2.
3. End-exhalation: The amount of CO_2 in exhaled air reaches a plateau during the last part of exhalation as all exhaled air is coming from the alveoli and lower airways. The CO_2 concentration measured at this plateau is reported by the instrument as $Etco_2$.
4. Inhalation: As exhalation ends, the next breath begins and atmospheric air rushes in past the sensor. During this phase, CO_2 levels rapidly drop and return the baseline to zero.

$Etco_2$ is used as an estimate of the pulmonary arterial CO_2 because CO_2 is highly diffusible, and the alveolar CO_2 concentration is normally close to the CO_2 in the pulmonary arterial blood. A gradient between $Etco_2$ and $Paco_2$ occurs because of the presence of dead space:

- Anatomic dead-space: There is usually a small difference (about 2–5 mm Hg) between $Etco_2$ and $Paco_2$ in normal animals. This difference is a result of some mixing of alveolar air with CO_2-poor air from anatomic dead space in larger airways.
- Physiologic dead-space: In animals with significant pulmonary disease, the gradient between $Etco_2$ and $Paco_2$ can be elevated because of increased physiologic dead space. This occurs because some regions of the lungs can have significant V/Q mismatch.

Clinically, capnography is an invaluable tool for monitoring ventilatory status. The most common applications of capnography in anesthesia, emergency, and critical care medicine include the following:

- Ventilatory monitoring in anesthetized intubated animals (**Fig. 10**).
- Monitoring ventilation in animals with tracheostomies.

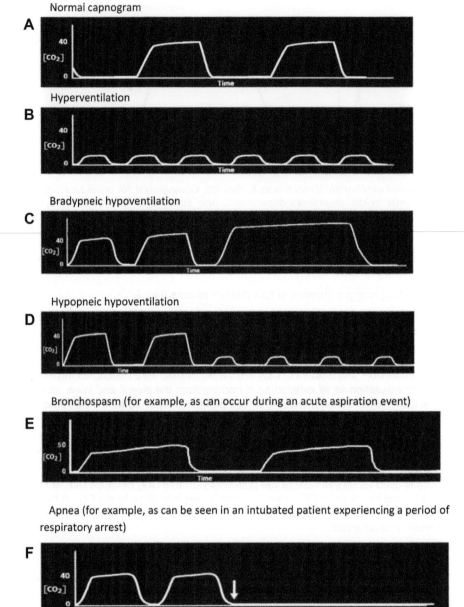

Fig. 10. Capnography during anesthetic monitoring. (*From* Krauss B, Hess DR. Capnography for procedural sedation and analgesia in the emergency department. *Ann Emerg Med* 2007;50(2):176–7; with permission.)

- Verification of endotracheal intubation during cardiopulmonary resuscitation (**Fig. 11**): Attachment of the capnometer to the endotracheal tube after an intubation attempt can help distinguish between accurate endotracheal intubation and a misplaced esophageal intubation because levels of CO_2 in the esophagus are

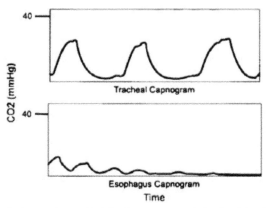

Fig. 11. Capnography in esophageal intubation versus endotracheal intubation. (*From* Roberts WA, Maniscalco WM, Cohen AR, et al. The use of capnography for recognition of esophageal intubation in the neonatal intensive care unit. *Pediatr Pulmonol* 1995;19(5):263; with permission.)

usually negligible, whereas endotracheal intubation should produce a normal capnogram with each breath (either spontaneous or positive pressure breath).

- Volumetric capnography: evaluates Etco$_2$ as a function of exhaled lung volume, allowing breath-by-breath quantification of the alveolar dead space and the volume of effective alveolar ventilation.[46] This method allows bedside measurement of dead space fraction in people who are receiving mechanical ventilation and may provide prognostic information in people with ARDS.[47] This diagnostic tool has yet to be fully evaluated in all respiratory diseases in people, and further studies are warranted to explore its use in veterinary medicine.

SUMMARY

PFTs are important diagnostic tools that have wide clinical applications in human and veterinary medicine. PFTs are becoming more readily available in veterinary medicine and may prove useful as a noninvasive diagnostic tool.

DISCLOSURE

The authors have nothing to disclose.

REFERENCES

1. Cooper BG. An update on contraindications for lung function testing. Thorax 2011;66(8):714–23.
2. Crapo RO. Pulmonary-function testing. N Engl J Med 1994;331(1):25–30.
3. Morris JF. Spirometry in the evaluation of pulmonary function. Q J Med 1976; 125(2):110.
4. Zibrak JD, O'Donnell CR, Marton K. Indications for pulmonary function testing. Ann Intern Med 1990;112(10):763–71.
5. Amis TC, Kurpershoek C. Tidal breathing flow-volume loop analysis for clinical assessment of airway obstruction in conscious dogs. Am J Vet Res 1986;47: 1002–6.

6. Amis TC, Smith MM, Gaber CE, et al. Upper airway obstruction: canine laryngeal paralysis. Am J Vet Res 1986;47:1007–10.

7. Pardali D, Adamama-Moraitou KK, Rallis TS, et al. Tidal breathing flow-volume loop analysis for the diagnosis and staging of tracheal collapse in dogs. J Vet Intern Med 2010;24(4):832–42.

8. Adamama-Moraitou KK, Pardali D, Menexes G, et al. Tidal breathing flow volume loop analysis of 21 healthy, unsedated, young adult male Beagle dogs. Aust Vet J 2013;91(6):226–32.

9. Adamama-Moraitou KK, Pardali D, Prassinos NN, et al. Analysis of tidal breathing flow volume loop in dogs with tracheal masses. Aust Vet J 2010;88(9):351–6.

10. McKiernan BC, Dye JA, Rozanski EA. Tidal breathing flow-volume loops in healthy and bronchitic cats. J Vet Intern Med 1993;7:388–93.

11. McKiernan BC, Johnson LR. Clinical pulmonary function testing in dogs and cats. Vet Clin North Am Small Anim Pract 1992;22:1087–99.

12. Dye JA, McKiernan BC, Rozanski EA, et al. Bronchopulmonary disease in the cat: historical, physical, radiographic, clinicopathologic, and pulmonary functional evaluation of 24 affected and 15 healthy cats. J Vet Intern Med 1996;10(6):385–400.

13. Rodarte JR, Rehder K. Dynamics of respiration. Comp Physiol 2011;131–44.

14. Stahl CA, Moller K, Schumann S, et al. Dynamic versus static respiratory mechanics in acute lung injury and acute respiratory distress syndrome. Crit Care Med 2006;34(8):2090–8.

15. Scanlan CL, Realey A, Earl L, et al, editors. Egan's fundamentals of respiratory care. 8th edition. St Louis (MO): Mosby-Year Book; 2003.

16. Ruppell GL, Enright PL. Pulmonary function testing. Respir Care 2012;57(1):165–75.

17. Hoffman AM. Airway physiology and clinical function testing. Vet Clin Small Anim 2007;37:829–43.

18. Bedenice D, Rozanski E, Bach J, et al. Canine awake head-out plethysmography (HOP): characterization of external resistive loading and spontaneous laryngeal paralysis. Respir Physiolo Neurobiol 2006;151:61–73.

19. Bedenice D, Bar-Yishay E, Ingenito EP, et al. Evaluation of head-out constant volume body plethysmography for measurement of specific airway resistance in conscious, sedated sheep. Am J Vet Res 2004;65:1259–64.

20. Lin C-H, Lee J-J, Liu C-H. Functional assessment of expiratory flow pattern in feline lower airway disease. J Feline Med Surg 2014;16(8):616–22.

21. Liu N-C, Sargan DR, Adams VJ, et al. Characterisation of brachycephalic obstructive airway syndrome in French bulldogs using whole-body barometric plethysmography. PLoS One 2015;10(6):e0130741.

22. Kirschvink N, Leemans J, Delvaux F, et al. Non-invasive assessment of airway responsiveness in healthy and allergen-sensitised cats by use of barometric whole body plethysmography. Vet J 2007;173(2):343–52.

23. García-Guasch L, Caro-Vadillo A, Manubens-Grau J, et al. Pulmonary function in obese vs non-obese cats. J Feline Med Surg 2015;17(6):494–9.

24. Bernaerts F, Talavera J, Leemans J, et al. Description of original endoscopic findings and respiratory functional assessment using barometric whole-body plethysmography in dogs suffering from brachycephalic airway obstruction syndrome. Vet J 2010;183(1):95–102.

25. Liu N-C, Adams VJ, Kalmar L, et al. Whole-body barometric plethysmography characterizes upper airway obstruction in 3 brachycephalic breeds of dogs. J Vet Intern Med 2016;30(3):853–65.

26. Hirt RA, Leinker S, Mosing M, et al. Comparison of barometric whole body plethysmography and its derived parameter enhanced pause (PENH) with conventional respiratory mechanics in healthy Beagle dogs. Vet J 2008;176(2):232–9.
27. Lin C-H, Wu H-D, Lo P-Y, et al. Simultaneous visual inspection for barometric whole-body plethysmography waveforms during pulmonary function testing in client-owned cats. J Feline Med Surg 2016;18(10):761–7.
28. Brashier B, Salvi S. Measuring lung function using sound waves: role of the forced oscillation technique and impulse oscillometry system. Breathe (Sheff) 2015;11(1):57–65.
29. Oostveen E, MacLeod D, Lorino H, et al. The forced oscillation technique in clinical practice: methodology, recommendations and future developments. Eur Respir J 2003;22(6):1026–41.
30. Faria AC, Lopes AJ, Jansen JM, et al. Evaluating the forced oscillation technique in the detection of early smoking-induced respiratory changes. Biomed Eng Online 2009;8(1):22.
31. Saydain G, Beck KC, Decker PA, et al. Clinical significance of elevated diffusing capacity. Chest 2004;125(2):446–52.
32. Sivova N, Launay D, Wémeau-Stervinou L, et al. Relevance of partitioning DLCO to detect pulmonary hypertension in systemic sclerosis. PLoS One 2013;8(10): 78001.
33. Proulx J. Respiratory monitoring: arterial blood gas analysis, pulse oximetry and end-tidal carbon dioxide analysis. Clin Tech Small Anim Pract 1999;14(4):227–30.
34. Wilkins PA, Otto CM, Baumgardner JE, et al. Acute lung injury and acute respiratory distress syndromes in veterinary medicine: consensus definitions: the Dorothy Russell Havemeyer Working Group on ALI and ARDS in Veterinary Medicine. J Vet Emerg Crit Care 2007;17(4):333–9.
35. Fanelli V, Vlachou A, Ghannadian S, et al. Acute respiratory distress syndrome: new definition, current and future therapeutic options. J Thorac Dis 2013;5(3): 326–34.
36. Schnapp LM, Cohen NH. Pulse oximetry: uses and abuses. Chest 1990;98: 1244–50.
37. Jubran A. Pulse oximetry. Crit Care 2015;19(1):272.
38. Rice TW, Wheeler AP, Bernard GR, et al. Comparison of the SpO2/FIO2 ratio and the PaO2/FIO2 ratio in patients with acute lung injury or ARDS. Chest 2007; 132(2):410–7.
39. Bilan N, Dastranji A, Ghalehgolab Behbahani A. Comparison of the Spo2/Fio2 ratio and the Pao2/Fio2 ratio in patients with acute lung injury or acute respiratory distress syndrome. J Cardiovasc Thorac Res 2015;7(1):28–31.
40. Calabro JM, Prittie JE, Palma DA. Preliminary evaluation of the utility of comparing SpO2/FiO2 and PaO2/FiO2 ratios in dogs. J Vet Emerg Crit Care (San Antonio) 2013;23(3):280–5.
41. Hendricks JC, King LG. Practicality, usefulness and limits of pulse oximetry in critical small animal patients. J Vet Emerg Crit Care 1993;3(1):5–12.
42. King GG. Cutting edge technologies in respiratory research: lung function testing. Respirology 2011;16:883–90.
43. Nagler J, Krauss B. Capnography: a valuable tool for airway management. Emerg Med Clin North Am 2008;26:881–97.
44. Sullivan KJ, Kissoon N, Goodwin SR. End–tidal carbon dioxide monitoring in pediatric emergencies. Pediatr Emerg Care 2005;21(5):327–32.

45. Kelmer E, Scanson LC, Reed A, et al. Agreement between values for arterial and end-tidal partial pressure of carbon-dioxide in spontaneously breathing, critically ill dogs. J Am Vet Med Assoc 2009;235:1314–8.

46. Verscheure S, Massion PB, Verschuren F, et al. Volumetric capnography: lessons from the past and current clinical applications. Crit Care 2016;20(1):184.

47. Zhang Y-J, Gao X-J, Li Z-B, et al. Comparison of the pulmonary dead-space fraction derived from ventilator volumetric capnography and a validated equation in the survival prediction of patients with acute respiratory distress syndrome. Chin J Traumatol 2016;19(3):141–5.

Laryngeal Disease in Dogs and Cats: An Update

Catriona M. MacPhail, DVM, PhD

KEYWORDS

- Upper airway obstruction • Laryngeal paralysis • Aspiration pneumonia
- Megaesophagus • Laryngeal collapse • Brachycephalic syndrome
- Laryngeal neoplasia

KEY POINTS

- The most common cause of laryngeal paralysis is a progressive generalized polyneuropathy in geriatric dogs.
- Functional laryngeal examination is required for definitive diagnosis of laryngeal paralysis and to rule out other obstructive diseases, such as laryngeal neoplasia.
- Surgical arytenoid lateralization improves respiration and quality of life in dogs with laryngeal paralysis, with guarded to good long-term prognosis.
- In varying degrees, laryngeal collapse is a common component of brachycephalic obstructive airway syndrome.
- Aspiration pneumonia is a common complication in animals with laryngeal disease before and after any surgical intervention.

 Video content accompanies this article at http://www.vetsmall.theclinics.com.

INTRODUCTION

Laryngeal disease in dogs and cats results in varying degrees of upper airway obstruction and can be life threatening. Conditions most commonly affecting the larynx include laryngeal paralysis, laryngeal collapse, and laryngeal masses. Differentials for laryngeal disease include nasal, nasopharyngeal, and tracheal conditions that also result in clinical signs of upper airway obstruction including stertor, stridor, wheezing, and gagging. Visual upper airway examination is the fundamental diagnostic tool for localizing the anatomic area involved in airway obstruction.

ANATOMY AND PHYSIOLOGY

The larynx is the collection of cartilages surrounding the rima glottidis. It is responsible for control of airflow during respiration. The 4 cartilages that constitute the larynx are

Small Animal Surgery, Department of Clinical Sciences, Colorado State University, 1601 Campus Delivery, Fort Collins, CO 80523-160, USA
E-mail address: Catriona.MacPhail@colostate.edu

Vet Clin Small Anim 50 (2020) 295–310
https://doi.org/10.1016/j.cvsm.2019.11.001
0195-5616/20/© 2019 Elsevier Inc. All rights reserved.
vetsmall.theclinics.com

the paired arytenoids and the unpaired epiglottis, cricoid, and thyroid cartilages. Each of the arytenoid cartilages has a cuneiform process rostrally, a corniculate process dorsally, a muscular process dorsolaterally, and a vocal process ventrally. The vocal processes are the attachment points for the vocal folds. The glottis consists of the vocal folds, the vocal process of the arytenoid cartilages, and the rima glottidis. The laryngeal saccules are mucosal diverticula that sit rostral and lateral to the vocal folds. The larynx of the cat differs from that of the dog because the arytenoid cartilage lacks cuneiform and corniculate processes. Also, true aryepiglottic folds are absent, and the sides of the epiglottis connect directly to the cricoid lamina by laryngeal mucosa.

The intrinsic muscles of the larynx (cricoarytenoideus dorsalis, cricoarytenoideus lateralis, thyroarytenoideus, vocalis, ventricularis, arytenoideus transversus, hyoepiglotticus, and cricothyroideus) are responsible for all laryngeal functions. These functions include regulation of airflow, protection of the lower airway from aspiration during swallowing, and control of phonation. The cricoarytenoideus dorsalis muscle is solely responsible for enlarging the glottis during inspiration. This muscle originates on the dorsolateral surface of the cricoid and inserts on the muscular process of the arytenoid cartilages. Contraction of this muscle results in external rotation and abduction of the arytenoid cartilages and then pulls the vocal processes laterally. The caudal laryngeal nerve is the terminal segment of the recurrent laryngeal nerve and is responsible for innervation of all intrinsic laryngeal muscles, except the cricothyroid muscle, which is innervated by the cranial laryngeal nerve.

CANINE LARYNGEAL PARALYSIS
Cause

Laryngeal paralysis is a common unilateral or bilateral respiratory disorder that primarily affects older (>9 years) large-breed and giant-breed dogs. A congenital form occurs in certain breeds such as Bouvier des Flandres, Siberian huskies, bull terriers, and white-coated German shepherd dogs.[1,2] An autosomal dominant trait has been documented in Bouvier des Flandres, resulting in wallerian degeneration of the recurrent laryngeal nerves and abnormalities of the nucleus ambiguus.[3] A hereditary predisposition has also been identified in Siberian husky dogs, Alaskan malamutes, and crosses of those two breeds.[4,5] From a recent study, an autosomal recessive mode of inheritance is suspected in Alaskan huskies based on pedigree analysis.[6] Laryngeal paralysis polyneuropathy disease complexes have been described in Dalmatians, Rottweilers, Leonberger dogs, Pyrenean mountain dogs, and American Staffordshire terriers.[7–11]

For the more frequently encountered acquired laryngeal paralysis, the Labrador retriever is the most common breed reported; golden retrievers, Saint Bernards, Newfoundlands, Irish setters, and Brittany spaniels are also overrepresented. Acquired laryngeal paralysis is caused by damage to the recurrent laryngeal nerve or intrinsic laryngeal muscles, most often attributed to polyneuropathy, polymyopathy, accidental or iatrogenic trauma, or intrathoracic or extrathoracic masses, although many other causes have been proposed (**Box 1**).

In many dogs the cause remains undetermined and these cases were traditionally classified as idiopathic; it has recently been shown that many of these dogs with acquired laryngeal paralysis develop systemic neurologic signs within 1 year following diagnosis of laryngeal paralysis, which is consistent with a progressive generalized neuropathy.[12] Abnormalities in results of electrodiagnostic tests and histopathologic analysis of nerve and muscle biopsy specimens reflecting generalized polyneuropathy have been documented in a small number of dogs with acquired laryngeal paralysis.[13] Therefore, it has been proposed that dogs previously described to have idiopathic

---

Box 1
Proposed causes of laryngeal paralysis

Congenital
  Genetic trait
  Laryngeal paralysis: polyneuropathy complex

Accidental trauma
  Cervical penetrating wounds
  Strangulating trauma

Iatrogenic surgical trauma
  Cranial thoracic surgery
  Correction of patent ductus arteriosus/vascular ring anomaly
  Thyroidectomy/parathyroidectomy
  Tracheal surgery
  Ventral slot surgery

Cervical/intrathoracic neoplasia
  Lymphoma
  Thymoma
  Thyroid carcinoma/ectopic thyroid carcinoma

Neuromuscular disease
  Geriatric-onset laryngeal paralysis polyneuropathy syndrome
  Endocrinopathy (hypothyroidism, hypoadrenocorticism)
  Immune mediated
  Infectious
  Myasthenia gravis
  Polymyopathy
  Systemic lupus erythematosus
  Toxins (lead, organophosphates)

Modified from MacPhail C. Laryngeal disease in dogs and cats. Vet Clin North Am Small Anim Pract. 2014;44(1):19-31; with permission.

---

acquired laryngeal paralysis may actually have a progressive generalized idiopathic polyneuropathy with laryngeal paralysis as one of the early clinical signs of this condition.[14] The abbreviation GOLPP (geriatric-onset laryngeal paralysis polyneuropathy) has been proposed as a more accurate term for dogs with acquired laryngeal paralysis when other causes have been ruled out (GOLPP Study Group. Michigan State University; Veterinary Medical Center. Available at: https://cvm.msu.edu/hospital/clinical-research/golpp-study-group).

Clinical Signs

With laryngeal paralysis, the arytenoid cartilages, and consequently the vocal folds, remain in a paramedian position during inspiration creating upper airway obstruction. Dogs typically present with noisy inspiratory respiration and exercise intolerance. Early clinical signs include voice change and mild coughing and gagging. Severe airway obstruction results in respiratory distress, cyanosis, and collapse. Dogs can also show dysphagia or develop rear limb weakness associated with peripheral neuropathy. The classic finding on physical examination is the presence of stridor over the upper airway, but this can be variable. A complete neurologic examination and assessment of proprioceptive placing should be performed in dogs suspected of laryngeal paralysis.

Progression of clinical signs is highly variable, and dogs can have clinical signs for several months to years before significant respiratory distress ensues. However, clinical signs are worsened by heavy exercise or increasing environmental temperature or humidity, which result in an acute exacerbation of a chronic condition. As respiratory rate increases, the mucosa covering the arytenoids becomes inflamed and edematous, which leads to further airway obstruction. A vicious cycle ensues that can become life threatening if not addressed.

Diagnosis

Routine diagnostic evaluation for dogs thought to have laryngeal paralysis includes physical examination, orthopedic and neurologic examination, complete blood count, biochemical profile, urinalysis, thyroid function screening, thoracic radiographs, and laryngeal examination. Dogs with bilateral laryngeal paralysis are at risk of aspiration pneumonia both before and after surgery, therefore thoracic radiographs are a necessary part of the diagnostic work-up in dogs suspected to have laryngeal dysfunction to rule out not only aspiration pneumonia (**Figs. 1** and **2**) but also overt megaesophagus, pulmonary edema, and concurrent cardiac or lower airway abnormalities.

For dogs that present with dysphagia or vomiting, positive contrast videofluoroscopy could be considered to rule out esophageal dysfunction or megaesophagus, which might not be apparent on survey thoracic radiographs. Severe progressive esophageal dysfunction has been reported in a set of dogs with idiopathic laryngeal

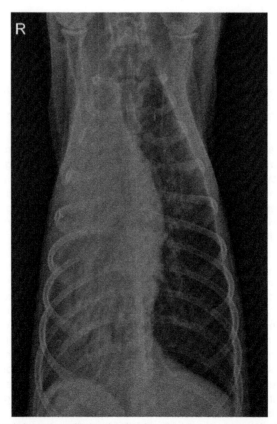

Fig. 1. Ventrodorsal thoracic radiograph of a dog showing a severe alveolar pattern in the right lung lobes indicating aspiration pneumonia.

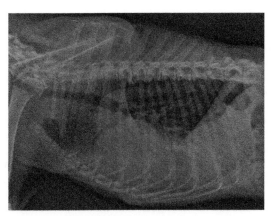

Fig. 2. Left lateral thoracic radiograph of the same dog from **Fig. 1**.

paralysis and likely reflects the progressive polyneuropathy that has been proposed as a cause of laryngeal dysfunction in most geriatric dogs.[12] However, acquiring information from esophagography should be weighed against the potential for risk of barium aspiration. It has recently been documented that a small subset of dogs with acquired laryngeal paralysis had an increased incidence of gastroesophageal reflux.[15]

Hypothyroidism occurs concurrently in approximately 30% of dogs with acquired laryngeal paralysis, although a direct causal link has not been established.[16,17] Regardless, thyroid function screening is performed routinely in the work-up for laryngeal paralysis. Thyroid supplementation should be instituted if indicated, although this does not resolve clinical signs associated with laryngeal paralysis.

Laryngeal examination under a light plane of anesthesia is required to provide a definitive diagnosis of laryngeal paralysis and to rule out other laryngeal abnormalities. This examination can be accomplished by direct visualization of the larynx with a simple laryngoscope, oral video-endoscopic laryngoscopy, transnasal laryngoscopy (TNL), ultrasonography (echolaryngography), or computed tomography (CT). Findings that indicate laryngeal paralysis on ultrasonography include asymmetry or absence of motion of the cuneiform processes, abnormal or paradoxic arytenoid movement, caudal displacement of the larynx, and collapse of the larynx.[18] CT findings in dogs with laryngeal paralysis included failure to abduct the arytenoid cartilages and collapse into the rima glottis on presumed inspiration, stenosis of the laryngeal inlet, and air-filled lateral ventricles.[19] Regardless of method, laryngoscopy can be confounding because false-positive results are common because of the influence of anesthetic agents and sedatives on laryngeal function. Echolaryngography, TNL, and CT avoid the need for heavy sedation and general anesthesia; however, none of these methods have been shown to be superior to traditional oral laryngeal examination for definitive diagnosis.[20]

Laryngeal paralysis is diagnosed based on the lack of arytenoid abduction during inspiration. Inflammation and swelling of the laryngeal cartilages can also be apparent. Diagnosis can be confounded by paradoxic movement of the arytenoids, resulting in a false-negative result (Video 1). In this scenario, the arytenoid cartilages move inward during inspiration because of negative intraglottic pressure created by increased respiratory effort against an obstruction. The cartilages then passively return to a normal position during expiration, which gives the impression of normal arytenoid movement. To avoid this situation, an assistant should state the phase of ventilation during laryngoscopy to distinguish normal from abnormal motion.

Intravenous thiopental administered to effect was thought to be the best anesthetic choice to allow assessment of laryngeal function; however, thiopental is no longer manufactured in the United States, which leaves propofol as the most often used induction agent for laryngeal examination in dogs, even though significant respiratory depression often occurs, with apnea related to dose, speed of injection, and use of concurrent premedications. Although ketamine has been shown to preserve laryngeal function better than thiopental in people, a study in dogs found no benefit for laryngeal examination when combining propofol and ketamine; no dose reduction in propofol was achieved and respiratory depression was more marked.[21] Alfaxalone can be used as an alternative to propofol, because it has been shown to be a safe and effective anesthetic induction agent in dogs.[22] Although alfaxalone still causes respiratory depression, apnea has been shown to be less likely compared with propofol.[23] In 1 direct comparison of propofol versus alfaxalone induction for laryngeal examination in healthy dogs, the addition of premedications (acepromazine and butorphanol) improved the quality of the laryngeal examination regardless of the induction agent.[24] This study did not recommend the use of propofol or alfaxalone alone for the evaluation of arytenoid motion. This finding is in contrast with a separate study[25] that showed alfaxalone alone resulted in the best respiratory function and quality of examination compared with propofol alone and alfaxalone or propofol used with premedications. Doxapram HCl (1 mg/kg IV) has been advocated for routine use during laryngoscopy to increase respiratory rate and effort and improve intrinsic laryngeal motion because it significantly improves the ability to determine normal versus abnormal function.[24]

Emergency Treatment

For dogs in acute respiratory distress associated with airway obstruction, initial treatment is directed at improving ventilation, reducing laryngeal edema, and minimizing the animal's stress. A typical treatment regimen involves oxygen supplementation and administration of short-acting steroids (eg, dexamethasone 0.1–1 mg/kg IV) and sedatives (eg, acepromazine 0.02 mg/kg IV). Additional administration of buprenorphine (0.005 mg/kg IV) or butorphanol (0.2 mg/kg IV) can also be considered to improve sedation. These dogs are often hyperthermic because of excessive respiratory effort, and appropriate cooling procedures should also be instituted, including wetting the fur with cool water and application of a fan until body temperature decreases to ∼38.9°C (102°F). If respiratory distress cannot be abated, intubation or a temporary tracheostomy should be considered. However, use of a temporary tracheostomy tube in dogs with laryngeal paralysis has been shown to be a negative prognostic indicator following definitive surgery, because dogs that received a temporary tracheostomy preoperatively were more likely to experience major complications.[17]

In addition, temporary tracheostomies involve complications. The presence of a tube within the tracheal lumen causes epithelial erosion, submucosal inflammation, and inhibition of the mucociliary apparatus. Mucus production dramatically increases, and the tube must be suctioned or cleaned at frequent intervals to prevent clogging. Therefore, a dog with a temporary tracheostomy tube requires intensive monitoring to avoid life-threatening complications. In a recent study, complications (clinical and incidental) were documented in 86% of cases receiving a temporary tracheostomy.[26] Sixteen types of complications were noted, but the most significant and frequent complications occurred in ∼25% of dogs and included airway obstruction, tube dislodgement, aspiration pneumonia, and stoma swelling.

Translaryngeal percutaneous arytenoid lateralization is currently under investigation as an alternative to temporary tracheostomy for dogs in severe respiratory distress from laryngeal paralysis. In this technique a mattress suture is placed through 1 arytenoid cartilage via an oral approach and exited through the skin ventral to the jugular vein.[27] Further studies are needed to determine the clinical utility of this method.

Medical Management

Often dogs are not severely affected clinically until they have bilateral laryngeal paresis or paralysis. Therefore, dogs with unilateral laryngeal dysfunction are typically not surgical candidates. For dogs with bilateral laryngeal paralysis, the decision to recommend surgery is based on the quality of life of the dog, severity of clinical signs, and time of year. The goal of conservative management of dogs with laryngeal paralysis is to improve the quality of life through environmental changes, reduction of daily exercise, owner education, weight loss, and consideration of antiinflammatory drugs to minimize laryngeal swelling. However, medical treatment is insufficient for long-term management. For dogs that are diagnosed with concurrent hypothyroidism, thyroid supplementation should be instituted. As noted earlier, this rarely improves clinical signs of laryngeal paralysis but it can assist with weight loss.

Surgical Treatment

Laryngeal paralysis is a surgical condition for severely affected dogs, and numerous techniques have been described. Unilateral arytenoid lateralization is the current technique of choice for most surgeons, but various types of partial laryngectomy (bilateral vocal fold resection, partial arytenoidectomy) are also performed. Bilateral arytenoid lateralization is not recommended because it results in unacceptable morbidity.[17] Permanent tracheostomy is considered a salvage procedure for dogs most at risk of aspiration pneumonia, but it is associated with a high rate of major and minor complications and requires diligent postoperative and long-term care. In a series of 21 dogs with permanent tracheostomies, 50% had major complications, 20% required revision surgery, and 26% acutely died at home, most likely from airway obstruction.[28]

Several variations of unilateral arytenoid lateralization have been described. The most common technique involves suturing the cricoid cartilage to the muscular process of the arytenoid cartilage, which mimics the directional pull of the cricoarytenoideus dorsalis muscle and rotates the arytenoid cartilage laterally. An alternative technique involves suture placement from the muscular process of the arytenoid cartilage to the caudodorsal aspect of the thyroid cartilage, which pulls the arytenoid cartilage laterally rather than rotating it and increases the area of the rima glottidis to a lesser degree than the cricoarytenoid suture. Differences in surgical technique and the degree of increase in surface area of the rima glottis do not seem to affect postoperative clinical signs and outcome. However, increasing the surface area of the rima glottidis beyond the edges of the epiglottis could put the animal at higher risk of aspiration. Limited lateral displacement of the arytenoid cartilage significantly reduces resistance to airflow within the larynx and might decrease the risk of postoperative aspiration pneumonia. This limited displacement can be accomplished by minimizing the degree of dissection; that is, separation of the cricothyroid articulation, transection of the sesamoid band connecting the paired arytenoids, and complete disarticulation of the cricoarytenoid joint are not necessary. A partial opening of the cricoarytenoid articulation allows accurate visualization of needle placement through the muscular process of the arytenoid but limits the degree of arytenoid cartilage abduction. Anatomic landmarks used to achieve limited abduction while reducing airway resistance were described in a cadaveric study.[29] A recent surgical description summarizes and advocates the less invasive approach that has been partially described previously to include less than 25% transection in length of the thyropharyngeus muscle and preservation of the cricopharyngeus muscle, cricothyroid articulation, and sesamoid bands.[30] However, in a separate study, there was no significant difference in risk of aspiration pneumonia or survival times between a standard technique and one that preserves laryngeal anatomy.[31]

Partial laryngectomy encompasses various techniques for vocal cord excision and partial arytenoidectomy to increase the diameter of the glottis. Partial laryngectomy has been associated with complications, including laryngeal webbing, laryngeal scarring, and aspiration pneumonia. High complication rates have been reported by some investigators; however, bilateral vocal fold resection alone resulted in fewer complications and better postoperative outcome than other partial laryngectomy techniques.[17,32,33] This finding is thought to be to the result of better laryngeal protection during swallowing and decreased laryngeal irritation because the corniculate processes of the arytenoid cartilages are left intact. Bilateral ventriculocordectomy via ventral laryngotomy was reported to have a reasonable long-term (>6 months) outcome with a low incidence of major complication (7%) in 1 study; however, a direct comparison of outcomes between dogs treated with either unilateral arytenoid lateralization or bilateral ventriculocordectomy found that dogs undergoing bilateral ventriculocordectomy were more likely to have chronic (lifelong) respiratory complications.[34,35] In addition, in a small cadaveric study of canine larynges, bilateral ventriculocordectomy did not seem to reduce laryngeal airway resistance.[36]

Prognosis

Aspiration pneumonia is the most common complication in dogs surgically treated for laryngeal paralysis; it occurs in 10% to 21% of dogs undergoing unilateral arytenoid lateralization. Although aspiration pneumonia is most likely in the first few weeks following surgery, it has been recognized that these dogs are at risk for this complication for the rest of their lives. Factors that have been found to be significantly associated with a higher risk of developing complications and that have a negative effect on long-term outcome include preoperative aspiration pneumonia, development of esophageal dysfunction, progression of generalized neurologic signs, temporary tracheostomy placement, and concurrent neoplastic disease. However, the most recent retrospective study identifying risk factors for the development of aspiration pneumonia found that preexisting aspiration pneumonia was not associated with an increased risk for development of aspiration pneumonia after surgery.[37] Postoperative megaesophagus and postoperative administration of opioid analgesics before discharge were significant risk factors for development of aspiration pneumonia.

The use of gastrointestinal motility modifiers has been suggested to reduce the risk of postoperative aspiration pneumonia. Metoclopramide increases lower esophageal sphincter (LES) tone and has been shown to reduce gastroesophageal reflux under anesthesia in normal dogs; however, a prospective multicenter clinical trial in dogs with laryngeal paralysis undergoing unilateral arytenoid lateralization found that perioperative administration of metoclopramide did not affect the incidence of aspiration pneumonia in the short-term postoperative period.[38] Based on a study in normal dogs, cisapride has been suggested for use to increase LES pressure, because cisapride administration, in contrast with metoclopramide and placebo drug, resulted in significant increases in LES pressure.[39] A retrospective evaluation of a cisapride constant-rate infusion suggested a positive effect on the incidence of postoperative aspiration pneumonia, but definitive conclusions could not be drawn because of low numbers of dogs in the study.[40]

Progressive neurologic signs can also affect outcome. In 1 study, 10 of 32 dogs had neurologic signs at the time of enrollment into the study, but all dogs had neurologic signs by 1 year after diagnosis.[12] In a separate study, dogs with neurologic comorbidities were at a greater risk for developing complications following surgical correction of laryngeal paralysis.[41]

In the absence of surgical complications, unilateral arytenoid lateralization results in reduced respiratory distress and stridor and improved exercise tolerance. Owner satisfaction with this procedure is excellent, with most owners believing that the quality of the dog's life was improved dramatically. One-year, 2-year, 3-year, and 4-year survival rates have been reported at 93.6%, 89.1%, 84.4%, and 75.2%, respectively; in dogs that developed aspiration pneumonia following surgery, the 1-year, 2-year, 3-year, and 4-year survival rates were 83.1%, 63.7%, 51.5%, and 25.8%, respectively.[37]

FELINE LARYNGEAL PARALYSIS

Laryngeal disease is uncommon in cats, but significant respiratory distress can result. Clinical presentation is similar to that in dogs in that it occurs most often in middle-aged to older cats (mean, 9–14 years), and both unilateral and bilateral conditions have been documented. There is also a prevalence of left-sided unilateral laryngeal paralysis in cats, which is similar to that reported in humans and horses (Video 2). Unlike dogs, cats with unilateral dysfunction can have significant clinical signs and require surgical intervention.

The specific cause of laryngeal paralysis in cats often remains undetermined, but several cases have been associated with trauma, neoplastic invasion, and iatrogenic damage (eg, following thyroidectomy or surgical correction of patent ductus arteriosus). Neoplastic infiltration can lead to fixed laryngeal obstruction with both inspiratory and expiratory respiratory difficulty and noise and should always be considered as a differential diagnosis of laryngeal paralysis in the cat. For assessment of laryngeal function, alfaxalone has been evaluated compared with propofol and midazolam/ketamine for effects on laryngeal function in normal cats (**Box 2**).[42] All 3 protocols provided similar conditions to evaluate laryngeal motion, although subjective arytenoid movement was present in all cats only when alfaxalone was used, which might allow improved functional evaluation of the larynx in a clinical setting.

Conservative management of cats with laryngeal paralysis consists of weight loss and minimization of excitement and rigorous exercise. Successful surgical treatment primarily using unilateral arytenoid lateralization has been described in several small studies.

LARYNGEAL COLLAPSE

Laryngeal collapse is a consequence of chronic upper airway obstruction, most often associated with brachycephalic obstructive airway syndrome (**Box 3**). However, laryngeal collapse can occur alone, or be associated with laryngeal paralysis, nasal and nasopharyngeal obstruction, or trauma in both brachycephalic and mesaticephalic breeds. Chronic upper airway obstruction causes increased airway resistance and increased negative intraglottic luminal pressure. Over time, this results in laryngeal collapse caused by cartilage fatigue and degeneration. Early onset of laryngeal collapse has been reported in brachycephalic dogs less than 6 months of age.

Concurrent laryngeal paralysis and laryngeal collapse has been reported in a small set of nonbrachycephalic small-breed dogs.[43] Norwich terriers have been identified as

---

Box 2
Drugs used during functional laryngeal examination

Premedications:
    Glycopyrrolate: 0.005 to 0.01 mg/kg IV, intramuscular (IM), subcutaneous (SC), and
    Butorphanol: 0.2 to 0.4 mg/kg IV, IM, SQ, or
    Buprenorphine: 0.005 to 0.02 mg/kg IV, IM, SC, or
    Hydromorphone: 0.1 to 0.2 mg/kg IV, IM, SC

Induction:
    Propofol: 4 to 8 mg/kg IV, administered slowly
    Alfaxalone: 2 to 4 mg/kg IV, administered slowly

To stimulate respiration:
    Doxapram HCl: 1 to 2 mg/kg IV

To decrease laryngeal swelling:
    Dexamethasone: 0.1 to 1.0 mg/kg IV

To mitigate anxiety:
    Acepromazine: 0.005 to 0.02 mg/kg IV
    Butorphanol: 0.2 to 0.4 mg/kg IV
    Buprenorphine: 0.005 to 0.02 mg/kg IV

Modified from MacPhail C. Laryngeal disease in dogs and cats. Vet Clin North Am Small Anim Pract. 2014;44(1):19-31; with permission.

---

a specific breed that can have laryngeal abnormalities consisting of redundant supra-arytenoid folds, laryngeal collapse, everted laryngeal saccules, and narrowed laryngeal openings.[44,45]

Diagnosis of laryngeal collapse requires oral laryngeal examination under heavy sedation or a light plane of general anesthesia without intubation. Functional and structural examination of the larynx should be performed. CT imaging and three-dimensional internal rendering have been used to document laryngeal collapse in 9 dogs with no sedation or general anesthesia required.[19]

The early stage of laryngeal collapse (**Fig. 3**) is amenable to surgical treatment. Resection of the everted laryngeal saccules is simple because each saccule is grasped with Allis tissue forceps and then sharply transected with Metzenbaum scissors. Options for treatment of advanced stages of laryngeal collapse are limited. Before considering any definitive surgery, underlying components of brachycephalic obstructive airway syndrome should be addressed, and the degree of improvement assessed. Dogs with stage 2 and 3 laryngeal collapse (**Fig. 4**) can markedly benefit from removal of everted laryngeal saccules, in addition to surgical correction of elongated soft palate and stenotic nares. However, in a recent study, brachycephalic dogs undergoing laryngeal sacculectomy in addition to staphylectomy and nares resection were more likely to develop complications compared with brachycephalic dogs receiving staphylectomy and nares resection alone.[46] Unilateral arytenoid

---

Box 3
Stages of laryngeal collapse

Stage 1: everted laryngeal saccules

Stage 2: aryepiglottic collapse with medial deviation of cuneiform processes

Stage 3: collapse of the corniculate processes

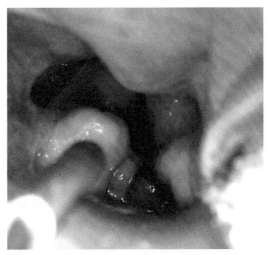

Fig. 3. Severely swollen and everted laryngeal saccules in a 6-year-old English bulldog. (*From* MacPhail C. Laryngeal disease in dogs and cats. Vet Clin North Am Small Anim Pract. 2014;44(1):19-31; with permission.)

laryngoplasty (cricoarytenoid lateralization combined with thyroarytenoid caudolateralization) has been reported to have reasonable long-term outcomes in a small number of brachycephalic dogs with laryngeal collapse, but this technique should be used with caution because the opposite cartilage may continue to collapse medially postoperatively leading to progressive airway obstruction. Permanent tracheostomy is the recommended treatment when dogs do not respond to other medical or surgical treatments, although many owners consider this an unacceptable option because of the high risk of complications and degree of maintenance required. In a study of 15 brachycephalic dogs with severe laryngeal collapse receiving permanent tracheostomy, there was a high risk of severe complications and postoperative death; however, a long-term (>5 years) good quality of life was reported in 5 of those dogs.[47]

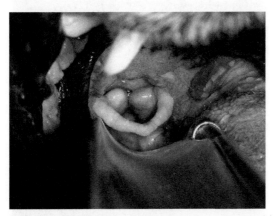

Fig. 4. Moderate to severe (stage 2–3) laryngeal collapse in a 7-year-old pug. (*From* MacPhail C. Laryngeal disease in dogs and cats. Vet Clin North Am Small Anim Pract. 2014;44(1):19-31; with permission.)

LARYNGEAL MASSES
Neoplasia

Tumors of the larynx are uncommon in dogs and cats. Numerous types of tumor have been reported in dogs, including rhabdomyosarcoma (oncocytoma), squamous cell carcinoma, adenocarcinoma, osteosarcoma, chondrosarcoma, chondroma, myxochondroma, lipoma, fibrosarcoma, undifferentiated carcinoma, extramedullary plasmacytoma, and mast cell tumor (**Fig. 5**). Squamous cell carcinoma and lymphoma are the most common tumors of the larynx in the cat, but adenocarcinoma and other poorly differentiated round cell tumors have been reported.

Small lesions can be removed by mucosal resection or partial laryngectomy through an oral approach or ventral laryngotomy. Cartilaginous tumors (eg, chondroma or chondrosarcoma) can be excised with reasonable success. Aggressive surgical intervention involves complete laryngectomy with permanent tracheostomy, but this has been reported only in isolated cases. Radioresponsive tumors can be treated with radiation therapy. Otherwise most treatment is palliative, consisting of airflow bypass of the laryngeal area through a permanent tracheostomy. Regardless, prognosis for laryngeal tumors is guarded because most cases are advanced at the time of diagnosis. There are only isolated reports of management of canine and feline laryngeal tumors. Treatment of 4 cats with laryngeal squamous cell carcinoma with tube tracheostomy alone resulted in a median survival of only 3 days; chemotherapeutic treatment of 5 cats with varying types of laryngeal masses resulted in a median survival of 141 days.[48] Two cats with laryngeal lymphoma were treated with chemotherapy, resulting in survival times of 60 and 1440 days.[49] In this same study, 1 cat with laryngeal squamous cell carcinoma was treated with prednisolone and had a survival time of 180 days.

A study reported on the placement of permanent tracheostomies in 5 cats with laryngeal carcinoma; survival at home ranged from 2 to 281 days, with 2 cats dying from tracheostomy site occlusion and 3 cats euthanized because of disease progression.[50]

Benign Growths

Inflammatory laryngeal disease is an uncommon nonneoplastic condition of the arytenoid cartilages of the larynx that has been reported in both dogs and cats. It can be

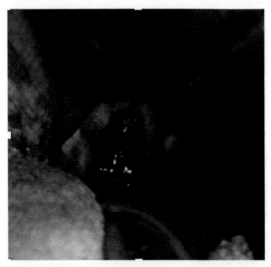

Fig. 5. A 10-year-old dog with laryngeal neoplasia.

granulomatous, lymphocytic-plasmacytic, or eosinophilic, with multiple factors likely contributing to the development of the disease. Severe cases can result in laryngeal stenosis and significant upper airway obstruction. Biopsy of the laryngeal mass is crucial to differentiate this disease from neoplasia, although it is still possible that inflammatory changes may represent a secondary response to underlying neoplasia. Treatment of inflammatory laryngeal disease is palliative and consists of debulking of the mass, steroid therapy, or permanent tracheostomy. Permanent tracheostomy may be considered, but this procedure has been associated with a higher mortality in cats with inflammatory laryngeal disease than in cats undergoing permanent tracheostomy for any other reason.

Benign laryngeal cysts also have been described in isolated canine and feline cases. Cysts are typically epithelial in origin and stem from the ventral aspect of the larynx. Some cysts are very large and can significantly obstruct airflow; however, surgical removal is usually curative.

SUMMARY

Diseases of the larynx can lead to life-threatening upper airway obstruction. Fundamental knowledge of laryngeal anatomy and use of appropriate sedation or anesthetic protocols are essential for thorough assessment of laryngeal structure and function. Prognosis is variable depending on the underlying cause.

DISCLOSURE

There are no commercial or financial conflicts of interest.

SUPPLEMENTARY DATA

Supplementary data related to this article can be found online at https://doi.org/10.1016/j.cvsm.2019.11.001.

REFERENCES

1. Monnet E, Tobias KM. Larynx. In: Tobias KM, Johnston SA, editors. Veterinary surgery small animal. St. Louis (MO): Elsevier; 2012. p. 1724.
2. Ridyard AE, Corcoran BM, Tasker S, et al. Spontaneous laryngeal paralysis in four white-coated German shepherd dogs. J Small Anim Pract 2000;41:558–61.
3. Venker-van Haagen AJ, Bouw J, Hartman W. Hereditary transmission of laryngeal paralysis in bouviers. J Am Anim Hosp Assoc 1981;18:75–6.
4. O'Brien JA, Hendriks J. Inherited laryngeal paralysis. Analysis in the husky cross. Vet Q 1986;8:301–2.
5. Polizopoulou ZS, Koutinas AF, Papadopoulos GC, et al. Juvenile laryngeal paralysis in three Siberian husky x Alaskan malamute puppies. Vet Rec 2003;153:624–7.
6. von Pfeil DJF, Zellner E, Fritz MC, et al. Congenital laryngeal paralysis in Alaskan Huskies: 25 cases (2009-2014). J Am Vet Med Assoc 2018;253:1057–65.
7. Braund KG, Shores A, Cochrane S, et al. Laryngeal paralysis-polyneuropathy complex in young Dalmatians. Am J Vet Res 1994;55:534–42.
8. Mahony OM, Knowles KE, Braund KG, et al. Laryngeal paralysis-polyneuropathy complex in young Rottweilers. J Vet Intern Med 1998;12:330–7.
9. Shelton GD, Podell M, Poncelet L, et al. Inherited polyneuropathy in Leonberger dogs: a mixed or intermediate form of Charcot-Marie-Tooth disease? Muscle Nerve 2003;27:471–7.

10. Gabriel A, Poncelet L, Van Ham L, et al. Laryngeal paralysis-polyneuropathy complex in young related Pyrenean mountain dogs. J Small Anim Pract 2006; 47:144–9.

11. Vandenberghe H, Escriou C, Rosati M, et al. Juvenile-onset polyneuropathy in American Staffordshire Terriers. J Vet Intern Med 2018;32:2003–12.

12. Stanley BJ, Hauptman JG, Fritz MC, et al. Esophageal dysfunction in dogs with idiopathic laryngeal paralysis: a controlled cohort study. Vet Surg 2010;39: 139–49.

13. Thieman KM, Krahwinkel DJ, Sims MH, et al. Histopathological confirmation of polyneuropathy in 11 dogs with laryngeal paralysis. J Am Anim Hosp Assoc 2010;46:161–7.

14. Shelton GD. Acquired laryngeal paralysis in dogs: evidence accumulating for a generalized neuromuscular disease. Vet Surg 2010;39:137–8.

15. Tarvin KM, Twedt DC, Monnet E. Prospective controlled study of gastroesophageal reflux in dogs with naturally occurring laryngeal paralysis. Vet Surg 2016; 45:916–21.

16. Jaggy A, Oliver JE, Ferguson DC, et al. Neurological manifestations of hypothyroidism: a retrospective study of 29 dogs. J Vet Intern Med 1994;8:328–36.

17. MacPhail CM, Monnet E. Outcome of and postoperative complications in dogs undergoing surgical treatment of laryngeal paralysis: 140 cases (1985–1998). J Am Vet Med Assoc 2001;218:1949–56.

18. Rudorf H, Barr FJ, Lane JG. The role of ultrasound in the assessment of laryngeal paralysis in the dog. Vet Radiol Ultrasound 2001;42:338–43.

19. Stadler K, Hartman S, Matheson J, et al. Computed tomographic imaging of dogs with primary laryngeal or tracheal airway obstruction. Vet Radiol Ultrasound 2011; 52:377–84.

20. Radlinsky MG, Williams J, Frank PM, et al. Comparison of three clinical techniques for the diagnosis of laryngeal paralysis in dogs. Vet Surg 2009;38:434–8.

21. McKeirnan KL, Gross ME, Rochat M, et al. Comparison of propofol and propofol/ketamine anesthesia for evaluation of laryngeal function in healthy dogs. J Am Anim Hosp Assoc 2014;50:19–26.

22. Maney JK, Shepard MK, Braun C, et al. A comparison of cardiopulmonary and anesthetic effects of an induction dose of alfaxalone or propofol in dogs. Vet Anaesth Analg 2013;40:237–44.

23. Amengual M, Flaherty D, Auckburally A, et al. An evaluation of anaesthetic induction in healthy dogs using rapid intravenous injection of propofol or alfaxalone. Vet Anaesth Analg 2013;40:115–23.

24. Radkey DI, Hardie RJ, Smith LJ. Comparison of the effects of alfaxalone and propofol with acepromazine, butorphanol and/or doxapram on laryngeal motion and quality of examination in dogs. Vet Anaesth Analg 2018;45:241–9.

25. Cheng E, Griffenhagen GM, MacPhail CM. Comparison of alfaxalone and propofol anesthesia for evaluation of laryngeal function in normal dogs. Vet Surg 2018; 47:E8–9.

26. Nicholson I, Baines S. Complications associated with temporary tracheostomy tubes in 42 dogs (1998 to 2007). J Small Anim Pract 2012;53:108–14.

27. Hardie RJ. Translaryngeal percutaneous arytenoid lateralization technique in a canine cadaveric study. J Vet Emerg Crit Care (San Antonio) 2016;26:659–63.

28. Occhipinti LL, Hauptman JG. Long-term outcome of permanent tracheostomies in dogs: 21 cases (2000-2012). Can Vet J 2014;55:357–60.

29. Gauthier CM, Monnet E. In vitro evaluation of anatomic landmarks for the placement of suture to achieve effective arytenoid cartilage abduction by means of unilateral cricoarytenoid lateralization in dogs. Am J Vet Res 2014;75:602–6.
30. von Pfeil DJ, Edwards MR, Déjardin LM. Less invasive unilateral arytenoid lateralization: a modified technique for treatment of idiopathic laryngeal paralysis in dogs: technique description and outcome. Vet Surg 2014;43:704–11.
31. Perez Lopez P, Barnes DC, Nelissen P, et al. Outcome of two variations of a surgical technique performed for canine unilateral arytenoid lateralisation. Vet Rec 2019. https://doi.org/10.1136/vr.105120.
32. Ross JT, Matthiesen DT, Noone KE, et al. Complications and long-term results after partial laryngectomy for the treatment of idiopathic laryngeal paralysis in 45 dogs. Vet Surg 1991;20:169–73.
33. Holt D, Harvey C. Idiopathic laryngeal paralysis: results of treatment by bilateral vocal fold resection in 40 dogs. J Am Anim Hosp Assoc 1994;30:389–95.
34. Zikes C, McCarthy T. Bilateral ventriculocordectomy via ventral laryngotomy for idiopathic laryngeal paralysis in 88 dogs. J Am Anim Hosp Assoc 2012;48: 234–44.
35. Bahr KL, Howe L, Jessen C, et al. Outcome of 45 dogs with laryngeal paralysis treated by unilateral arytenoid lateralization or bilateral ventriculocordectomy. J Am Anim Hosp Assoc 2014;50:264–72.
36. Regier PJ, McCarthy TC, Monnet E. Effect of bilateral ventriculocordectomy via ventral laryngotomy on laryngeal airway resistance in larynges of canine cadavers. Am J Vet Res 2017;78:1444–8.
37. Wilson D, Monnet E. Risk factors for the development of aspiration pneumonia after unilateral arytenoid lateralization in dogs with laryngeal paralysis: 232 cases (1987-2012). J Am Vet Med Assoc 2016;248:188–94.
38. Milovancev M, Townsend K, Spina J, et al. Effect of metoclopramide on the incidence of early postoperative aspiration pneumonia in dogs with acquired idiopathic laryngeal paralysis. Vet Surg 2016;45:577–81.
39. Kempf J, Lewis F, Reusch CE, et al. High-resolution manometric evaluation of the effects of cisapride and metoclopramide hydrochloride administered orally on lower esophageal sphincter pressure in awake dogs. Am J Vet Res 2014;75: 361–6.
40. Ogden J, Ovbey D, Saile K. Effects of preoperative cisapride on postoperative aspiration pneumonia in dogs with laryngeal paralysis. J Small Anim Pract 2019;60:183–90.
41. Bookbinder LC, Flanders J, Bookbinder PF, et al. Idiopathic canine laryngeal paralysis as one sign of a diffuse polyneuropathy: an observational study of 90 cases (2007-2013). Vet Surg 2016;45:254–60.
42. Nelissen P, Corletto F, Aprea F, et al. Effect of three anesthetic induction protocols on laryngeal motion during laryngoscopy in normal cats. Vet Surg 2012;41: 876–83.
43. Nelissen P, White RA. Arytenoid lateralization for management of combined laryngeal paralysis and laryngeal collapse in small dogs. Vet Surg 2012;41:261–5.
44. Johnson LR, Mayhew PD, Steffey MA, et al. Upper airway obstruction in Norwich Terriers: 16 cases. J Vet Intern Med 2013;27:1409–15.
45. Koch DA, Rosaspina M, Wiestner T, et al. Comparative investigations on the upper respiratory tract in Norwich terriers, brachycephalic and mesaticephalic dogs. Schweiz Arch Tierheilkd 2014;156:119–24.
46. Hughes JR, Kaye BM, Beswick AR, et al. Complications following laryngeal sacculectomy in brachycephalic dogs. J Small Anim Pract 2018;59:16–21.

47. Gobbetti M, Romussi S, Buracco P, et al. Long-term outcome of permanent tracheostomy in 15 dogs with severe laryngeal collapse secondary to brachycephalic airway obstructive syndrome. Vet Surg 2018;47:648–53.
48. Guenther-Yenke CL, Rozanski EA. Tracheostomy in cats: 23 cases (1998-2006). J Feline Med Surg 2007;9:451–7.
49. Jakubiak MJ, Siedlecki CT, Zenger E, et al. Laryngeal, laryngotracheal, and tracheal masses in cats: 27 cats (1998-2003). J Am Anim Hosp Assoc 2005; 41:310–6.
50. Stepnik MW, Mehl ML, Hardie EM, et al. Outcome of permanent tracheostomy for treatment of upper airway obstruction in cats: 21 cases (1990-2007). J Am Vet Med Assoc 2009;234:638–43.

Chronic Rhinitis in the Cat

An Update

Nicki Reed, BVM&S, Cert VR, MRCVS

KEYWORDS

- Feline chronic rhinitis • Nasal • Inflammation • Herpesvirus • Bacteria • Treatment

KEY POINTS

- Feline chronic rhinitis/rhinosinusitis is the second most common cause of feline nasal disease, accounting for approximately 35% of cases.
- Proposed etiology relates to initial turbinate damage by feline herpesvirus 1 (FHV-1). The role of *Bordetella bronchiseptica* and *Mycoplasma* spp, as well as inhaled allergens as primary agents, is unclear at this time.
- Repeated short courses of antibacterials to treat secondary bacterial infection (typically oropharyngeal commensals) may result in selection for *Pseudomonas* spp or other resistant organisms.
- Treatment is primarily supportive comprising antibacterials, mucolytics or decongestants, antiviral therapies, and in severe cases surgery. Nasal flushing to remove mucus often is beneficial.
- Owners need to be counseled that cure is unlikely. Treatment aims to reduce the frequency and severity of episodes.

INTRODUCTION

Feline chronic rhinitis can be defined as inflammation of the nasal cavity that has been present for 4 weeks or longer, either intermittently or continuously.[1] Because the frontal sinuses also can be involved, the condition may be called chronic rhinosinusitis (CRS). The diagnosis accounts for approximately 35% of cases of feline rhinitis[2,3] and after neoplasia is the second most common cause of chronic nasal discharge in cats.[3] Despite being a relatively common condition in feline practice, it can be a frustrating disease to manage.

ETIOLOGY

It has been proposed that primary viral infection, especially by feline herpesvirus 1 (FHV-1), causes damage to the mucosal epithelium and underlying turbinate bones, thereby predisposing to recurrent bacterial rhinitis.[4–6] One study used a polymerase

Veterinary Specialists, Scotland, 1 Deer Park Road, Livingston, West Lothian, Scotland, EH54 8AF, UK
E-mail address: nicki@vetscotland.com

Vet Clin Small Anim 50 (2020) 311–329
https://doi.org/10.1016/j.cvsm.2019.10.005
0195-5616/20/© 2019 Elsevier Inc. All rights reserved.

chain reaction (PCR) technique to identify FHV-1 DNA in nasal biopsy samples but failed to show a difference in isolation rates between cats with CRS and healthy control cats.[6] This suggests that recrudescence of viral disease per se may be less important in the role of CRS than other factors, such as structural damage, secondary bacterial infection, and impaired immune function.[7-10]

Although bacterial infection has been identified in 69% to 90% of cases,[1,6] primary bacterial infection is thought to be rare. Mixed growth of commensal organisms frequently is identified; more significance might be attached to a heavy pure growth of 1 organism, especially one considered pathogenic[6] (**Box 1**). Rarer bacteria isolated from cases of CRS include *Haemophilus* spp[11] and *Capnocytophaga* spp.[12]

One study[10] attempted to evaluate the role of *Bartonella* spp in CRS but failed to identify these organisms by culture of blood samples or PCR of nasal biopsies, with the exception of 1 case that had a nasopharyngeal abscess. Serologic testing did not identify differences in seropositivity to *Bartonella* spp between cats with CRS and 3 control groups. Although the study was underpowered, it did not support a role for these organisms in CRS.

The role of *Mycoplasma* spp in rhinitis remains uncertain, because these organisms have been considered to be part of the commensal flora in the upper respiratory tract. *Mycoplasma* spp were detected in cats affected by CRS but not in control cats, suggesting that they may play a role in this disease complex.[6] Use of PCR may facilitate identification of *Mycoplasma* spp, which can be difficult to culture.[13]

Retroviral infection was previously suggested to be associated with CRS,[14] because in 1 study 55% of cats were positive for feline leukemia virus infection.[15] Subsequent studies, however, showed a reduced prevalence of retroviral infection (0%–7%).[1,16,17] This mirrored the declining prevalence of infection in the feline population subsequent to the introduction of feline leukemia virus vaccination.

A recent case report identified the presence of *Tritrichomonas foetus* organisms in nasal cavity swabs from a cat with chronic rhinitis; however, because *Mycoplasma felis* was concurrently identified, the role of this protozooal organism in this disease is uncertain.[18]

Box 1
Potentially pathogenic bacteria in feline chronic rhinosinusitis

Pseudomonas aeruginosa

Escherichia coli

Viridans streptococci

Staphylococcus pseudintermedius

Pasteurella multocida

Corynebacterium spp

Actinomyces spp

Bordetella bronchiseptica

Mycoplasma spp

All anaerobes

Data from Johnson LR, Foley JE, De Cock HE, et al. Assessment of infectious organisms associated with chronic rhinosinusitis in cats. J Amer Vet Med Assoc. 2005; 227(4): 579-85.

The role of allergens has not been extensively investigated in cats. This is a common cause of rhinitis in people, estimated to affect 1.4 million people worldwide[19]; therefore, the prevalence of allergic rhinitis may be underestimated in the feline population, particularly in cats exhibiting concurrent signs of asthma or conjunctivitis.

PATIENT HISTORY

- Usually identified in young to middle-aged cats, although there is a wide age range affected (0.5–16 years)[3,10]
- Might have had a history of cat flu as a kitten, although this is often difficult to establish
- Recurrent episodes of nasal discharge (**Fig. 1**), which can be
  - Serous (initially)
  - Mucoid
  - Mucopurulent
  - Sanguineous (less common)
  - Unilateral, bilateral, or unilateral progressing to bilateral
- Sneezing
- Stertorous respiration
- Episodes may be associated with stressors, such as boarding, breeding, or neutering.
- Cats can become inappetent at times of clinical signs due to
  - Inability to smell food
  - Difficulty breathing
  - Pyrexia
- Episodes often respond to antibacterials but relapse is common.
- Gagging, choking, or reverse sneezing is more commonly seen with nasopharyngeal diseases, rather than rhinitis, but could be observed with accumulation of discharges in the nasopharynx.

PHYSICAL EXAMINATION

In addition to a complete physical examination, particular attention should be made to examining the specific features listed in **Table 1**. In order to perform a thorough oral examination, general anesthesia invariably is required.

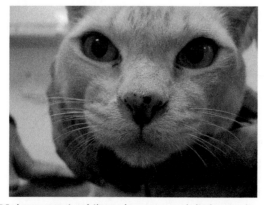

Fig. 1. Cat with CRS demonstrating bilateral serous nasal discharge. (*From* Reed N. Chronic rhinitis in the cat. Vet Clin North Am Small Anim Pract. 2014;44(1):33-50; with permission.)

Table 1
Salient features of physical examination in chronic rhinosinusitis

Assessment	Significance
Nasal airflow Can be assessed by observing condensation on a cold microscope slide or by holding wisps of cotton wool in front of nares	Decreased nasal airflow often is due to obstruction with mass lesions (neoplastic, fungal, or foreign body related)
Presence of nasal discharge Unilateral or bilateral; nature	Unilateral discharge is more common with foreign body or neoplasia than CRS. Discharge typically is mucoid, becoming mucopurulent with secondary bacterial infection.
Facial symmetry	Facial asymmetry is seen more commonly with neoplasia or fungal infection but can be seen with CRS.
Facial pain May be appreciated on palpation or if the cat demonstrates head aversion when approached.	Can be seen with CRS, neoplasia, fungal infections, foreign bodies or dental disease and indicates that analgesia should be provided
Conjunctivitis	Can indicate infection with certain organisms, such as FHV-1, FCV, C felis, or Mycoplasma spp, which may or may not be related to rhinitis.
Epiphora Fluorescein staining can be used to assess patency of nasolacrimal duct.	May have concurrent keratitis or ocular ulceration Chronic inflammation can cause blockage of the nasolacrimal system.
Retinal examination	Can identify chorioretinitis associated with cryptococcal infection or lymphoma.
Oral examination	Used to identify cleft palate, oronasal fistula, and mass lesions causing ventral deviation of the soft palate. Visualization of the nasopharynx can be facilitated by retracting the soft palate with a spay hook and using a dental mirror.
Otic examination	Mass lesions or bowing of the tympanic membrane can be seen in association with nasopharyngeal polyps.
Lymph node palpation The submandibular and retropharyngeal lymph nodes should be evaluated.	Lymph node enlargement is a nonspecific finding, although asymmetry can suggest disease, such as neoplasia, fungal infection, or foreign body, is more likely than CRS.

From Reed N. Chronic rhinitis in the cat. Vet Clin North Am Small Anim Pract. 2014;44(1):33-50; with permission.

DIAGNOSTIC TESTING

A diagnosis of CRS is usually based on excluding other conditions that could cause signs of upper respiratory tract disease. Differential diagnoses to consider for the clinical presentation of sneezing and nasal discharge are given in **Box 2**. In order to eliminate these other conditions, several tests generally are required. Investigations typically progress from the least invasive to the most invasive.

Box 2
Differential diagnoses for chronic sneezing and nasal discharge
Neoplasia (lymphoma, adenocarcinoma, sarcoma)
Nasopharyngeal polyp
Foreign body
Fungal infection (*Cryptococcosis, Aspergillosis, Penicillium* spp)
Nasopharyngeal stenosis
Trauma
Congenital (cleft palate; extreme brachycephalic conformation)
Dental disease (oronasal fistula; tooth root infection/abscess)
Inflammatory polyps of the nasal turbinates (mesenchymal nasal hamartoma)
From Reed N. Chronic rhinitis in the cat. Vet Clin North Am Small Anim Pract. 2014;44(1):33-50; with permission.

Laboratory Analysis

Routine hematology, biochemistry, and urinalysis findings are nonspecific but give information about the general health of the cat prior to administration of general anesthesia or therapeutics. Retroviral testing does not assist with the diagnosis but contributes toward the overall health status of the cat and may have an effect on prognosis. Serologic evaluation for respiratory viruses is of no use due to the high prevalence of seropositivity in healthy cats.[20] In cases of suspected *Cryptococcus* infection, performance of a latex cryptococcal antigen test is useful for both diagnosis and monitoring.[21] See Vanessa R. Barrs and Jessica J. Talbot's article, "Fungal Rhinosinusitis and Disseminated Invasive Aspergillosis in Cats," in this issue for further information on feline aspergillosis.

Oropharyngeal/Conjunctival Swabbing

In cats with acute upper respiratory tract disease, oropharyngeal and conjunctival swabs can be submitted for bacterial culture (*Chlamydia felis, Bordetella bronchiseptica,* and *Mycoplasma* spp), virus isolation (FHV-1), feline calicivirus (FCV), and PCR (FHV-1, FCV, *C felis, B bronchiseptica,* and *Mycoplasma* spp). Special transport media are required, particularly for virus isolation. Interpretation of results can be problematic. A negative result does not necessarily exclude the infection as the cause of the disease, particularly with fragile organisms that are difficult to culture (eg, *Mycoplasma*) or if the organism is intermittently shed (eg, FHV-1). Conversely identifying FHV-1 or FCV does not always explain the clinical signs, due to the high prevalence of these infections in the healthy cat population and inability to differentiate positive test results from presence of vaccinal strains.[22–24]

Nasal Swabbing

Swabbing nasal discharge for culture is of minimal benefit, because it is likely that only commensal bacteria of the oropharynx will be cultured.[25] Cytology is likely to reveal degenerate neutrophils as the predominant cell type, and, again, although bacteria may be identified, their significance is questionable. The finding of encapsulated yeast organisms would be supportive of *Cryptococcus* infection; use of Romanowsky stains, new methylene blue, or Gram stain enables the organism to be seen surrounded by a clear halo.[26]

Special Considerations for Epistaxis

If frank hemorrhage from the nose is part of the presenting complaint, a coagulation panel should be assessed in addition to a platelet count. If the nasal discharge is sanguineous in nature, if the cat is older than 8 years old, or if concurrent kidney disease is identified, systolic blood pressure also should be measured.

Diagnostic Imaging

Accurate positioning requires general anesthesia, and several radiographic views should be taken to fully evaluate the nasal cavity and sinuses.[27] Superimposition of the mandible in the dorsoventral views necessitates use of dental film or performance of a ventro 30° rostral-dorsocaudal view.[27] Radiological interpretation is given elsewhere,[28] but findings consistent with CRS include unilateral or bilateral soft tissue/fluid opacification of the nasal cavity and/or frontal sinuses with blurring of turbinate structures. Erosion of the turbinate bones and mass lesions can be identified radiographically in cats with neoplasia or chronic rhinitis,[29] making a definitive diagnosis by radiological assessment impossible.

Computed tomography (CT) is considered superior to radiography for imaging the nasal cavity and paranasal sinuses in dogs[30–32] and the same is likely true in the cat. The CT appearance of the normal feline nasal cavity and paranasal sinuses has been described.[33] Studies comparing the CT appearance of nasal neoplasia and inflammatory disease in cats identified that many imaging findings overlapped between these conditions[34,35] (**Fig. 2**). Features occurring significantly more often in cats with neoplasia included lysis of the ventral aspect of the maxilla or vomer bone, unilateral lysis of the ethmoturbinates or dorsal and lateral aspects of the maxilla, bilateral lysis of the orbital lamina and unilateral soft tissue opacification of the frontal sinus, sphenoid sinus, and retrobulbar space.[35] In addition, where the medial retropharyngeal lymph nodes are also evaluated, the presence of an abnormal hilum, asymmetry in height of the lymph nodes, and decreased precontrast heterogeneity were significantly associated with the presence of neoplasia.[36]

Nasal Flush

Nasal flushes can be performed to collect diagnostic material; however, flushing may also be used as a therapeutic technique. The procedure should be performed under general anesthesia with a cuffed endotracheal tube in place. The cat is in sternal recumbency with the head angled down to facilitate drainage of fluid.

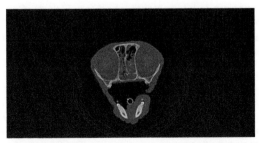

Fig. 2. CT scan of a cat with CRS demonstrating loss of turbinate structure and accumulation of fluid within the nasal cavity. Deviation of the septum can be a normal finding in cats. (*From* Reed N. Chronic rhinitis in the cat. Vet Clin North Am Small Anim Pract. 2014;44(1):33-50; with permission.)

- Diagnostic flush: a 6F–8F sterile catheter is inserted into the rostral nasal cavity (not beyond the level of the medial canthus of the eye). The nasopharynx is occluded by dorsal digital pressure on the soft palate; 2mL to 4 mL of sterile saline then is gently flushed down the catheter followed by aspiration of the fluid to obtain a sample for aerobic and anaerobic culture. Fungal culture and PCR testing for viral agents or Mycoplasma may also be performed where indicated.
- Therapeutic flush: the oropharynx is packed with a gauze swab or surgical laparotomy pad to prevent aspiration of material and allow collection of any foreign material that is flushed from the nasal cavity. A 10-mL to 35-mL syringe is filled with sterile saline and the tip inserted into the nostril. The naris is compressed around the syringe tip and the contralateral naris occluded. The syringe is then depressed with steady pulsations of pressure to force material caudally onto the swab (**Fig. 3**). The process is repeated until all the mucopurulent material is flushed through and then performed on the contralateral side. Mass lesions and foreign bodies also can be dislodged by this technique.

Although good agreement has been reported between bacterial cultures from nasal flush samples compared with biopsy samples,[6] discordant results were reported between these 2 methods in 32%, 10%, and 18% of cases, when culture of aerobic, anaerobic, and *Mycoplasma* organisms were respectively considered.[37] The increased recovery of organisms from nasal flushes could be due to culture of superficial organisms not involved in the disease process or could reflect increased difficulty in culturing representative bacteria from tissue samples compared with flush fluid, because the latter is directly inoculated onto culture media while maceration of biopsy material is required.[37]

Endoscopy

The nasopharynx can be evaluated with a flexible endoscope (eg, 3–5 mm bronchoscope) capable of 180° flexion. Endoscopic evaluation of the nasal cavity can be performed in a normograde fashion using either a rigid endoscope with a viewing angle of 0° to 30° or a flexible endoscope of 2-mm to 3-mm diameter. Saline flushing via the biopsy channel can remove mucus and facilitate visualization of the mucosa. A throat pack or swabs should be placed in the pharynx to prevent aspiration of material. The nasal mucosa overlying the turbinates should appear pink and smooth and the vessels

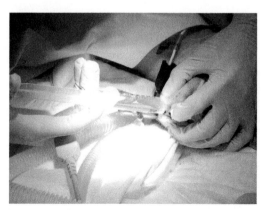

Fig. 3. A nasal flush being performed to remove mucus and potentially foreign bodies. (*From* Reed N. Chronic rhinitis in the cat. Vet Clin North Am Small Anim Pract. 2014;44(1):33-50; with permission.)

should be clearly seen. Abnormalities seen with chronic rhinitis include congestion and decreased visibility of the capillaries, hyperemia, increased fragility, ulceration, and increased mucus. In addition, turbinate destruction can give rise to increased space when trying to navigate the meati.

Endoscopy allows collection of targeted cytology or biopsy samples. Evaluation of the frontal sinuses cannot normally be undertaken in cats, although extensive turbinate destruction from fungal infection permitted passage of a small endoscope in 1 case.[38]

Brush Cytology

An endoscopic cytology brush can be passed down the biopsy channel or passed adjacent to the endoscope to allow direct visualization,[2] although samples can be nondiagnostic due to poor cellularity.[2,39] Comparison between cytologic and histologic samples has shown poor agreement, with only 25% of samples having the same predominant cell type[2]; neoplasia was incorrectly diagnosed as inflammatory in 27% of cases.[39] Because histopathology is likely to give a more accurate diagnosis, this technique is rarely used.

Nasal Biopsy

Before taking nasal biopsy samples, the author recommends evaluation of coagulation status. As a minimum, prothrombin time, activated partial thromboplastin time, and fibrinogen should be measured, but performance of a buccal mucosal bleeding time also allows assessment of function of platelets and von Willebrand factor. Samples can be obtained via the biopsy channel of the endoscope; however, biopsy samples obtained are very small. Targeted sampling of focal lesions also can be achieved by passing the biopsy instrument alongside the rigid telescope, or, for diffuse disease, blind biopsies can be diagnostic. These can be performed with 3-mm biopsy cups (**Fig. 4**) and both right and left nasal cavities should be biopsied. The nasopharynx also can be biopsied via the biopsy channel of a flexible endoscope.

Where endoscopic equipment is not available, a suction biopsy can be obtained with a plastic catheter, the tip of which has been angled to 45° and suction applied with a 10-mL to 20-mL syringe.[40] Biopsy material should be submitted in plain tubes for bacterial and fungal culture as well as fixed in formalin for histopathology.

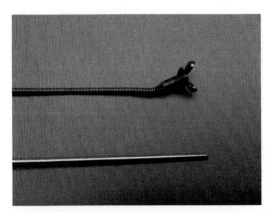

Fig. 4. Biopsy cups, 3-mm (*top*), allow for larger biopsy samples than can be obtained alongside a rigid endoscope (*bottom*). (*From* Reed N. Chronic rhinitis in the cat. Vet Clin North Am Small Anim Pract. 2014;44(1):33-50; with permission.)

Inflammatory infiltrate is classified according to the predominant cell type and is often described as lymphoplasmacytic, neutrophilic (suppurative), or mixed.[2,6] Neutrophilic infiltrate appears to be twice as common as lymphoplasmacytic infiltrate[2,17,41] and associated with more severe inflammatory changes.[38] Although neutrophilic infiltrate has been classified as acute rhinitis by some investigators,[3] and lymphoplasmacytic infiltrate considered the most common form of chronic rhinitis by others,[42] these differences may simply reflect the spectrum of 1 disease. The nature of the inflammatory infiltrate might depend on the presence or absence of bacterial infection at the time of sampling, because many cats with neutrophilic infiltrate have a chronic rather than acute history.

Other features that can be identified on histopathology include epithelial ulceration, fibrosis, turbinate destruction or remodeling, necrosis, and glandular hyperplasia.[43] The poor correlation between rhinoscopic appearance and histopathology indicates the need to obtain biopsy material bilaterally for histopathology.[41]

Eosinophilic infiltrate could suggest an allergic or parasitic origin, although this is unproved. Eosinophilic infiltrate in nasal biopsies from cats with rhinitis and concurrent signs of asthma has been identified on occasion by this author and also in a study of nasal histology in cats with experimentally induced allergic asthma,[44] which could support a role of allergy in eosinophilic rhinitis.

TREATMENT

Treatment of feline CRS is frustrating. No definitive therapy exists, and treatment is aimed at controlling episodes of clinical signs and preventing extension of disease. Owners need to be counseled regarding the recurrent nature of this condition and that treatment will not be curative. Multimodal therapy can be used to address different aspects of the disease.

Antibacterials

Ideally, choice of antibacterial agent should be based on culture and sensitivity results from nasal biopsies and/or nasal flush fluid.[6] Due to the recurrent nature of this disease, however, owners may be unwilling to subject the cat to repeated general anesthesia every time there is recurrence of clinical signs. As such, empiric prescribing often has to be used, with the choice of antibiotic based on the spectrum of infectious agents typically identified (see **Box 1**). In addition, the antibacterial chosen should have good penetration to bone and cartilage. Suggested antibacterial choices are given in **Table 2**. Due to the chronic, deep nature of these infections, this author normally prescribes therapy for a 6-week to 8-week period.

Although a few studies have assessed the efficacy of antibacterials in the treatment of acute rhinitis and *Chlamydia* infections,[46–51] these studies are based on culture of superficial ocular, nasal or oropharyngeal swabs. *Pseudomonas* spp were not identified in these studies, yet this is a commonly identified organism when deeper nasal samples are obtained.[6,8] *Pseudomonas* spp are resistant to the commonly used antibacterials listed in **Table 2**; hence, repeated antibacterial courses that eliminate other commensal organisms are likely to contribute to selection for this organism. Culture can identify appropriate sensitivity to veterinary licensed antibacterials, such as marbofloxacin or pradofloxacin. Alternatively, a licensed human antibacterial, such as a third-generation cephalosporin (eg, ceftazidime or cefoperazone) or aminoglycoside (eg, amikacin or tobramycin), might be required, although due consideration must be given to renal and ototoxicity with the aminoglycosides.[52] Efficacy of antibacterials might be enhanced by supportive therapies, discussed later.

Table 2
Oral antibacterial drugs used for management of chronic rhinosinusitis

Antibacterial	Spectrum	Dose	Comments
Amoxicillin-clavulanate	*Staphylococci* *Streptococci* *Chlamydia* *Escherichia coli* *Pasteurella* *Bordetella* Anaerobes	10–20 mg/kg q 8 h	Not effective against *Pseudomonas*
Azithromycin	*Staphylococci* *Streptococci* *Chlamydia* *Mycoplasma* *Bordetella* Anaerobes	10–15 mg/kg q 24 h	Inconsistent efficacy against *Chlamydia*.[44] Not effective against *Pseudomonas*
Chloramphenicol	*Staphylococci* *Streptococci* *Chlamydia* *E coli* *Bordetella* Anaerobes	20–40 mg/kg q 12 h	Can be ineffective, or resistance can develop with *Pseudomonas* Monitor hematology weekly due to risk of myelosuppression
Clindamycin	*Staphylococci* *Streptococci* *Chlamydia* *Actinomyces* Anaerobes *Mycoplasma*— variable efficacy	10–12 mg/kg q 12–24 h	Not effective against *Pseudomonas* or other gram- negative organisms Can cause esophagitis and esophageal strictures
Doxycycline	*Chlamydia* *Pasteurella* *Bordetella* *Mycoplasma* *Actinomyces*	10 mg/kg q 24 h	Good penetration into frontal sinuses Not effective against *Pseudomonas* or *Ecoli* Only effective against a few *Staphylococcus* and *Streptococcus* spp Can cause esophagitis and esophageal strictures May also have an immunomodulatory effect
Marbofloxacin	*Staphylococci* *Streptococci* *E coli* *Pasteurella* *Mycoplasma* (*Pseudomonas*)	5 mg/kg q 24 h	Could be less likely to cause retinal toxicity than enrofloxacin *Pseudomonas* may develop resistance.
Metronidazole	Anaerobes	15–20 mg/kg	Unpalatable Narrow spectrum, therefore, typically combined with other drugs

(continued on next page)

Table 2 (continued)			
Antibacterial	**Spectrum**	**Dose**	**Comments**
Pradofloxacin	*Staphylococci* *Streptococci* *E coli* *Pasteurella* *Mycoplasma* *(Pseudomonas)*	5 mg/kg q 24 h 10 mg/kg q 24 h[45]	Greater activity against anaerobes than other quinolones Less likely to cause retinal toxicity than enrofloxacin *Pseudomonas* may develop resistance

Data from Greene CE and Calpin J. Antimicrobial drug formulary In: Greene CE, editor. Infectious Diseases of the Dog and Cat 4th edition. St. Louis, Missouri: Elsevier Saunders; 2012. p. 1207-320; and Plumb DC. In: Plumb's Veterinary Drug Handbook 6th edition. Ames, Iowa: Blackwell Publishing Professional; 2008.

Improvement to Air Flow

Nasal flushing

The presence of tenacious mucopurulent discharge within the nasal cavity not only can result in difficulty breathing but also may occlude the ostia, impairing drainage of fluid from the frontal sinuses. This in turn results in sinusitis, which can cause frontal sinus pain, contributing to lethargy and inappetence. Periodic nasal flushing, discussed previously, may provide clinical relief by removing this mucopurulent material. Use of hypertonic saline may be beneficial over isotonic saline, but this has not been studied in feline patients.[53]

Nebulization

Nebulization involves suspension of droplets of a liquid (usually saline) within a propellant gas (usually air or oxygen) (**Fig. 5**). Smaller droplets ($0.5\ \mu$–$5.0\ \mu$) are deposited within the lower airways, whereas larger droplets (20.0μ) are deposited within the nasopharynx.[54] Although there are no studies demonstrating efficacy, nebulization could be beneficial in making secretions less viscous and promoting ciliary clearance. A suggested regime is 15 minutes every 8 hours to 12 hours. Nebulization can also be used to deliver antibacterial agents topically (primarily aminoglycosides) or mucolytic agents, such as N-acetylcysteine. Again, there are no studies demonstrating efficacy of drugs delivered by this route, and inhaled *N*-acetylcysteine can cause bronchospasm and epithelial toxicity attributed to its hypertonicity[55,56]; therefore, caution is warranted. If nebulization is not available, instillation of saline drops can improve hydration of the nasal passages. This therapeutic modality does not appear particularly well tolerated by cats; therefore, placing the cat in a steamy environment (eg, shower room) is an alternate option, although use of a standard humidifier is more likely to be beneficial.

Mucolytics

Mucolytics, such as bromhexine, can be considered[56]; however, their primary action is to facilitate mucociliary clearance within the tracheobronchial tree; therefore, their role in sinonasal disease is unknown (**Table 3**).

Decongestants

Decongestants might improve nasal airflow by reducing mucosal edema through vasoconstriction (see **Table 3**). Unfortunately, this often is followed by rebound vasodilation and worsening signs; therefore, it is recommended that topical use of these

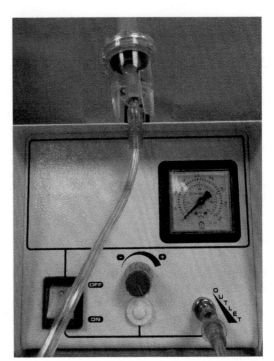

Fig. 5. A hospital nebulizer can be used to humidify the upper airways and facilitate removal of nasal discharges.

drugs is limited to 3 days.[22] As with mucolytics, there is no published evidence of benefit in the management of CRS.

Antivirals

The rationale for using antiviral therapy is based on the presumed association between recrudescence of chronic FHV-1 infection and episodes of clinical signs. The lack of evidence to support current active infection with FHV-1 in association with signs of rhinitis likely accounts for the weak evidence to support use of these treatments.

Interferon

Although FHV-1 is susceptible to interferon (IFN) in vitro, clinical trials have yet to demonstrate a clear benefit. Although IFN-α can be used topically for ocular lesions, systemic administration is more logical for respiratory disease hence feline recombinant IFN-ω is more appropriate for administration by this route. A suggested dose is 1 MU/kg sq every 24 hours for 5 days.[57] No clear efficacy in feline rhinitis has been reported to date.

Famciclovir

Famciclovir is a prodrug of the deoxyguanosine analog penciclovir.[58] As such it is virostatic rather than virocidal. Although controlled clinical trials have not been performed, improvement in clinical signs was reported in 2 cats with CRS.[59] The optimal dose is not yet known, and dose ranges have varied from 62.5 mg/cat[59] every 24 hours to 90 mg/kg every 8 hours,[60] with a protracted course (up to 4 months) appearing to be well tolerated.

Table 3
Mucolytics and decongestants for clinical management of chronic rhinosinusitis

Drug	Dose	Comment
Acetylcysteine	50 mg diluted in saline to 2% solution	Mucolytic Nebulize for 30–60 min Can cause bronchospasm and is toxic to respiratory epithelial cells
Bromhexine	3 mg/cat IM q 12 h 1 mg/kg po q 24 h	Bronchial secretolytic
Dimenhydrinate	4 mg/cat po q 8 h	Antihistamine, antiemetic, anticholinergic. The last of these contributes to decongestant effect
Ephedrine hydrochloride 0.5% nasal drops	1 drop each nostril q 12–24 h	Only administer for 72 h to avoid rebound congestion
Oxymetazoline	1 drop each nostril q 12 h 1 drop each nostril q 24 h	Maximum 48 h Maximum 72 h
Phenylephrine hydrochloride	1 drop each nostril q 24 h	Maximum 72 h
Pseudoephedrine	1 mg/kg po q 8 h	Administration facilitated by use of 6-mg/mL syrup rather than tablets
Xylometazoline	1 drop each nostril q 24 h	Maximum 72 h

Data from Refs.[45,57,66]

Lysine

Lysine is thought to have an antiviral effect by competing for arginine, an essential amino acid for viral replication.[58] Studies have demonstrated decreased conjunctivitis and viral shedding in cats experimentally infected with FHV-1 that are treated with lysine.[61,62] Unfortunately, this has not translated into decreased clinical signs of upper respiratory tract disease in shelter cats administered oral lysine or lysine-supplemented diets.[63–65] Although no clinical benefit has been proved in the shelter situation, client-owned cats are likely subjected to less stress than shelter cats, and it could be of use in this population, provided the stress of administering the drug does not outweigh any benefit. The recommended dose is 500 mg/cat twice daily.[58]

Antihistamines

Antihistamines have been proposed to be beneficial by some investigators,[42,66] although they could have the unwanted side effect of further drying out inspissated secretions. The nature of the cellular infiltrate might guide the decision to use antihistamines, which could be more likely to be beneficial with an eosinophilic or possibly lymphoplasmacytic infiltrate, rather than a neutrophilic or suppurative infiltrate. The individual response to antihistamines is variable; therefore, it can be beneficial to try different classes of antihistamine before considering they are of no benefit (**Table 4**).

Anti-inflammatories

Johnson and colleagues[67] identified increased levels of gene transcription for the inflammatory cytokines interleukin (IL)-6, IL-10, IL-12p40, IFN-γ, and regulated on activation, normal T-cell expression and secretion in nasal biopsies with an inflammatory infiltrate compared with normal biopsies. There was no alteration in gene transcription

Table 4
Antihistamine options for chronic rhinosinusitis

Antihistamine Class	Drug	Dose (Oral)
Alkylamines	Chlorpheniramine; chlorphenamine	1–2 mg/cat q 8–12 h
Ethanolamine	Diphenhydramine	2–4 mg/kg q 8 h
	Clemastine	0.1 mg/kg q 12 h
Piperazines	Ceterizine	5 mg/cat q 12 h
	Hydroxyzine	2 mg/kg q 8–12 h
Piperidines	Loratadine	0.5 mg/kg q 24 h
	Fexofenadine	10 mg/cat q 12 h
Phenothazines	Trimeprazine; alimemazine	0.5–1.0 mg/kg q 8–12 h
Antiserotonergic	Cyproheptadine	1 mg/cat q 12 h

Data from Refs.[42,57,66]

of Il-4, IL-5, IL-16, and IL-18. This indicates a predominantly type 1 T helper cell response to inflammatory stimuli, which could lead to more targeted therapies to modify this inflammatory response.

Glucocorticoids

Glucocorticoids have several effects on the immune system, and, by reducing mucosal edema and migration of inflammatory cells, they could be considered beneficial in CRS. There are no studies, however, demonstrating benefit in cats with CRS, and they could potentially be detrimental in the presence of bacterial infection and a suppurative infiltrate. In addition, they could initiate recrudescence of herpes virus infection. Glucocorticoids can be administered orally or by inhalational therapy. If the latter route is used, it is likely to be more effective if mucus build-up has been cleared first, for example, by nasal flushing or nebulization.

Nonsteroidal anti-inflammatory drugs

Nonsteroidal anti-inflammatory drugs might reduce sinus pain associated with CRS, thereby improving appetite and demeanor. There are no studies assessing the efficacy of the anti-inflammatory effect, and they should not be considered in cats that are not well hydrated or in cats with renal insufficiency.

Leukotriene inhibitors

Leukotrienes are produced from arachidonic acid through the action of 5-lipoxygenase. They exert a chemoattractant effect on inflammatory cells, contributing to nasal edema, increased vascular permeability, and mucus production. Levels of leukotrienes can be reduced through blockade of 5-lipoxygenase (zileuton), thereby inhibiting production. Alternatively, the action of leukotrienes can be inhibited through blockade of the cysteinyl-leukotrienetype 1 receptor (zafirlukast or montelukast). Although leukotriene inhibition has been shown to be beneficial in humans with chronic rhinitis (in particular, allergic rhinitis, concurrent nasal polyps, or aspirin intolerance),[68] the benefit in cats is unknown.

Immunomodulation

One study attempted to demonstrate immunomodulation of the inflammatory response after intraperitoneal injection of liposome-IL-2 DNA complex to stimulate the innate immune response.[8] This demonstrated a reduction in sneezing in older cats with chronic rhinitis and a progressive decrease in tumor necrosis factor-α mRNA expression; however, the clinical utility of this experimental treatment is uncertain at this time.

Surgery

Surgical intervention in the management of CRS has been described.[16,69,70] Turbinectomy can be performed via a dorsal or ventral approach, and the latter is promoted as more cosmetically acceptable to owners.[69,70] A procedure that allows débridement of chronically infected material from the frontal sinuses is likely beneficial over turbinectomy alone. After stripping of affected periosteum, the ablated sinus can be packed with an autogenous fat graft,[16] polymethylmethacrylate bone cement,[70] or polymethylmethacrylate infused with gentamicin.[70] Although good outcomes were reported, with compete resolution of signs in 4 of 6 cases[16] and good to excellent outcome in 9 of 19[70] cases, no comparison was made with medical management in the studies. Complications of surgery reported include failure to remove all the periosteal lining, surgical site abscessation, ataxia, death, and ongoing nasal discharge.[16,70]

Laser therapy also has been suggested to be beneficial in the management of chronic rhinitis in cats, but there are no clinical studies into this.[71,72]

PROGNOSIS

The prognosis for CRS should be considered guarded. The condition is rarely cured, which can result in cats being euthanized if owners cannot cope with the expense of ongoing treatment or the presence of persistent nasal discharge. There is the potential for persistent inflammation to lead to development of nasal or nasopharyngeal polyps or nasopharyngeal stricture formation.[73,74] These structural abnormalities also can lead to the development of chronic rhinitis; therefore, it can be difficult to evaluate which condition came first. In addition, chronic obstruction of the eustachian tubes by purulent discharge can lead to otitis media. In some cases, extensive bone lysis can occur, resulting in facial deformity or potentially erosion through the cribriform plate and involvement of the brain.[75]

Where owners are committed to administering medications and adjunct therapies, quality of life can be substantially improved, even though the condition is not cured. Surgical management can potentially affect a cure or a substantial improvement.

SUMMARY

Feline chronic rhinitis presents as recurring clinical signs of nasal discharge, sneezing, and stertor that can be accompanied by lethargy and inappetence. Diagnosis of this condition involves exclusion of other conditions that result in similar clinical signs and identification of an inflammatory infiltrate on nasal biopsy. Treatment is not curative and can involve prolonged courses of antibacterials in combination with adjunctive therapies and in some cases surgery. Prognosis is affected by owner commitment and can vary from excellent, where surgery is curative, to poor, where owners elect euthanasia.

DISCLOSURE

The author declares no funding sources or conflicts of interest.

REFERENCES

1. Cape L. Feline idiopathic chronic rhinosinusitis: a retrospective study of 30 cases. J Am Anim Hosp Assoc 1992;28(2):149–55.
2. Michiels L, Day MJ, Snaps F, et al. A retrospective study of non-specific rhinitis in 22 cats and the value of nasal cytology and histopathology. J Feline Med Surg 2003;5(5):279–85.
3. Henderson SM, Bradley K, Day MJ, et al. Investigation of nasal disease in the cat – a retrospective study of 77 cases. J Feline Med Surg 2004;6(4):245–57.
4. Ford RB. Pathogenesis and sequelae of feline viral respiratory infection. Supplement to the Compendium on Continuing Education for the Practicing Veterinarian 1997;19(3):21–7.
5. Hawkins EC. Chronic viral upper respiratory disease in cats: differential diagnosis and management. The Compendium on Continuing Education for the Practicing Veterinarian 1988;10(9):1003–12.
6. Johnson LR, Foley JE, De Cock HE, et al. Assessment of infectious organisms associated with chronic rhinosinusitis in cats. J Am Vet Med Assoc 2005;227(4):579–85.
7. Johnson LR, Maggs DJ. Feline herpesvirus type-1 transcription is associated with increased nasal cytokine gene transcription in cats. Vet Microbiol 2005;108(3–4):225–33.
8. Veir JK, Lappin MR, Dow SW. Evaluation of a novel immunotherapy for treatment of chronic rhinitis in cats. J Feline Med Surg 2006;8(6):400–11.
9. Gaskell R, Dawson S, Radford A, et al. Feline herpesvirus. Vet Res 2007;38(2):337–54.
10. Berryessa NA, Johnson LR, Kasten RW, et al. Microbial culture of blood samples and serologic testing for bartonellosis in cats with chronic rhinosinusitis. J Am Vet Med Assoc 2008;233(7):1084–9.
11. Milner RJ, Horton JH, Crawford PC, et al. Suppurative rhinitis associated with Haemophilus species infection in a cat. J S Afr Vet Assoc 2004;75(2):103–7.
12. Frey E, Pressler B, Guy J, et al. Capnocytophaga sp isolated from a cat with chronic sinusitis and rhinitis. J Clin Microbiol 2003;41(11):5321–4.
13. Johnson LR, Drazenovich N, Foley JE. A comparison of routine culture with polymerase chain reaction technology for the detection of *Mycoplasma* species in feline nasal samples. J Vet Diagn Invest 2004;16(4):347–51.
14. Van Pelt DR, Lappin MR. Pathogenesis and treatment of feline rhinitis. Vet Clin North Am Small Anim Pract 1994;24(5):807–23.
15. Hardy WD. Feline leukemia virus non-neoplastic diseases. J Am Anim Hosp Assoc 1981;17(6):941–9.
16. Anderson GI. The treatment of chronic sinusitis in six cats by ethmoid conchal curettage and autogenous fat graft sinus ablation. Vet Surg 1987;16(2):131–4.
17. Demko JL, Cohn LA. Chronic nasal discharge in cats: 75 cases (1993-2004). J Am Vet Med Assoc 2007;230(7):1032–7.
18. Pazzini L, Mugnaini L, Mancianti F, et al. *Tritrichomonas foetus* and *Mycoplasma felis* coinfection in the upper respiratory tract of a cat with chronic purulent nasal discharge. Vet Clin Pathol 2018;47:294–6.
19. Settipane RA, Schwindt C. Chapter 15: allergic rhinitis. Am J Rhinol Allergy 2013;27(Suppl 1):S52–5.
20. Maggs DJ, Lappin MR, Reif JS, et al. Evaluation of serologic and viral detection methods for diagnosing feline herpesvirus-1 infection in cats with acute respiratory and chronic ocular disease. J Am Vet Med Assoc 1999;214(4):502–7.

21. Malik R, McPetrie R, Wigney DI, et al. A latex cryptococccal antigen agglutination test for diagnosis and monitoring of therapy for cryptococcosis. Aust Vet J 1996; 74(5):358–64.
22. Thiry E, Addie D, Belak S, et al. Feline herpesvirus infection: ABCD guidelines on prevention and management. J Feline Med Surg 2009;11(7):547–55.
23. Radford AD, Addie D, Belak S, et al. Feline calicivirus infection: ABCD guidelines on prevention and management. J Feline Med Surg 2009;11(7):556–64.
24. Maggs DJ, Clarke HE. Relative sensitivity of polymerase chain reaction assays used for detection of feline herpesvirus type 1 DNA in clinical samples and commercial vaccines. Am J Vet Res 2005;66(9):1550–5.
25. Schulz BS, Wolf G, Hartmann K. Bacteriological and antibiotic sensitivity test results in 271 cats with respiratory tract infections. Vet Rec 2006;158(8):269–70.
26. Sykes JE, Malik R. Cryptococcosis. In: Green CE, editor. Infectious diseases of the dog and cat. 4th edition. St Louis (MO): Elsevier Saunders; 2012. p. 621–34.
27. Reed N, Gunn-Moore D. Nasopharyngeal disease in cats: 1. Diagnostic investigation. J Feline Med Surg 2012;14(5):306–15.
28. Farrow CS, Green R, Shively M. The head. In: Farrow CS, editor. Radiology of the cat. St Louis (MO): Mosby; 1994. p. 1–29.
29. O'Brien RT, Evans SM, Wortman JA, et al. Radiographic findings in cats with intranasal neoplasia or chronic rhinitis: 29 cases (1982-1988). J Am Vet Med Assoc 1996;208(3):385–9.
30. Thrall DE, Robertson ID, McLeod DA, et al. A comparison of radiographic and computed tomographic findings in 31 dogs with malignant nasal cavity tumors. Vet Radiol Ulltrasound 1989;30(2):59–65.
31. Park RD, Beck ER, LeCouteur RA. Comparison of computed tomography and radiography for detecting changes induced by malignant nasal neoplasia in dogs. J Am Vet Med Assoc 1992;201(11):1720–4.
32. Codner EC, Lurus AG, Miller JB, et al. Comparison of computed tomography with radiography as a non-invasive diagnostic technique for chronic nasal disease in dogs. J Am Vet Med Assoc 1993;202(7):1106–10.
33. Losonsky JM, Abbott LC, Kuriashkin IV. Computed tomography of the normal feline nasal cavity and paranasal sinuses. Vet Radiol Ultrasound 1997;38(4):251–8.
34. Schoenborn WC, Wisner ER, Kass PP, et al. Retrospective assessment of computed tomographic imaging of feline sinonasal disease in 62 cats. Vet Radiol Ulltrasound 2003;44(2):185–95.
35. Tromblee TC, Jones JC, Etue AE, et al. Association between clinical characteristics, computed tomography characteristics, and histologic diagnosis for cats with sinonasal disease. Vet Radiol Ultrasound 2006;47(3):241–8.
36. Nemanic S, Hollars K, Nelson NC, et al. Combination of computed tomographic imaging characteristics of medial retropharyngeal lymph nodes and nasal passages aids discrimination between rhinitis and neoplasia in cats. Vet Radiol Ultrasound 2015;56(6):617–27.
37. Johnson LR, Kass PH. Effect of sample collection methodology on nasal culture results in cats. J Feline Med Surg 2009;11(8):645–9.
38. Tomsa K, Glaus TM, Zimmer C, et al. Fungal rhinitis and sinusitis in three cats. J Am Vet Med Assoc 2003;222(10):1380–4.
39. Caniatti M, Roccabianca P, Ghisleni G, et al. Evaluation of brush cytology in the diagnosis of chronic intranasal disease in cats. J Small Anim Pract 1998; 39(2):73–7.
40. Elie M, Sabo M. Basics in canine and feline rhinoscopy. Clin Tech Small Anim Pract 2006;21(2):60–3.

41. Johnson LR, Clarke HE, Bannasch MJ, et al. Correlation of rhinoscopic signs of inflammation with histologic findings in nasal biopsy specimens of cats with or without upper respiratory tract disease. J Am Vet Med Assoc 2004;225(3): 395–400.
42. Scherk M. Snots and snuffles. Rational approach to chronic feline upper respiratory syndromes. J Feline Med Surg 2010;12(7):548–57.
43. Kuehn N. Chronic rhinitis in cats. Clin Tech Small Anim Pract 2006;21(2):69–75.
44. Venema CM, Williams KJ, Gershwin LJ, et al. Histopathologic and morphometric evaluation of the nasal and pulmonary airways of cats with experimentally induced asthma. Int Arch Allergy Immunol 2013;160(4):365–76.
45. Plumb DC. In: Plumb's veterinary drug handbook. 6th edition. Ames (IA): Blackwell Publishing Professional; 2008.
46. Sturgess CP, Gruffydd-Jones TJ, Harbour DA, et al. Controlled study of the efficacy of clavulanic acid-potentiated amoxycillin in the treatment of Chlamydia psittaci in cats. Vet Rec 2001;149(3):73–6.
47. Sparkes AH, Caney SMA, Sturgess CP, et al. The clinical efficacy of topical and systemic therapy for the treatment of feline ocular chlamydiosis. J Feline Med Surg 1999;1(1):31–5.
48. Owen WMA, Sturgess CP, Harbour DA, et al. Efficacy of azithromycin for the treatment of feline chlamydophilosis. J Feline Med Surg 2003;5(6):305–11.
49. Hartmann AD, Helps CR, Lapin MR, et al. Efficacy of pradofloxacin in cats with feline upper respiratory tract disease due to Chlamydophila felis or Mycoplasma infections. J Vet Intern Med 2008;22(1):44–52.
50. Spindel ME, Veir JK, Radecki S, et al. Evaluation of pradofloxacin for the treatment of feline rhinitis. J Feline Med Surg 2008;10(5):472–9.
51. Ruch-Gallie RA, Veir JK, Spindel ME, et al. Efficacy of amoxicillin and azithromycin for the empirical treatment of shelter cats with suspected bacterial upper respiratory infections. J Feline Med Surg 2008;10(6):542–50.
52. Koenig A. Gram-negative bacterial infections. In: Greene CE, editor. Infectious diseases of the dog and cat. 4th edition. St Louis (MO): Elsevier Saunders; 2012. p. 349–59.
53. Kanjanawasee D, Seresirikachorn K, Chitsuthipakonrn W, et al. Hypertonic saline versus isotonic saline nasal irrigation: systematic review and meta-analysis. Am J Rhinol Allergy 2018;32(4):269–79.
54. Court MH, Dodman NH, Seeler DC. Inhalation therapy. Oxygen administration, humidification and aerosol therapy. Vet Clin North Am Small Anim Pract 1985; 15(5):1041–59.
55. Portel L, Turion de Lara JM, Vernejoux JM, et al. Osmolarity of solutions used in nebulisation. Rev Mal Respir 1998;15(2):191–5 [in French].
56. Ramsey I. In: BSAVA small animal formulary. 7th edition. Quedgley (Gloucester): BSAVA; 2011.
57. Hartmann K. Antiviral and immunomodulatory chemotherapy. In: Greene CE, editor. Infectious diseases of the dog and cat. 4th edition. St Louis (MO): Elsevier Saunders; 2012. p. 10–24.
58. Maggs DJ. Antiviral therapy for feline herpesvirus infections. Vet Clin North Am Small Anim Pract 2010;40(6):1055–62.
59. Malik R, Lessels NS, Webb S, et al. Treatment of feline herpesvirus-1 associated disease in cats with famciclovir and related drugs. J Feline Med Surg 2009; 11(1):40–8.
60. Thomasy SM, Lim CC, Reiley CM, et al. Evaluation of famciclovir in cats experimentally infected with feline herpesvirus-1. Am J Vet Res 2011;72(1):85–95.

61. Stiles J, Townsend WM, Rogers QR, et al. Effect of oral administration of L-lysine on conjunctivitis caused by feline herpesvirus in cats. Am J Vet Res 2002;63(1): 99–103.
62. Maggs DJ, Nasisse MP, Kass PH. Efficacy of oral supplementation with L-lysine in cats latently infected with feline herpesvirus. Am J Vet Res 2003;64(1):37–42.
63. Maggs DJ, Sykes JE, Clarke HE, et al. Effects of dietary lysine supplementation in cats with enzootic upper respiratory disease. J Feline Med Surg 2007;9:97–108.
64. Rees TM, Lubinski JL. Oral supplementation with L-lysine did not prevent upper respiratory infection in a shelter population of cats. J Feline Med Surg 2008;10(5): 510–3.
65. Drazenovich TL, Fascetti AJ, Westermeyer HD, et al. Effects of dietary lysine supplementation on upper respiratory and ocular disease and detection of infectious organisms in cats within an animal shelter. Am J Vet Res 2009;70(11):1391–400.
66. Sturgess K. Chronic nasal discharge and sneezing in cats. In Pract 2013;35: 67–74.
67. Johnson LR, De Cock HEV, Sykes JE, et al. Cytokine gene transcription in feline nasal tissue with histologic evidence of inflammation. Am J Vet Res 2005;66(6): 996–1001.
68. Parnes SM. The role of leukotriene inhibitors in patients with paranasal sinus disease. Curr Opin Otolaryngol Head Neck Surg 2003;11(3):184–91.
69. Holmberg DL, Fries C, Cockshutt J, et al. Ventral rhinotomy in the dog and cat. Vet Surg 1989;18(6):446–9.
70. Norsworthy GD. Surgical treatment of chronic nasal discharge in 17 cats. Vet Med 1993;88(6):526–37.
71. Gorman C. Equipment review: companion therapy laser CTL-6 and CTL-10. UK Vet Companion Animal 2011;16(2):61–6.
72. Arza RA. Upper and lower respiratory conditions. In: Riegel RJ, Godbold JC Jr, editors. Laser therapy in veterinary medicine: photobiomodulation. John Wiley and Sons; 2017. p. 150–60.
73. Mitten RW. Nasopharygeal stenosis in four cats. J Small Anim Pract 1988;29(6): 341–5.
74. Mitten R. Acquired nasopharyngeal stenosis in cats. In: Kirk RW, Bonagura JD, editors. Current veterinary therapy X. Philadelphia: WB Saunders; 1992. p. 801–3.
75. Hecht S, Adams WH. MRI of brain disease in veterinary patients. Part 2: acquired brain disorders. Vet Clin North Am Small Anim Pract 2010;40(1):39–63.

Fungal Rhinosinusitis and Disseminated Invasive Aspergillosis in Cats

Vanessa R. Barrs, BVSc (Hons), PhD, MVetClinStud, FANZCVSc (Feline Medicine), GradCertEd (Higher Ed)[a],*, Jessica J. Talbot, BVSc (Hons), BSc (Vet), PhD[b]

KEYWORDS

- Aspergillosis • Sinonasal aspergillosis • Sino-orbital aspergillosis • *Aspergillus felis*
- Fungal rhinosinusitis • Antifungals

KEY POINTS

- There are 2 forms of fungal rhinosinusitis (FRS): sinonasal aspergillosis (SNA) and sino-orbital aspergillosis (SOA). Both infections start in the nasal cavity, and SOA is the most common form (65% of cases).
- Brachycephalic breeds of cats, especially Persian and Himalayan, are predisposed to FRS.
- Feline SNA is usually noninvasive and resembles SNA in dogs. The most common causes of SNA are *Aspergillus fumigatus* and *Aspergillus niger*.
- The most common cause of SOA is *Aspergillus felis*, followed by *Aspergillus udagawae*, both close relatives of *A fumigatus*. Molecular identification is required to differentiate these species from *A fumigatus*.
- The prognosis for SNA is favorable with topical antifungal therapy alone or combined with systemic antifungals but is guarded to poor for SOA.

INTRODUCTION

Aspergillosis is a mycosis of a diverse range of human and animal hosts, including mammals and birds. Among the most common molds on earth, *Aspergillus* species are filamentous ascomycetes distributed primarily in soil and decaying vegetation that have an important role in recycling environmental carbon and nitrogen.[1,2]

Feline fungal rhinosinusitis (FRS) was first described in the early 1980s; however, most cases have been reported in the past decade.[3–20] Other forms of aspergillosis

[a] City University of Hong Kong, Department of Infectious Diseases & Public Health, Jockey Club College of Veterinary Medicine, Kowloon, Hong Kong SAR, China; [b] Faculty of Veterinary Science, University Veterinary Teaching Hospital, Sydney, University of Sydney, Faculty of Science, Sydney School of Veterinary Science, Camperdown, New South Wales 2006, Australia
* Corresponding author.
E-mail address: vanessa.barrs@cityu.edu.hk

Vet Clin Small Anim 50 (2020) 331–357
https://doi.org/10.1016/j.cvsm.2019.10.006
0195-5616/20/© 2019 Elsevier Inc. All rights reserved.

in cats, including disseminated[7,9,21–25] and focal (non-FRS) invasive infections,[21,23,24,26–39] are reported less commonly and little is known about the etiological agents that cause them.

CLASSIFICATION SCHEMES

Aspergillosis can be classified by body system involvement, duration of infection, pathology, and pathogenesis. Disease is defined as invasive if there is hyphal invasion into tissues.[40] The respiratory tract is the most common site of disease in humans and animals, reflecting the primary inhalational route of infection.

Invasive aspergillosis (IA) in humans occurs predominantly in the sino-pulmonary tract of immunocompromised individuals as a consequence of inhalation of A spp conidia, and invasive pulmonary aspergillosis (IPA) accounts for more than 90% of IA cases.[41] Upper respiratory tract aspergillosis occurs less commonly and is classified as invasive or noninvasive FRS. By contrast, FRS is the most common form of aspergillosis reported in immunocompetent cats and dogs.[15,42] FRS in cats is also referred to as feline upper respiratory tract aspergillosis. In this review, the term FRS is used, in line with nomenclature used for classification of human aspergillosis syndromes. FRS can be further subdivided into sinonasal aspergillosis (SNA), which is usually noninvasive, and sino-orbital aspergillosis (SOA), which is invasive. In dogs, SNA accounts for more than 99% of cases, whereas in cats SOA is the most common form (65% of cases).[3,8,9,11,12,15,18,20,43–49]

Disseminated IA typically occurs in immunocompromised hosts and is defined as active infection in 2 or more noncontiguous sites or the hematogenous spread of disease.[50] There are few reports of disseminated IA in cats and most cases had pulmonary involvement.[7,21–25] Focal (non–upper respiratory tract; URT) invasive infections have also been reported in cats involving lung,[21,23,24,26–29,32,38] gastrointestinal tract,[24,33–35] urinary bladder, brain, or ear.[30,31,36,37]

ETIOLOGY

The genus Aspergillus contains several hundred species. Those that cause aspergillosis in cats are mostly from 2 subgenera; Circumdati and Fumigati (**Table 1**). Each subgenus can be further divided into sections.[51] Groups of related species within each section are informally termed "species complexes." In section Fumigati, which contains approximately 70 species, those associated with feline aspergillosis include the A viridinutans species complex and the A fumigatus species complex (**Table 1**).[52,53] Many species of Aspergillus cannot be reliably identified based on phenotypic features alone, especially "cryptic species," which is the term used to describe closely related species within a species complex or section that have similar macromorphology and micromorphology. Accurate identification of these species requires additional tests, such as molecular methods, for example, polymerase chain reaction (PCR) and comparative DNA sequence analysis.[15,54,55] Other techniques, such as those that use mass spectrometry, including matrix-assisted laser desorption ionization–time of flight (MALDI-TOF), are also being used increasingly for accurate identification of clinical Aspergillus isolates.[56]

Fungal Rhinosinusitis

The most common isolates that cause FRS in cats and dogs are from section Fumigati.[15,57–61] In addition to A fumigatus, which causes approximately 95% of cases of SNA in dogs,[62] a more diverse range of Aspergillus species has been identified to cause feline SNA, including several cryptic species in section Fumigati, as well as A *niger* (subgenus *Circumdati* section *Nigri*) (**Table 1**).[13,15,16,45] Section *Nigri* isolates, known as the black aspergilli, are phenotypically distinct from section *Fumigati* (**Fig. 1**).[63]

SOA is most commonly caused by 2 species in the *A viridinutans* complex in section *Fumigati, A felis* and *A udagawae* (see **Table 1**).[16,19,20,63] A third species in the complex, *A wyomingensis* also can cause SOA. Another member, *A viridinutans* was reported to cause SOA in a cat from Japan,[20] but on subsequent phylogenetic analysis was correctly identified as *A felis*.[64] Soon after its discovery in 2013 in cats with aspergillosis,[16] *A felis* was split into 4 species comprising *A felis, A parafelis, A pseudofelis,* and *A pseudoviridinutans*.[65] This classification was premature, and analysis of a large number of isolates showed that *A felis, A parafelis,* and *A pseudofelis,* are the same species (*A felis*), whereas *A pseudoviridinutans* is a separate species.[6,53]

Although *A fumigatus* has previously been reported as the cause of several cases of SOA, isolates in these cases were identified from phenotypic features alone, which is unreliable.[14,46–48] Misidentification of at least some of these isolates was likely based on their high minimum inhibitory concentrations (MICs) of amphotericin.[14,46,47] Compared with *A fumigatus*, the MICs of amphotericin for cryptic species such as *A lentulus* and *A udagawae* are high.[15,16,19,20,60,66] *A felis* has been reported in only one case of SNA, which would likely have progressed to SOA if it had not received aggressive systemic antifungal therapy.[16]

Disseminated and Focal Invasive Aspergillosis

The *Aspergillus* species that cause disseminated IA and focal IA in cats remain largely unknown because most cases were diagnosed postmortem based on histologic findings alone.[21–25] *A fumigatus* was identified from fungal culture morphology in 2 cats with mycotic pneumonia,[29,32] 1 cat with mycotic cystitis,[30] 1 cat with disseminated IA,[22] and 1 case of mycotic otitis.[36] *A nidulans* was identified from fungal culture morphology in 1 cat with mycotic cystitis.[27] Molecular confirmation of isolate identity was not performed in any of these cases.

Table 1
Causative agents of feline FRS based on reports in which the isolate was definitively identified using PCR and DNA sequencing

Subgenus	Section	Species Complex	Species	Form of Disease
Fumigati	*Fumigati*	*Aspergillus fumigatus*	*Aspergillus fumigatus*	SNA
			Aspergillus fischeri	SOA
			Aspergillus lentulus	SNA
Fumigati	*Fumigati*	-	*Aspergillus thermomutatus*[a]	SNA, SOA
Fumigati	*Fumigati*	*Aspergillus viridinutans*	*Aspergillus felis*	SNA, SOA, disseminated IA
			Aspergillus udagawae	SOA
			Aspergillus wyomingensis	SOA
Circumdati	*Nigri*	*Aspergillus niger*	*A. niger*	SNA
Circumdati	*Flavi*	*Aspergillus flavus*	*A. flavus*	SNA, focal (keratomycosis)

Abbreviations: IA, invasive aspergillosis; PCR, polymerase chain reaction; SNA, sinonasal aspergillosis; SOA, sino-orbital aspergillosis.
[a] Previously known as *Neosartorya pseudofischeri*.

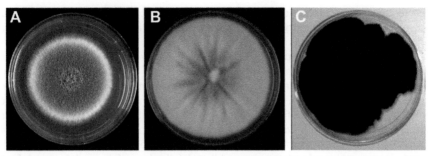

Fig. 1. Isolates of *Aspergillus fumigatus* (*A*), *Aspergillus felis* (*B*) and *Aspergillus niger* (*C*) on malt extract agar, from cats with URT aspergillosis. The black aspergilli (section *Nigri* [*C*]) are phenotypically distinct from Section *Fumigati* (*A, B*). Species within section *Fumigati* cannot be reliably identified from phenotypic features. Some, like *A felis* (*B*) are generally slow to sporulate. (*From* Barrs VR, Talbot JJ. Feline aspergillosis. Vet Clin North Am Small Anim Pract. 2014;44(1):51-73; with permission.)

Isolates from section *Nigri* were identified from fungal culture morphology in 3 cats with invasive pulmonary aspergillosis. *A* spp were identified from fungal culture morphology in cats with otitis.[36] Molecular confirmation of isolate identity was not performed in these cases. One case of chronic SOA in a cat due to *A felis* progressed to disseminated IA.[7] Molecular methods (PCR) have been applied to the affected tissue of hosts where fungal culture was not available or was negative, identifying *A* as a cause of subcutaneous mycosis in the ear of a cat using formalin-fixed, paraffin-embedded biopsy tissue, and *A flavus* in a corneal cytology sample from a cat with keratomycosis.[37,39]

Aspergillus Life-Stages and Taxonomy

- All *Aspergillus* species reproduce asexually (by mitosis). Some *Aspergillus* species also reproduce sexually (by meiosis) under certain conditions.
- The asexual form (*anamorph*) is mouldlike and composed of filamentous hyphae bearing mitotic spores (conidia).
- The sexual form (*teleomorph*) is characterized by the production of meiotic spores (*ascospores*) that develop within sacs (*asci*) inside enclosed fruiting bodies (*cleistothecia*).[54]
- The *Aspergillus* species that reproduce sexually are mostly *heterothallic*, with 2 complementary mating-types (eg, *A fumigatus, A felis, A udagawae*). Some are *homothallic*, with only 1 mating-type, and are able to self-fertilize (eg, *A thermomutatus*).
- The anamorph and teleomorph of a fungal species together comprise the *holomorph*.

In 2011, a controversial dual nomenclature system that used different genus names to describe the anamorphic and teleomorphic phases of the same fungus was abandoned. Previously, the anamorph was assigned to the genus *Aspergillus*, whereas the teleomorph of the same organism was assigned to the genus *Neosartorya*. The teleomorph name received taxonomic precedence, that is, species with known sexual stages were referred to by their teleomorph names.[67] Although this system of dual nomenclature provided a practical solution for distinguishing organisms that produce ascospores, confusion arose for organisms such as *A fumigatus* because its teleomorph (*Neosartorya fumigata*) was only discovered in 2009 and the taxon continued to be referred to by its anamorph name.[68]

In reforms to the *International Code of Nomenclature for Algae, Fungi and Plants,* a "one-fungus, one-name" principle was adopted in 2011[69] and the genus *Neosartorya* is now included in the genus *Aspergillus.*[70]

EPIDEMIOLOGY

Feline FRS occurs worldwide, with cases reported in Australia,[3,5,7,15–17,43] the United States,[11–14,44,45,48] the United Kingdom/Europe,[8,12,18,46,71] Japan,[4,19,20] and South America.[49] No age or sex predilection is apparent. The median age at diagnosis is 6.5 years (range 16 months to 13 years).[3,8,9,11,12,15,18,20,43–48]

Of cases in which serologic testing for feline immunodeficiency virus (FIV) and feline leukemia virus (FeLV) was performed, only 1 cat tested positive for FeLV.[8] Diabetes mellitus, a recognized risk factor for aspergillosis in humans, is likely a risk factor for both SNA and SOA in cats. More than 10 cases of FRS have been described in cats with diabetes, including several seen by the authors.[4,7,43,45,72] As has been reported in canine SNA,[42,73,74] feline FRS occurs occasionally in association with facial trauma, nasal neoplasia, and nasal foreign bodies.

In contrast to canine SNA, where dolichocephalic and mesaticephalic breeds are overrepresented,[42] purebred brachycephalic cats of Persian ancestry, including Persians, Himalayans, British or Scottish Shorthairs, and Ragdolls, account for more than a third of all feline FRS cases.[3,8,9,11,12,15,18,20,43–48]

No sex or breed predisposition has been recorded for disseminated and focal IA in cats. Affected cats are usually young to middle-aged. There is often evidence of systemic immunocompromise present, especially in cases of disseminated IA, including coinfections with FeLV, feline infectious peritonitis, or prolonged corticosteroid therapy.[21–25,33–35]

PATHOGENESIS
Route of Infection

The route of infection in both forms of FRS is inhalational. SOA is the result of extension of a primary sinonasal infection to involve paranasal structures including, but not limited to, the orbit. Lysis of the thin orbital bone allows direct communication of the nasal cavity or frontal sinuses with the orbit. Other factors are likely involved in the establishment of orbital infections, because orbital lysis, albeit more subtle, is often identified on computed tomographic (CT) studies of cats and dogs with SNA.[75,76]

Immunity and Mechanisms of Infection

The ability of fungi to cause disease depends on a complex interplay between the pathogen (virulence factors) and the host (innate and adaptive immune responses). Elimination of infection requires recruitment and activation of phagocytes and the development of T-helper (Th)1-type adaptive immunity. The production of Th1 cytokines is essential for host protection against invasive infection, whereas a Th2 response permits persistence of infection.[77] A balance among Th1, Th17, and Treg subsets is required for CD4$^+$ T-cell-mediated clearance of *Aspergillus* with limited tissue damage.[78] After inhalation, *A* conidia that escape mucociliary clearance are mostly phagocytosed by macrophages and dendritic cells.[41] Phagocytic host cells express *pattern recognition receptors (PRRs)* that recognize specific fungal epitopes known as *pathogen-associated molecular patterns (PAMPs)* and damaged host cell components known as *damage-associated molecular patterns (DAMPs).* The main PRRs involved in *Aspergillus* detection are the toll-like receptors (TLRs) TLR2 and TLR4, the C-type lectin receptors (CLRs) dectin-1, DC-SIGN, mannose-binding lectin, dectin-2, and melanin-sensing C-type lectin receptor (MelLEc), and the Nucleotide Oligomerization Domain-like receptors (NOD-like receptors) P3 and NOD2. The major PAMPs of filamentous fungi are cell-wall components including β-glucans, chitin, and mannans, whereas DAMPS include nucleic acids and alarmins.[79–82]

In humans, disorders of innate immunity that predispose individuals to IA include reduced mucociliary clearance (eg, cystic fibrosis), decreased numbers of phagocytic cells (ie, neutropenia), and phagocytic cell dysfunction (eg, chronic granulomatous disease, in which there is impaired production of oxidative intermediates).[80]

Mechanisms by which immunocompetent hosts can develop aspergillosis include environmental exposure to a heavy burden of fungal spores that overwhelms innate immune defenses, heritable defects in innate immune genes specific for fungal epitope recognition (eg, polymorphisms in PRR genes), and anatomic defects that predispose to fungal colonization. In addition, virulence factors of some opportunistic *Aspergillus* species, such as toxins or other secondary metabolites, can enable the establishment of infection.[83]

Is Feline Fungal Rhinosinusitis Associated with a Disorder of Innate Immunity?

Cats with FRS appear to be systemically immunocompetent based on a typical history of previous good health, seronegativity to the retroviral infections FIV and FeLV, and a robust humoral immune-response. High titers of anti-*Aspergillus* immunoglobulin (Ig)G and IgA are typically detected in the sera of affected cats compared with healthy cats and cats with nonfungal respiratory disease.[5,84] Given the predisposition of purebred cats of Persian lineage to FRS, an inherited defect in innate immunity has been proposed as a risk factor for FRS.[7,12] Persian cats also appear to be overrepresented for other fungal infections, including invasive dermatophytosis (pseudomycetoma), mucormycosis, and phaeohyphomycosis[85–89]

In immunocompromised humans, for example, stem cell and organ transplant recipients, single nucleotide polymorphisms (SNPs) in TLRs (1–6), Dectin-1, pentraxin-3, and DC-SIGN increase susceptibility to invasive pulmonary aspergillosis.[79,90–94] In systemically immunocompetent humans with preexisting lung damage, SNPs in the genes encoding the soluble PRRs mannose-binding lectin and SP-A are associated with chronic necrotizing pulmonary aspergillosis.[95–98]

Prompted by the identification of upregulation in mRNA expression of some TLRs in the nasal mucosa of dogs with SNA,[99] investigators sequenced the coding regions of TLR2, 4, and 9, in dogs with SNA to identify nonsynonymous SNPs. Although 14 nonsynonymous SNPs were identified, genotyping of 31 dogs with SNA from 4 different breeds and 31 breed-matched controls found no significant differences in the prevalence of these SNPs.[100] In a similar investigation, the allelic frequency of 23 nonsynonymous SNPs identified in TLRs 1, 2, and 4 of 14 cats with SNA or SOA was compared with those identified in the same genes in 20 healthy controls, and no significant differences were found.[101] Both canine and feline studies involved small case numbers, and future investigations using larger sample sizes, deep sequencing methods, and interrogation of other immune genes are warranted.

Is Fungal Rhinosinusitis Associated with Impaired Mucociliary Clearance?

Mucociliary clearance is an important component of innate immunity, acting to expel inhaled fungal spores before germination. The increased risk of FRS observed in brachycephalic cats could reflect impaired mucociliary clearance from abnormal sinonasal cavity conformation. In brachycephalic cats, horizontal rotation of the nasal passages and abnormal nasolacrimal drainage results from fore-shortening of the muzzle and cranium.[102] A decrease in sinus aeration and drainage of respiratory secretions secondary to infection, polyps, and allergic rhinosinusitis is a risk factor for invasive FRS in humans.[103] However, because brachycephalic dogs are underrepresented for SNA, additional risk factors for disease in cats, such as previous viral URT infection or recurrent antimicrobial therapy, also could be involved.[8,12,15]

Fungal Virulence Factors

An important virulence factor of *A* spp is their thermotolerant nature that enables survival in mammals.[104] Toxic secondary metabolites are associated with host immunosuppression or evasion of the immune system.[105] Gliotoxin, a mycelial-derived product, prevents phagocytosis by macrophages, reduces T-cell proliferation and activation, and induces macrophage apoptosis.[105–107] Species-specific fungal virulence factors could be involved in the development of invasive FRS because different fungal species are implicated in SNA and SOA in cats.[16] *A felis* produces a large number of secondary metabolites, including antifumicins/clavatols, aszonalenins, cytochalasin E, fumagillin, helvolic acid, kotanins, and viriditoxin.[108] The role of these metabolites as virulence factors is not known, although viriditoxin is lethal in mice after intraperitoneal administration and also inhibits growth of some bacterial species.[109,110]

Other putative fungal virulence factors include the ability to adhere to host tissue via conidia and laminin-binding components; factors interfering with fungal cell opsonization; and the production of proteases capable of macromolecule degradation for provision of fungal nutrients.[105]

In humans, *A fumigatus* is the most common cause of aspergillosis, and its small conidial size (2.5–3 μm diameter) favors pulmonary localization after inhalation. By contrast, *A flavus* is the most common cause of invasive FRS in immunocompetent humans in North Africa, Pakistan, and India.[111] Although environmental conditions promote high aerosolized burdens of *A flavus* in the region, the increased conidial size of *A flavus* (3–6 μm) is thought to favor deposition in the sinonasal cavity rather than the lungs after inhalation.[112] Although the conidia of *A felis* are smaller (1.5–2.5 μm) than *A fumigatus,* this species also readily produces large sexual spores (5–7 μm), which would enhance sinonasal deposition after inhalation.[16]

Exposure to High Environmental Fungal Spore Burdens

Environmental factors identified to increase the risk of FRS in immunocompetent dogs on the west coast of the United States include low environmental temperature differences, high differences in wind velocity, and locations with high composting activity.[113] In cats, behaviors leading to overwhelming pathogen exposure, such as digging in soil to bury feces or grooming, might be associated with the development of invasive FRS.[83] *A* spp spores have been identified in the coat of a high proportion of healthy cats.[114]

CLINICAL PRESENTATION
Fungal Rhinosinusitis

Clinical findings in feline SNA (outlined in **Box 1**) are similar to those reported for chronic rhinosinusitis (see Nicki Reed's article, "Chronic Rhinitis in the Cat: An Update," in this issue). Most cats with SOA are presented for clinical signs associated with an invasive retrobulbar fungal granuloma (**Box 2, Fig. 2**).[3,11,14,15,18–20,46–48] In most cats, exophthalmos is unilateral, but in severe, chronic infections, bilateral exophthalmos can occur.[3,15,46] Nasal signs are absent

---

Box 1
Clinical signs in sinonasal aspergillosis

Common Signs

- Sneezing

- Stertor

- Unilateral or bilateral serous to mucopurulent nasal discharge

- Ipsilateral mild mandibular lymphadenopathy

Less Common Signs

- Epistaxis (30% of cases)

- Fever

- Discharge from the frontal sinus

- Soft tissue mass involving the nasal bone or frontal sinus

Modified from Barrs VR, Talbot JJ. Feline aspergillosis. Vet Clin North Am Small Anim Pract. 2014;44(1):51-73; with permission.

---

in 40% of SOA cases at presentation; however, the medical history usually reveals sneezing or nasal discharge in the preceding 6 months. Pain on opening the mouth and neurologic signs are uncommon at initial presentation. However, cats with advanced disease are often euthanized because of the development of neurologic signs, which can include seizures, nystagmus, circling, facial muscle fasciculation, hyperesthesia, and blindness.[15,47,48]

Box 2
Clinical signs in sino-orbital aspergillosis

Common Signs

- Unilateral exophthalmos with dorsolateral deviation of the globe

- Unilateral conjunctival hyperemia

- Unilateral prolapse of the nictitating membrane

- Unilateral corneal ulceration (central)

- Oral mass or ulcer in the ipsilateral pterygopalatine fossa

- Paranasal soft tissue swelling

- Nasal signs (clinical or historical finding within the previous 6 months)

- Mild mandibular lymphadenopathy

Less Common Signs

- Fever

- Bilateral exophthalmos

- Ulceration of the hard palate

- Neurologic signs, for example, seizures, hyperesthesia

- Discharge from the frontal sinus

Modified from Barrs VR, Talbot JJ. Feline aspergillosis. Vet Clin North Am Small Anim Pract. 2014;44(1):51-73; with permission.

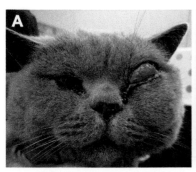 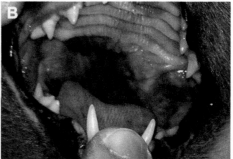

Fig. 2. British shorthair cat with SOA. Infection was caused by *Aspergillus felis.* Note the left-sided third eyelid prolapse, hyperemia, and edema, and the paranasal soft tissue swelling (*A*), and the pterygopalatine fossa mass (*B*), caused by an invasive retrobulbar fungal granuloma. (*From* Barrs VR, Talbot JJ. Feline aspergillosis. Vet Clin North Am Small Anim Pract. 2014;44(1):51-73; with permission.)

DIFFERENTIAL DIAGNOSES

Differential diagnoses for cats presenting with chronic nasal signs are listed in **Box 3** and for cats presenting with exophthalmos are listed in **Box 4**. Brachycephalic conformation should increase suspicion for aspergillosis, although these cats can be over-represented for viral URT infections or chronic rhinosinusitis. When epistaxis is present, neoplasia, mycotic rhinitis, foreign body disease, or severe chronic rhinosinusitis are more likely than other conditions. Inability to retropulse the globe and measurement of intraocular pressure enables differentiation of exophthalmos from buphthalmos (abnormal enlargement of the globe).[48] Other infectious or neoplastic processes extending from the nasal cavity to the orbit can have a similar presentation to SOA, including cryptococcosis, nasal lymphoma, and nasal carcinoma.

DIAGNOSIS

Diagnosis of feline FRS requires various combinations of serology, advanced imaging, rhinosinuscopy, cytology, histology, fungal culture, and molecular identification.

Box 3
Differential diagnoses for nasal signs

Neoplasia (lymphoma, carcinoma, other)

Inflammatory (chronic rhinosinusitis, nasal/nasopharyngeal polyp, nasopharyngeal stenosis)

Infectious
  Viral (FHV-1, FCV)
  Mycotic rhinitis (Cryptococcosis, Aspergillosis, Sporotrichosis, Phaeohyphomycoses, other)
  Bacterial (Bordetella, Mycoplasma, Chlamydophila felis, Actinomycetes)

Foreign body

Congenital (choanal atresia, palatine defects)

Dental disease (oronasal fistula)

Modified from Barrs VR, Talbot JJ. Feline aspergillosis. Vet Clin North Am Small Anim Pract. 2014;44(1):51-73; with permission.

Box 4
Differential diagnoses for orbital mass lesions

Neoplasia
  Lymphoma
  Adenocarcinoma/undifferentiated carcinoma
  Squamous cell carcinoma
  Fibrosarcoma,
  Osteoma/osteosarcoma
  Other

Infectious
  Bacterial abscess/granuloma (odontogenic, penetrating bite wound, hematogenous)
  Mycotic granuloma
    Aspergillosis
    Cryptococcosis
    Penicilliosis
    Phaeohyphomycosis
    Hyalohyphomycosis
  Pythiosis

Inflammatory
  Orbital myofascitis
  Orbital pseudotumor (idiopathic sclerosing inflammation)
  Zygomatic or lacrimal adenitis

Foreign body (eg, grass awn)

Orbital fat prolapse

From Barrs VR, Talbot JJ. Feline aspergillosis. Vet Clin North Am Small Anim Pract. 2014;44(1):51-73; with permission.

Definitive diagnosis is based on identification of fungal hyphae on cytologic or histologic examination of tissue biopsies or sinonasal fungal plaques. Similar to canine SNA, diagnosis can also be made by visualization of sinonasal fungal plaques on endoscopy.[8,45] However, given the more diverse range of fungal pathogens that can cause feline FRS, identification of fungal pathogens always should be attempted.

Hematology and Biochemistry

- Hematology is unremarkable or there is evidence of a stress or inflammatory leukogram.
- Peripheral eosinophilia is uncommon (10% of cases).[11,12,14,15,20,45–48]
- Mild to severe hyperglobulinemia is the most common abnormality on serum biochemistry. This was reported in 9 of 16 cats with SOA and 1 cat with SNA due to *A felis* infection.[11,14,15,48] This finding suggests that in cats with confirmed FRS, the presence of hyperglobulinemia is a marker for invasive disease; however, prospective studies are required to investigate this.

Serology

Aspergillus antigen detection in FRS

Galactomannan (GM), a polysaccharide component of the cell wall of *Aspergillus* and other filamentous fungal species, is released into the circulation during hyphal invasion into tissue.[115,116] Detection of GM in serum or bronchoalveolar lavage fluid is a commonly used test for the diagnosis of aspergillosis in humans. However, test sensitivity is heavily influenced by systemic immunocompetence and is highest in immunocompromised patients. A commercial enzyme-linked immunosorbent assay (ELISA) to detect GM in serum (Platelia *Aspergillus* EIA; Bio-Rad, Hercules, CA) has a sensitivity of up to 90% in neutropenic human patients with pulmonary aspergillosis and dogs with disseminated IA.[117,118] In non-neutropenic patients with pulmonary aspergillosis and in immunocompetent dogs with SNA, GM is detectable in fewer than 30% of cases.[117,119–121] In immunocompetent patients, GM is cleared by neutrophils, which possess mannose-binding receptors, or by antibody complexing.[122,123] Also, lack of tissue invasion in noninvasive mycoses such as SNA, likely contributes to lack of detectable circulating GM. In cats the sensitivity of GM detection was found to be low for both noninvasive (SNA) and invasive (SOA) forms of FRS with an overall sensitivity of only 23%.[116] Test specificity was also low (78% overall) with false-positives more likely in young cats (<1 year old) and cats treated with beta-lactam antibiotics, which can contain small amounts of GM introduced during the manufacturing process.[124]

Serology: antibody tests

Serum anti-*Aspergillus* antibodies can be detected by numerous methods, including counter-immunoelectrophoresis, agar gel immunodiffusion (AGID), or ELISA. Detection of *Aspergillus*-specific IgG by ELISA has high sensitivity in immunocompetent patients with aspergillosis, including dogs with SNA (88%) and humans with chronic pulmonary aspergillosis (>90%).[121,125] Specificity is also high (>90%), and optimal cutoff values can generally differentiate between exposure and infection.[121,125,126] Similar results were found in cats using an indirect ELISA to diagnose FRS (sensitivity 95%, specificity 93%). Most cats in the study had infections with *A felis, A thermomutatus, A lentulus,* or *A udagawae,* demonstrating antibody cross-reactivity with the commercial antigen preparation used in the assay, which was derived from mycelial elements of *A fumigatus, A flavus,* and *A niger.*[84] The same study evaluated a commercial precipitin test (AGID) and found a low sensitivity of 43%. Human patients with chronic pulmonary aspergillosis that test negative for IgG may test positive for IgA because *Aspergillus*-specific IgA can bind different fungal antigens than IgG.[125] Most cats with FRS also have detectable *Aspergillus*-specific IgA titers, but paired measurement of serum *Aspergillus*-specific IgA and IgG is of no benefit for diagnosis of FRS over IgG alone.[5]

Diagnostic imaging: computed tomography and MRI

CT or MRI is recommended for all cases of suspected feline FRS because evidence of invasive disease, including paranasal soft tissue infiltration and orbital involvement is often not apparent on physical examination, and determination of orbital involvement will affect subsequent case management.[15] The presence and extent of cribriform plate integrity should be assessed before treatment with topical sinonasal antifungal preparations, although damage to the cribriform plate does not preclude treatment in dogs. In cats with suspected intracranial extension of infection, MRI after intravenous contrast administration is superior to CT for evaluation of intracranial soft tissues.

CT features of feline SNA (**Box 5**) are similar to canine SNA, including turbinate lysis, which can be severe and cause a cavitated effect (**Fig. 3**).[75] Nasal cavity involvement, including increased soft tissue attenuation, is frequently bilateral and asymmetric, whereas frontal sinus involvement is usually unilateral. Other common findings in SNA include punctate areas of orbital bone lysis, which may be bilateral, and reactive change (sclerosis) of the nasal and frontal bones. Cats with SOA have similar signs of sinonasal cavity involvement, although turbinate lysis is less severe and sphenoid

---

Box 5
Computed tomography (CT) findings in sinonasal aspergillosis (SNA)

- Nasal cavity involvement is usually bilateral and asymmetric
- Frontal sinus involvement is usually unilateral
- Increased nasal cavity soft tissue attenuation
- Turbinate lysis
- Reactive thickening of the nasal and paranasal bones
- Increased soft tissue attenuation within frontal and sphenoid sinuses

Additional CT findings in sino-orbital aspergillosis (SOA)

- Ventromedial orbital mass
- Dorsolateral displacement of the globe
- Heterogeneous and peripheral rim postcontrast enhancement of orbital mass
- Paranasal soft tissue mass-effect - pterygopalatine fossa, adjacent maxilla
- Lytic lesions in paranasal bones

Modified from Barrs VR, Talbot JJ. Feline aspergillosis. Vet Clin North Am Small Anim Pract. 2014;44(1):51-73; with permission.

---

sinus involvement is more common. In SOA, lysis and reactive change of the paranasal bones also is common. Orbital masses cause dorsolateral displacement of the globe and extend laterally into paranasal maxillary soft tissues and ventrally into the pterygopalatine fossa of the oral cavity. Masses show heterogeneous contrast enhancement, including central coalescing hypoattenuating foci with peripheral rim enhancement (**Fig. 4**). Mass lesions within the nasal cavity, nasopharynx, or paranasal sinuses are also more commonly observed in cryptic species infections than in those caused by *A fumigatus,* which typically cause cavitated turbinate lysis.[75] Changes seen in FRS are not pathognomonic for the disease and can be similar to other mycotic, chronic inflammatory, or neoplastic diseases (**Fig. 5**). MRI is the imaging

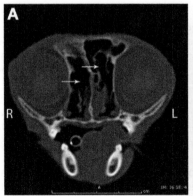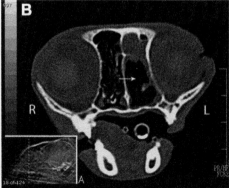

Fig. 3. Transverse skull CT images (bone algorithm) of 2 cats with SNA due to *A. fumigatus* infection showing severe "cavitated" turbinate lysis (*A*) bilaterally (*arrows*) and (*B*) in the left nasal cavity (*arrow*). (*From* Barrs VR, Beatty JA, Dhand NK, et al. Computed tomographic features of feline sino-nasal and sino-orbital aspergillosis. Vet J. 2014; 201(2):215-222; with permission.)

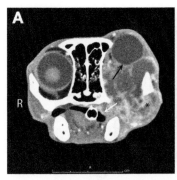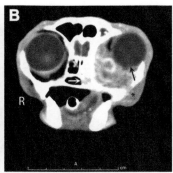

Fig. 4. Transverse postcontrast soft tissue images of the head reconstructed using a soft tissue algorithm showing left orbital masses in 2 cats with SOA and *A felis* infection. There is heterogeneous contrast enhancement, with central coalescing hypoattenuating foci and peripheral rim enhancement. There is (*A, B, black arrow*) compression and dorsal displacement of the globe, and (*A, white arrow*) extension into the oral cavity (*B, white arrow*), nasopharynx, and (*A, B, black asterisk*) adjacent paranasal maxillary soft tissues. (*From* Barrs VR, Beatty JA, Dhand NK, et al. Computed tomographic features of feline sino-nasal and sino-orbital aspergillosis. Vet J. 2014; 201(2):215-222; with permission.)

modality of choice for patients with SOA presenting with neurologic signs to assess central nervous system (CNS) involvement. On MRI, feline SOA orbital masses are T2-hyperintense.

Calcified nasal cavity masses or sinus concretions were reported in 1 case of feline SNA and 1 case of SOA.[12,75] Calcification of fungal plaques is common in humans with noninvasive FRS due to deposition of calcium oxalate or phosphate crystals that are thought to be fungal metabolites.[127]

Biopsy procedures

Endoscopic visualization of the sinonasal cavity can be performed using nasopharyngoscopy, rhinoscopy, and sinuscopy. Biopsy specimens are obtained for cytology and/or histology and culture. Biopsy specimens can be stored frozen for PCR if FRS is suspected but fungal culture is negative. Nasal cavity lavage might also yield fungal plaques for cytology and culture and assists in debridement of mucosal plaques (**Fig. 6**).

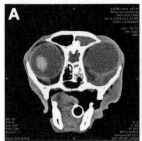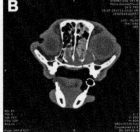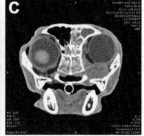

Fig. 5. CT features of SOA (*A*), including nasal cavity soft tissue attenuation, lysis of paranasal bones, and mass-effect (ventromedial orbital mass), overlap those of other mycoses for example, cryptococcosis (*B*), and neoplasia, for example, lymphoma (*C*). (*From* Barrs VR, Talbot JJ. Feline aspergillosis. Vet Clin North Am Small Anim Pract. 2014;44(1):51-73; with permission.)

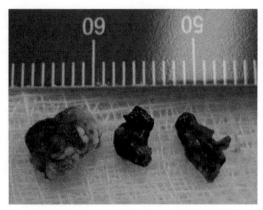

Fig. 6. Plaques of *A fumigatus* retrieved from the nasopharynx of a cat after nasal lavage under general anesthesia, with sterile saline. (*From* Barrs VR, Talbot JJ. Feline aspergillosis. Vet Clin North Am Small Anim Pract. 2014;44(1):51-73; with permission.)

Sinuscopy is indicated when CT findings indicate sinus involvement and fungal plaques are not visualized on rhinoscopy. Anatomic landmarks have been defined for sinus trephination in cats.[128] Trephine openings are made slightly lateral to the midline on a line that joins the anterior borders of the supra-orbital processes.

For cats with SOA, biopsies of retrobulbar masses can be obtained via the oral cavity when there is pterygopalatine invasion.[15] CT-guided biopsies of orbital or other paranasal mass lesions also can be performed.[48]

Fungal culture

Fungal pathogens that cause feline FRS can be readily cultured from tissue biopsies or fungal plaques using commercial culture media, for example, Sabouraud's dextrose agar (SDA) or malt extract agar. In one study in which samples from suspected cases of FRS were cultured on SDA, 22 of 23 were culture positive.[15]

Molecular identification of fungal isolates that cause fungal rhinosinusitis

Accurate identification requires a combination of phenotypic methods, such as culture morphology, plus molecular or metabolomic methods (eg, MALDI-TOF). Molecular testing has been used most extensively for identification of veterinary *Aspergillus* isolates, and comparative DNA sequence analysis is available at fungal reference laboratories and some commercial veterinary laboratories.[16,129] Fungal DNA is extracted for PCR and sequencing, preferably from fungal culture material. If the fungal culture is negative, DNA can be extracted from fresh or frozen clinical specimens or from formalin-fixed paraffin-embedded tissues (FFPET), although the latter yields shorter DNA fragments, which limits the gene targets for amplification.

The genome of all fungi contains multiple copies of the ribosomal DNA (rDNA) gene complex, consisting of highly variable regions (the internal transcribed spacer [ITS] regions), which are flanked by highly conserved gene sequences that are suitable targets for primers. The rDNA gene complex includes 3 genes: the 18s rDNA gene, also known as the small-subunit (SSU) rDNA gene, the 5.8S gene (159 base pairs) and the 28S rDNA, also known as the large-subunit (LSU) rDNA gene (**Fig. 7**).[130] PCRs that target one or both of the ITS regions are known as panfungal PCRs or universal DNA barcodes and they enable identification of most fungal genera, including yeasts and molds. Because some *Aspergillus* species have little or no variation in

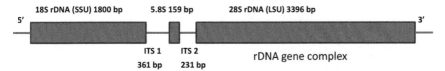

Fig. 7. Representation of the rDNA gene complex in fungi denoting gene order of small-subunit (SSU) and large-subunit (LSU) and position of internal transcribed spacer (ITS) regions. Bp, base pairs. (*From* Barrs VR, Talbot JJ. Feline aspergillosis. Vet Clin North Am Small Anim Pract. 2014;44(1):51-73; with permission.)

this region, a second genetic marker, such as calmodulin, ß-tubulin, or the RNA polymerase II second largest subunit (*RPB2*), is required for identification to the species level.[131] Calmodulin is best for identification of clinical isolates because amplification of *RPB2* is more difficult, and amplification of ß-tubulin can be complicated by the presence of paralogue genes that are preferentially amplified.[132]

The entire ribosomal DNA ITS1-5.8S-ITS2 region of approximately 600 nucleotides is readily amplified from DNA extracted from fungal culture material using primers ITS1 and ITS4.[16] For FFPET, amplification of the shorter ITS1 region (290 nucleotides) using primers ITS1 and ITS2 or the ITS2 region (330 nucleotides) using primers ITS3 and ITS4 is often possible.[15,55] One study used amplification of the ITS2 region from FFPET to identify fungi visualized on histologic sections from veterinary biopsies and was able to identify these fungi to the genus level in 65% of samples. In 96% of these, the identified fungus was the same as that diagnosed morphologically on histologic examination.[55]

Histopathology

Sinonasal aspergillosis

Histologic changes in canine SNA are characterized by an ulcerated and severely inflamed mucosa, often covered by a plaque of necrotic tissue containing hyphae, and/or luminal exudates containing hyphae.[13,45,133] Fungal hyphae do not penetrate the mucosal epithelium, and the underlying lamina propria is typically heavily infiltrated by a dense lymphoplasmacytic infiltrate. Histologic changes in feline SNA are similar, including severe inflammatory rhinitis with lymphoplasmacytic or mixed-cell inflammatory cell infiltrates, necrosis, and mats of fungal hyphae.[7,12,13,15,45] Because SNA is typically noninvasive, fungal plaques colonize but do not invade the sinonasal mucosa. A thorough histopathological assessment for the presence of tissue invasion by fungal hyphae should be performed because invasive infections indicate the likely presence of cryptic species of fungi and orbital or other paranasal involvement. The histologic detection of invasion will inform treatment decisions (see the Treatment and prognosis section).[12]

Sino-orbital aspergillosis

Cats with SOA have lymphoplasmacytic, eosinophilic, or granulomatous mycotic rhinosinusitis with variable submucosal invasion and bony lysis.[3,7,15,46] Granulomas are composed of central necrotic cellular debris within which parallel-walled, dichotomously branching, septate fungal hyphae are confined and visualized using special stains, for example, periodic acid-Schiff, Grocott methenamine silver, or Gridley stain (see **Fig. 8**).[3,11,14,15,46,48] Surrounding the central area of coagulative necrosis are zones of inflammatory cells and peripheral fibrosis that wall off the hyphae. In some lesions, eosinophilic inflammation is prolific, whereas in others neutrophilic inflammation is predominant. Adjacent to inflammatory infiltrates are

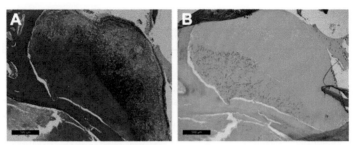

Fig. 8. Nasal mucosa from a cat with SOA, hematoxylin-eosin (A) and Groccott (B) stain, demonstrating granulomatous rhinitis (A) and submucosal invasion by septate branching fungal hyphae (B).

activated and epithelioid macrophages with vacuolated cytoplasm that variably form sheets. Peripherally there is a zone of fibroblasts and a cuff of lymphocytes and plasma cells. Inflammatory lesions can efface adjacent skeletal muscle and bone.[15] The globe is resistant to infiltration by fungal hyphae; however, invasion of adjacent structures including the nictitating membrane and eyelid can occur.[14,47] In cats that developed blindness, mycotic invasion of the optic nerve and optic chiasm was reported.[15] The development of CNS signs in some cases implies fungal invasion of CNS tissue, however brain histology was not performed in the 2 cats in which seizures were described.[47,48]

TREATMENT AND PROGNOSIS
Sinonasal Aspergillosis

Results of multiple retrospective comparative, experimental, and prospective treatment trials have shaped key principles for the treatment of canine SNA, which include endoscopic debridement of all visible fungal plaques, infusion of a topical azole antifungal preparation, and follow-up endoscopic assessment to determine whether repeat debridement and topical azole therapy are required.[134–140] Similar studies are lacking in cats with FRS. However, prognosis of SNA appears favorable based on the small numbers of cases for which treatment outcomes have been reported. Signs resolved in 12 of 15 treated cases with follow-up available.[4,8,12,13,15,45,71] Successful treatment regimens included systemic antifungal therapy in 6 cases (itraconazole or posaconazole monotherapy or combined with amphotericin B), systemic triazole therapy (itraconazole or posaconazole) combined with topical intranasal clotrimazole or enilconazole infusion in 2 cases, and topical intranasal clotrimazole infusion alone in 2 cases. As for canine SNA, debridement of fungal lesions in the nasal cavity was an integral component of therapy for most cases. In humans with noninvasive FRS due to *A fumigatus* infection, sinus fungal plaques form tangled masses of hyphae termed "fungal balls."[141] Aggressive endo-surgical debridement is usually curative, and postoperative or perioperative antifungal treatment is not prescribed. Similarities of this type of noninvasive FRS in humans with canine and feline SNA highlight the importance of endoscopic debridement of all visible fungal elements in the therapeutic approach to noninvasive FRS. **Box 6** outlines a suggested therapeutic strategy for the treatment of feline SNA that is based on previous reports, treatment of canine SNA, and considering whether infection is invasive or noninvasive. If submucosal hyphal invasion is identified or if *A felis,* a species highly correlated with invasive disease, has been identified, concurrent topical and systemic therapy is recommended.

Box 6
Therapeutic approach for treatment of feline SNA

- Determine the identity of the fungal isolate and its antifungal susceptibility.

- Assess whether infection is invasive or noninvasive based on histopathology.

- If infection is invasive on histopathology; CT findings should be evaluated to rule out orbital or other paranasal tissue involvement.

- Determine the integrity of the cribriform plate on CT.

- Debride fungal plaques/lesions from the nasal cavity and frontal sinuses using endoscopic techniques and saline irrigation.

- For noninvasive infections instill an intranasal infusion of 1% clotrimazole in polyethylene glycol (1 h soak under general anesthesia). Ensure drainage of the infusion from the nasal cavities at the end of the procedure by tilting the head downward.

- For invasive infections and/or where A felis is identified, give additional systemic antifungal therapy (see SOA treatment).

Modified from Barrs VR, Talbot JJ. Feline aspergillosis. Vet Clin North Am Small Anim Pract. 2014;44(1):51-73; with permission.

Techniques for intranasal clotrimazole infusion are adapted from procedures used to treat canine SNA and are described in detail elsewhere.[12,42,45] Polyethylene glycol should be used as the vehicle for 1% intranasal clotrimazole infusions, not polypropylene glycol, because the latter can cause severe mucosal edema and ulceration.[142] The use of depot azole preparations, such as clotrimazole cream has decreased anesthesia times for treatment of canine SNA; however, cream preparations tend to cause temporary obstruction of the nasal passages and cats are reluctant to open-mouth breathe. Therefore, use of cream preparations in cats is not recommended routinely. Response to therapy can be assessed by repeat CT and endoscopy. As for canine SNA, repeat endoscopic debridement and topical clotrimazole infusions may be required to resolve infection and nasal discharge may persist when turbinate destruction is severe.[15,71]

Sino-Orbital Aspergillosis

Overall, the prognosis for SOA remains poor, even with aggressive treatment. No clear benefit of surgical treatment, in the form of orbital exenteration, has been demonstrated. In one study of 12 cats with SOA, all were treated with systemic triazoles and 5 also had orbital exenteration. Only 1 cat, which did not have surgery, was cured.[15]

Based on treatment responses in case reports,[11,14,15,20,48] the recommended therapeutic approach is to commence oral posaconazole monotherapy empirically until antifungal susceptibility test results are available. Itraconazole is no longer recommended for empirical therapy because antifungal susceptibility testing of 90 clinical and environmental isolates from the A viridinutans complex showed that most species demonstrated high MICs of voriconazole and itraconazole.[143] Overall, the MICs of posaconazole and the minimum effective concentrations of 3 echinocandins (anidulafungin, micafungin, and caspofungin) were low. The study also found that a commercial broth microdilution method of antifungal susceptibility testing (Sensititre YeastOne; Trek Diagnostic Systems Ltd, East Grinstead, UK), commonly fails to detect high MICs of itraconazole compared with the EUCAST reference method.

Voriconazole and posaconazole are structurally similar to fluconazole and itraconazole, respectively. These fungicidal triazoles were developed as more efficacious agents for treatment and prophylaxis of IA in humans and to improve on the absorption, tolerability, and drug interaction profile of itraconazole. Posaconazole is well tolerated in cats after oral administration and liver enzyme elevations are infrequent.[14,15,47,144] Administration of voriconazole to cats has been associated with severe adverse neurologic effects, including hindlimb paraplegia and blindness, as well as anorexia.[15,48,145] Voriconazole has a long oral half-life in cats (>43 hours) and nonlinear pharmacokinetics are suspected to be the cause of toxicosis at higher drug doses due to saturation of metabolizing enzymes and decreased drug clearance.[146] In one pharmacokinetic study of voriconazole, cats were

Table 2
Dosages of antifungals used in the treatment of feline aspergillosis

Drug/Formulation	Dosage/Route of Administration	Adverse Effects/Comments
Itraconazole 100-mg capsules 10-mg/mL oral suspension (Sporanox)	Capsules (administer with food): 5 mg/kg q 12 h or 10–12.5 mg/kg q 24 h PO[149] Oral suspension (administer with or without food): 4 mg/kg q 24 h PO	Gastrointestinal: anorexia, vomiting Hepatotoxicity: elevated liver enzymes, jaundice. Monitor ALP/ALT monthly. If hepatotoxicity occurs, reduce dosage to 5 mg/kg q 24 h or 10 mg/kg q 48 h PO (capsules) or 2–3 mg/kg q 24 h PO (suspension) and perform TDM.
Posaconazole 40-mg/mL liquid (Noxafil)	15 mg/kg PO loading dose[144] 7.5 mg/kg q 24 h; administer with food	Hepatotoxicity TDM recommended
Voriconazole 50-mg tablets 40-mg/mL powder for oral suspension (Vfend)	Loading dose 25 mg/cat Suggested dose 12.5 mg/cat q 72 h PO[146]	Gastrointestinal: anorexia Neurologic: blindness, ataxia, stupor, hindlimb paraplegia. Use only when other therapies have failed. TDM recommended
Terbinafine 250-mg tablets (Lamisil)	30 mg/kg q 24 h PO	Gastrointestinal: anorexia, vomiting, diarrhea
Amphotericin B deoxycholate 50-mg vial (Fungizone)	0.5 mg/kg of 5 mg/mL stock solution in 250–350 mL per cat of 0.45% NaCl + 2.5% dextrose SC 2 or 3 times weekly to a cumulative dose of 10–15 mg/kg	Nephrotoxicity: Monitor urea/ creatinine every 2 wk. Discontinue for 2–3 wk if azotemic.
Liposomal amphotericin (AmBisome)	1–1.5 mg/kg IV q 48 h to a cumulative dose of 12–15 mg/kg Give as a 1–2 mg/mL solution in 5% dextrose by IV infusion over 1–2 h	Nephrotoxicity: Less nephrotoxic than Amphotericin B, but azotemia can occur. Monitor urea/creatinine 1–2 times weekly.

Abbreviations: ALP/ALT, alkaline phosphatase/alanine aminotransferase; IV, intravenous; PO, per os; q, every; SC, subcutaneous; TDM, therapeutic drug monitoring.
From Barrs VR, Talbot JJ. Feline aspergillosis. Vet Clin North Am Small Anim Pract. 2014;44(1):51-73; with permission.

administered a loading dose of 25 mg orally then given 12.5 mg every 48 hours for 14 days.[146] At the end of this period, plasma drug concentrations were still increasing and steady state had not been reached. Thus, the optimal dose rate of voriconazole for long-term treatment in cats is unknown. Voriconazole is not recommended for treatment of feline SOA unless other therapies have failed, and if used should be accompanied by therapeutic drug monitoring (TDM). TDM involves measurement of trough plasma drug concentrations and is also useful for cats that are not responding to posaconazole or voriconazole but where in vitro MICs indicate susceptibility.

The importance of antifungal susceptibility testing in guiding therapy is illustrated by 1 case of feline SOA that failed sequential treatment with itraconazole and amphotericin B but was subsequently cured with posaconazole. The section *Fumigati* isolate from this cat, which was not identified molecularly, had high MICs of amphotericin and itraconazole and a low MIC of posaconazole.[14]

Two weeks after commencement of oral posaconazole for treatment of SOA, if there is no clinical response to treatment, consideration should be given to TDM and/or to the use of adjunctive parenteral antifungal drugs, including amphotericin B or caspofungin, and as guided by the antifungal susceptibility profile. The pharmacokinetics of caspofungin were recently established in cats and it is well tolerated with minimal side effects.[147] Echinocandins are semisynthetic amphiphilic lipopeptides that inhibit synthesis of the fungal cell-wall component 1,3-β-glucan. As with other polypeptides, echinocandins can cause histamine release. They are fungistatic and are used for treatment of refractory IA in humans.[148]

The authors have used caspofungin in combination with posaconazole and oral terbinafine to treat several cats with SOA successfully, including 1 cat with SOA that failed treatment with AMB and posaconazole.[15] Administration of oral antifungals for 6 months or longer may be necessary in some cases and reinfection or relapse of infection can occur.[15,20] Dose rates and considerations for antifungal therapy are listed in **Table 2**. Establishing pretreatment renal function and baseline liver enzymes is important because nephrotoxicity and hepatotoxicity are common with some antifungal drugs.

SUMMARY

Feline FRS, the most commonly reported form of aspergillosis in cats, occurs after nasal inhalation of *A* conidia, which colonize the sinonasal cavity. In SNA, infection is usually noninvasive, whereas in SOA, infection is always invasive and extends beyond the nasal cavity to involve paranasal structures, including the orbit. SNA is mostly caused by *A fumigatus* but also can be caused by cryptic species in section *Fumigati*, such as *A lentulus* and *A thermomutatus,* as well as by *A niger* in section *Nigri*. SOA is caused by cryptic species in section *Fumigati,* especially *A felis* or *A udagawae*. Accurate identification of the fungi that cause FRS and antifungal susceptibility testing are important because many infecting isolates have high MICs of antifungal drugs. PCR and sequencing is usually required in addition to cultural morphologic examination to determine fungal species identity. SNA carries a favorable prognosis with treatment, whereas the prognosis for SOA is poor, overall.

DISCLOSURE

The authors have nothing to disclose.

REFERENCES

1. Latge JP. Aspergillus fumigatus and aspergillosis. Clin Microbiol Rev 1999; 12(2):310–50.
2. Bennett JW. Aspergillus: a primer for the novice. Med Mycol 2009;47:S5–12.
3. Wilkinson GT, Sutton RH, Grono LR. *Aspergillus* spp infection associated with orbital cellulitis and sinusitis in a cat. J Small Anim Pract 1982;23(3):127–31.
4. Kano R, Takahashi T, Hayakawa T, et al. The first case of feline sinonasal aspergillosis due to *Aspergillus fischeri* in Japan. J Vet Med Sci 2015;77(9):1183–5.
5. Taylor A, Peters I, Dhand NK, et al. Evaluation of serum *Aspergillus*-specific immunoglobulin A by indirect ELISA for diagnosis of feline upper respiratory tract aspergillosis. J Vet Intern Med 2016;30(5):1708–14.
6. Talbot JJ, Houbraken J, Frisvad JC, et al. Discovery of *Aspergillus frankstonensis* sp. nov. during environmental sampling for animal and human fungal pathogens. PLoS One 2017;12(8):e0181660.
7. Whitney JL, Krockenberger MB, Day MJ, et al. Immunohistochemical analysis of leucocyte subsets in the sinonasal mucosa of cats with upper respiratory tract aspergillosis. J Comp Pathol 2016;155(2–3):130–40.
8. Goodall SA, Lane JG, Warnock DW. The diagnosis and treatment of a case of nasal aspergillosis in a cat. J Small Anim Pract 1984;25(10):627–33.
9. Davies C, Troy GC. Deep mycotic infections in cats. J Am Anim Hosp Assoc 1996;32(5):380–91.
10. Halenda RM, Reed AL. Ultrasound computed tomography diagnosis - fungal, sinusitis and retrobulbar myofascitis in a cat. Vet Radiol Ultrasound 1997; 38(3):208–10.
11. Hamilton HL, Whitley RD, McLaughlin SA. Exophthalmos secondary to aspergillosis in a cat. J Am Anim Hosp Assoc 2000;36(4):343–7.
12. Tomsa K, Glaus TA, Zimmer C, et al. Fungal rhinitis and sinusitis in three cats. J Am Vet Med Assoc 2003;222(10):1380–4.
13. Whitney BL, Broussard J, Stefanacci JD. Four cats with fungal rhinitis. J Feline Med Surg 2005;7(1):53–8.
14. McLellan GJ, Aquino SM, Mason DR, et al. Use of posaconazole in the management of invasive orbital aspergillosis in a cat. J Am Anim Hosp Assoc 2006; 42(4):302–7.
15. Barrs VR, Halliday C, Martin P, et al. Sinonasal and sino-orbital aspergillosis in 23 cats: aetiology, clinicopathological features and treatment outcomes. Vet J 2012;191(1):58–64.
16. Barrs VR, van Doorn TM, Houbraken J, et al. *Aspergillus felis* sp. nov., an emerging agent of invasive aspergillosis in humans, cats, and dogs. PLoS One 2013;8(6):e64871.
17. Katz ME, Dougall AM, Weeks K, et al. Multiple genetically distinct groups revealed among clinical isolates identified as atypical *Aspergillus fumigatus*. J Clin Microbiol 2005;43(2):551–5.
18. Declercq J, Declercq L, Fincioen S. Unilateral sino-orbital and subcutaneous aspergillosis in a cat. Vlaams Diergeneeskd Tijdschr 2012;81(6):357–62.
19. Kano R, Itamoto K, Okuda M, et al. Isolation of *Aspergillus udagawae* from a fatal case of feline orbital aspergillosis. Mycoses 2008;51(4):360–1.
20. Kano R, Shibahashi A, Fujino Y, et al. Two cases of feline orbital aspergillosis due to *A. udagawae* and *A. virdinutans*. J Vet Med Sci 2013;75:7–10.
21. Fox JG, Murphy JC, Shalev M. Systemic fungal infections in cats. J Am Vet Med Assoc 1978;173(9):1191–5.

22. Vogler GA, Wagner JE. What's your diagnosis. Lab Anim 1975;5:14.
23. Köhler H, Kuttin E, Kaplan W, et al. Occurrence of systemic mycoses in animals in Austria. Zentralblatt für Veterinärmedizin B 1978;25(10):785–99.
24. Ossent P. Systemic aspergillosis and mucormycosis in 23 cats. Vet Rec 1987; 120(14):330–3.
25. Burk RL, Joseph R, Baer K. Systemic aspergillosis in a cat. Veterinary Radiology 1990;31(1):26–8.
26. Sautter JH, Steele DS, Henry JF. Symposium on granulomatous diseases. II. J Am Vet Med Assoc 1955;127:518.
27. Pakes SP, New AE, Benbrook SC. Pulmonary aspergillosis in a cat. J Am Vet Med Assoc 1967;151(7):950–3.
28. McCausland IP. Systemic mycoses of two cats. N Z Vet J 1972;20(1–2):10–2.
29. Hazell KLA, Swift IM, Sullivan N. Successful treatment of pulmonary aspergillosis in a cat. Aust Vet J 2011;89(3):101–4.
30. Kirkpatrick RM. Mycotic cystitis in a male cat. Vet Med Small Anim Clin 1982;77: 1365–71.
31. Adamama-Moraitou KK, Paitaki CG, Rallis TS, et al. Aspergillus species cystitis in a cat. J Feline Med Surg 2001;3:31–4.
32. Degi J, Radbea G, Balaban S, et al. Aspergillus pneumonia in a Burmese cat - case study. Lucrari Stiintifice Medicina Veterinara 2011;44(2):278–81.
33. Weiland F. Intestinal mycosis in a cat. Dtsch Tierarztl Wochenschr 1970;77(10): 232–3.
34. Bolton GR, Brown TT. Mycotic colitis in a cat. Vet Med Small Anim Clin 1972; 67(9):978–81.
35. Stokes R. Letter: intestinal mycosis in a cat. Aust Vet J 1973;49(10):499–500.
36. Goodale EC, Outerbridge CA, White SD. Aspergillus otitis in small animals–a retrospective study of 17 cases. Vet Dermatol 2016;27(1). 3-e2.
37. Bernhardt A, von Bomhard W, Antweiler E, et al. Molecular identification of fungal pathogens in nodular skin lesions of cats. Med Mycol 2015;53(2):132–44.
38. Leite-Filho RV, Fredo G, Lupion CG, et al. Chronic invasive pulmonary aspergillosis in two cats with diabetes mellitus. J Comp Pathol 2016;155(2–3):141–4.
39. Labelle AL, Hamor RE, Barger AM, et al. Aspergillus flavus keratomycosis in a cat treated with topical 1% voriconazole solution. Vet Ophthalmol 2009;12(1): 48–52.
40. Ascioglu S, Rex JH, de Pauw B, et al. Defining opportunistic invasive fungal infections in immunocompromised patients with cancer and hematopoietic stem cell transplants: an international consensus. Clin Infect Dis 2002;34(1):7–14.
41. Segal BH. Medical progress aspergillosis. N Engl J Med 2009;360(18):1870–84.
42. Peeters D, Clercx C. Update on canine sinonasal aspergillosis. Vet Clin North Am Small Anim Pract 2007;37(5):901–16, vi.
43. Malik R, Vogelnest L, O'Brien CR, et al. Infections and some other conditions affecting the skin and subcutis of the naso-ocular region of cats - clinical experience 1987-2003. J Feline Med Surg 2004;6(6):383–90.
44. Karnik K, Reichle JK, Fischetti AJ, et al. Computed tomographic findings of fungal rhinitis and sinusitis in cats. Vet Radiol Ultrasound 2009;50(1):65–8.
45. Furrow E, Groman RP. Intranasal infusion of clotrimazole for the treatment of nasal aspergillosis in two cats. J Am Vet Med Assoc 2009;235(10):1188–93.
46. Barachetti L, Mortellaro CM, Di Giancamillo M, et al. Bilateral orbital and nasal aspergillosis in a cat. Vet Ophthalmol 2009;12(3):176–82.

47. Giordano C, Gianella P, Bo S, et al. Invasive mould infections of the naso-orbital region of cats: a case involving *Aspergillus fumigatus* and an aetiological review. J Feline Med Surg 2010;12(9):714–23.

48. Smith LN, Hoffman SB. A case series of unilateral orbital aspergillosis in three cats and treatment with voriconazole. Vet Ophthalmol 2010;13(3):190–203.

49. da Costa FV, Spanamberg A, Araujo R, et al. Feline sino-orbital fungal infection caused by aspergillus and scopulariopsis. Acta Scientiae Veterinariae 2019; 47(383):8.

50. Hope WW, Walsh TJ, Denning DW. The invasive and saprophytic syndromes due to *Aspergillus* spp. Med Mycol 2005;43:S207–38.

51. Houbraken J, Samson RA. Phylogeny of Penicillium and the segregation of Trichocomaceae into three families. Stud Mycol 2011;(70):1–51.

52. Barrs VR. Feline aspergillosis. In: Seyedmousavi S, de Hoog S, Guillot J, et al, editors. Emerging and epizootic fungal infections in animals. Cham (Switzerland): Springer International Publishing AG; 2018. p. 337–56.

53. Hubka V, Barrs V, Dudova Z, et al. Unravelling species boundaries in the *Aspergillus viridinutans* complex (section Fumigati): opportunistic human and animal pathogens capable of interspecific hybridization. Persoonia 2018;41:142–74.

54. Samson RA, Hong S, Peterson SW, et al. Polyphasic taxonomy of *Aspergillus* section *Fumigati* and its teleomorph *Neosartorya*. Stud Mycol 2007;(59): 147–203.

55. Meason-Smith C, Edwards EE, Older CE, et al. Panfungal polymerase chain reaction for identification of fungal pathogens in formalin-fixed animal tissues. Vet Pathol 2017;54(4):640–8.

56. Masih A, Singh PK, Kathuria S, et al. Identification by molecular methods and matrix-assisted laser desorption ionization-time of flight mass spectrometry and antifungal susceptibility profiles of clinically significant rare aspergillus species in a Referral Chest Hospital in Delhi, India. J Clin Microbiol 2016;54(9): 2354–64.

57. Pomrantz JS, Johnson LR. Update on the efficacy of topical clotrimazole in the treatment of canine nasal aspergillosis. J Vet Intern Med 2007;21(3):608.

58. Pomrantz JS, Johnson LR. Repeated rhinoscopic and serologic assessment of the effectiveness of intranasally administered clotrimazole for the treatment of nasal aspergillosis in dogs. J Am Vet Med Assoc 2010;236(7):757–62.

59. Peeters D, Peters IR, Helps CR, et al. Whole blood and tissue fungal DNA quantification in the diagnosis of canine sinonasal aspergillosis. Vet Microbiol 2008; 128:194–203.

60. Balajee SA, Nickle D, Varga J, et al. Molecular studies reveal frequent misidentification of *Aspergillus fumigatus* by morphotyping. Eukaryot Cell 2006;5(10): 1705–12.

61. Balajee SA, Houbraken J, Verweij PE, et al. Aspergillus species identification in the clinical setting. Stud Mycol 2007;59:39–46.

62. Talbot JJ, Johnson LR, Martin P. What causes sino-nasal aspergillosis in dogs? A molecular approach to species identification. Vet J 2014;200(1):17–21.

63. Varga J, Frisvad JC, Kocsube S, et al. New and revisited species in *Aspergillus* section *Nigri*. Stud Mycol 2011;(69):1–17.

64. Novakova A, Hubka V, Dudova Z, et al. New species in *Aspergillus* section *Fumigati* from reclamation sites in Wyoming (U.S.A) and revision of A. *viridinutans* complex. Fungal Diversity 2014;64(1):253–74.

65. Sugui JA, Peterson SW, Figat A, et al. Genetic relatedness versus biological compatibility between *Aspergillus fumigatus* and related species. J Clin Microbiol 2014;52(10):3707–21.

66. Alcazar-Fuoli L, Mellado E, Aslastruey-Izquierdo A, et al. *Aspergillus* section *fumigati*: antifungal susceptibility patterns and sequence-based identification. Antimicrob Agents Chemother 2008;52(4):1244–51.

67. Pitt JI, Samson RA. Nomenclatural considerations in naming species of *Aspergillus* and its teleomorphs. Stud Mycol 2007;(59):67–70.

68. O'Gorman CM, Fuller HT, Dyer PS. Discovery of a sexual cycle in the opportunistic fungal pathogen *Aspergillus fumigatus*. Nature 2009;457:471–4.

69. Miller JS, Funk VA, Wagner WL, et al. Outcomes of the 2011 Botanical Nomenclature Section at the XVIII International Botanical Congress. Phytokeys 2011; 5:1–3.

70. Hawksworth DL, Crous PW, Redhead SA, et al. The Amsterdam declaration on fungal nomenclature. Mycotaxon 2011;116:491–500.

71. Tamborini A, Robertson E, Talbot JJ, et al. Sinonasal aspergillosis in a British shorthair cat in the UK. JFMS Open Rep 2016;2(1). 2055116916653775.

72. Sykes JE. Aspergillosis. In: Sykes JE, editor. Canine and feline infectious diseases. St Louis (MO): Elsevier; 2014. p. 633–48.

73. Sharp NJ, Harvey CE, Sullivan M. Canine nasal aspergillosis and penicilliosis. Compendium on Continuing Education for the Practicing Veterinarian 1991; 13(1):41.

74. Day MJ. Canine sino-nasal aspergillosis: parallels with human disease. Med Mycol 2009;47:S315–23.

75. Barrs VR, Beatty JA, Dhand NK, et al. Computed tomographic features of feline sino-nasal and sino-orbital aspergillosis. Vet J 2014;201(2):215–22.

76. Saunders JH, Zonderland JL, Clercx C, et al. Computed tomographic findings in 35 dogs with nasal aspergillosis. Vet Radiol Ultrasound 2002;43(1):5–9.

77. Lass-Florl C, Roilides E, Loffler J, et al. Minireview: host defence in invasive aspergillosis. Mycoses 2013;56(4):403–13.

78. Verma A, Wüthrich M, Deepe G, et al. Adaptive immunity to fungi. Cold Spring Harb Perspect Med 2015;5:a019612.

79. Romani L. Immunity to fungal infections. Nat Rev Immunol 2011;11(4):275–88.

80. Shoham S, Levitz SM. The immune response to fungal infections. Br J Haematol 2005;129(5):569–82.

81. Li ZZ, Tao LL, Zhang J, et al. Role of NOD2 in regulating the immune response to *Aspergillus fumigatus*. Inflamm Res 2012;61(6):643–8.

82. Stappers MHT, Clark AE, Aimanianda V, et al. Recognition of DHN-melanin by a C-type lectin receptor is required for immunity to *Aspergillus*. Nature 2018; 555(7696):382–6.

83. Talbot JJ, Barrs VR. One-health pathogens in the *Aspergillus viridinutans* complex. Med Mycol 2018;56(1):1–12.

84. Barrs VR, Ujvari B, Dhand NK, et al. Detection of *Aspergillus*-specific antibodies by agar gel double immunodiffusion and IgG ELISA in feline upper respiratory tract aspergillosis. Vet J 2015;203(3):285–9.

85. Chang SC, Liao JW, Shyu CL, et al. Dermatophytic pseudomycetomas in four cats. Vet Dermatol 2011;22(2):181–7.

86. Miller RI. Nodular granulomatous fungal skin diseases of cats in the United Kingdom: a retrospective review. Vet Dermatol 2010;21(2):130–5.

87. Cunha SCS, Aguero C, Damico CB, et al. Duodenal perforation caused by *Rhizomucor* species in a cat. J Feline Med Surg 2011;13(3):205–7.

88. Dillehay DL, Ribas JL, Newton JC, et al. Cerebral pheohyphomycosis in 2 dogs and a cat. Vet Pathol 1987;24(2):192–4.

89. Grau-Roma L, Galindo-Cardiel I, Isidoro-Ayza M, et al. A case of feline gastro-intestinal eosinophilic sclerosing fibroplasia associated with Phycomycetes. J Comp Pathol 2014;151(4):318–21.

90. Gresnigt MS, Netea MG, van de Veerdonk FL. Pattern recognition receptors and their role in invasive aspergillosis. Ann NY Acad Sci 2012;1273:60–7.

91. Cunha C, Aversa F, Lacerda JF, et al. Genetic PTX3 deficiency and *Aspergillosis* in stem-cell transplantation. N Engl J Med 2014;370(5):421–32.

92. Fisher CE, Hohl TM, Fan WH, et al. Validation of single nucleotide polymor-phisms in invasive aspergillosis following hematopoietic cell transplantation. Blood 2017;129(19):2693–701.

93. Skonieczna K, Styczynski J, Krenska A, et al. Massively parallel targeted rese-quencing reveals novel genetic variants associated with aspergillosis in paedi-atric patients with haematological malignancies. Pol J Pathol 2017;68(3):210–7.

94. White PL, Parr C, Barnes RA. Predicting invasive aspergillosis in hematology pa-tients by combining clinical and genetic risk factors with early diagnostic bio-markers. J Clin Microbiol 2018;56(1) [pii:e01122-17].

95. Woodworth BA, Neal JG, Newton D, et al. Surfactant protein A and D in human sinus mucosa: a preliminary report. ORL J Otorhinolaryngol Relat Spec 2007; 69(1):57–60.

96. Crosdale DJ, Poulton KV, Ollier WE, et al. Mannose-binding lectin gene polymor-phisms as a susceptibility factor for chronic necrotizing pulmonary aspergillosis. J Infect Dis 2001;184(5):653–6.

97. Harrison E, Singh A, Morris J, et al. Mannose-binding lectin genotype and serum levels in patients with chronic and allergic pulmonary aspergillosis. Int J Immu-nogenet 2012;39(3):224–32.

98. Vaid M, Kaur S, Sambatakou H, et al. Distinct alleles of mannose-binding lectin (MBL) and surfactant proteins A (SP-A) in patients with chronic cavitary pulmo-nary aspergillosis and allergic bronchopulmonary aspergillosis. Clin Chem Lab Med 2007;45(2):183–6.

99. Mercier E, Peters IR, Day MJ, et al. Toll- and NOD-like receptor mRNA expres-sion in canine sino-nasal aspergillosis and idiopathic lymphoplasmacytic rhinitis. Vet Immunol Immunopathol 2012;145(3–4):618–24.

100. Mercier E, Peters IR, Farnir F, et al. Assessment of Toll-like receptor 2, 4 and 9 SNP genotypes in canine sino-nasal aspergillosis. BMC Vet Res 2014;10:187.

101. Whitney J, Haase B, Beatty J, et al. Genetic polymorphisms in Toll-like receptors 1, 2 and 4 in feline upper respiratory tract aspergillosis. Vet Immunol Immuno-pathol 2019;217:109921. https://doi.org/10.1016/j.vetimm.2019.109921.

102. Schlueter C, Budras KD, Ludewig E, et al. Brachycephalic feline noses - CT and anatomical study of the relationship between head conformation and the naso-lacrimal drainage system. J Feline Med Surg 2009;11(11):891–900.

103. Siddiqui AA, Shah AA, Bashir SH. Craniocerebral aspergillosis of sinonasal origin in immunocompetent patients: clinical spectrum and outcome in 25 cases. Neurosurgery 2004;55(3):602–11.

104. Latge JP. The pathobiology of *Aspergillus fumigatus*. Trends Microbiol 2001; 9(8):382–9.

105. Tomee JFC, Kauffman HF. Putative virulence factors of *Aspergillus fumigatus*. Clin Exp Allergy 2000;30(4):476–84.

106. Sugui JA, Pardo J, Chang YC, et al. Gliotoxin is a virulence factor of *Aspergillus fumigatus*: gliP deletion attenuates virulence in mice immunosuppressed with hydrocortisone. Eukaryot Cell 2007;6(9):1562–9.

107. Hogan LH, Klein BS, Levitz SM. Virulence factors of medically important fungi. Clin Microbiol Rev 1996;9(4):469–88.

108. Talbot JJ, Frisvad JC, Meis JF, et al. *Cyp51*A mutations, extrolite profiles, and antifungal susceptibility in clinical and environmental isolates of the *Aspergillus viridinutans* species complex. Antimicrob Agents Chemother 2019;63(11) [pii: e00632-19].

109. Lillehoj EB, Ciegler A. A toxic substance from *Aspergillus viridi-nutans*. Can J Microbiol 1972;18(2):193–7.

110. Lillehoj EB, Milburn MS. Viriditoxin production by *Aspergillus viridi-nutans* and related species. Appl Microbiol 1973;26(2):202–5.

111. Webb BJ, Vikram HR. Chronic invasive sinus aspergillosis in immunocompetent hosts: a geographic comparison. Mycopathologia 2010;170(6):403–10.

112. Pasqualotto AC. Differences in pathogenicity and clinical syndromes due to *Aspergillus fumigatus* and *Aspergillus flavus*. Med Mycol 2009;47:S261–70.

113. Magro M, Sykes J, Vishkautsan P, et al. Spatial patterns and impacts of environmental and climatic factors on canine sinonasal aspergillosis in Northern California. Front Vet Sci 2017;4:104.

114. Ivaskiene M, Siugzdaite J, Matusevicius A, et al. Isolation of fungal flora from the hair coats of clinically healthy dogs and cats. Veterinarija Ir Zootechnika 2009; 45(67):13–9.

115. Hope WW, Walsh TJ, Denning DW. Laboratory diagnosis of invasive aspergillosis. Lancet Infect Dis 2005;5(10):609–22.

116. Whitney J, Beatty JA, Dhand N, et al. Evaluation of serum galactomannan detection for the diagnosis of feline upper respiratory tract aspergillosis. Vet Microbiol 2013;162(1):5.

117. Pfeiffer CD, Fine JP, Safdar N. Diagnosis of invasive aspergillosis using a galactomannan assay: a meta-analysis. Clin Infect Dis 2006;42(10):1417–27.

118. Garcia RS, Wheat LJ, Cook AK, et al. Sensitivity and specificity of a blood and urine galactomannan antigen assay for diagnosis of systemic aspergillosis in dogs. J Vet Intern Med 2012;26(4):911–9.

119. Hachem RY, Kontoyiannais DP, Chemaly RF, et al. Utility of galactomannan enzyme immunoassay and (1,3) B-D-glucan in diagnosis of invasive fungal infections: low sensitivity for *Aspergillus fumigatus* infection in hematologic malignancy patients. J Clin Microbiol 2009;47(1):129–33.

120. Kitasato Y, Tao Y, Hoshino T, et al. Comparison of *Aspergillus galactomannan* antigen testing with a new cut-off index and *Aspergillus* precipitating antibody testing for the diagnosis of chronic pulmonary aspergillosis. Respirology 2009;14(5):701–8.

121. Billen F, Peeters D, Peters IR, et al. Comparison of the value of measurement of serum galactomannan and *Aspergillus*-specific antibodies in the diagnosis of canine sino-nasal aspergillosis. Vet Microbiol 2009;133(4):358–65.

122. Mennink-Kersten M, Donnelly JP, Verweij PE. Detection of circulating galactomannan for the diagnosis and management of invasive aspergillosis. Lancet Infect Dis 2004;4(6):349–57.

123. Herbrecht R, Letscher-Bru V, Oprea C, et al. *Aspergillus galactomannan* detection in the diagnosis of invasive aspergillosis in cancer patients. J Clin Oncol 2002;20(7):1898–906.

124. Zandijk E, Mewis A, Magerman K, et al. False-positive results by the platelia *Aspergillus galactomannan* antigen test for patients treated with Amoxicillin-Clavulanate. Clin Vaccine Immunol 2008;15(7):1132–3.

125. Richardson M, Page I. Role of serological tests in the diagnosis of mold infections. Curr Fungal Infect Rep 2018;12(3):127–36.

126. Page ID, Richardson MD, Denning DW. Siemens immulite *Aspergillus*-specific IgG assay for chronic pulmonary aspergillosis diagnosis. Med Mycol 2019; 57(3):300–7.

127. Lenglinger FX, Krennmair G, MullerSchelken H, et al. Radiodense concretions in maxillary sinus aspergillosis: pathogenesis and the role of CT densitometry. Eur Radiol 1996;6(3):375–9.

128. Winstanley EW. Trephining frontal sinuses in the treatment of rhinitis and sinusitis in the cat. Vet Rec 1974;95:289–92.

129. Talbot JJ, Johnson LR, Martin P, et al. What causes canine sino-nasal aspergillosis? A molecular approach to species identification. Vet J 2014;200(1):17–21.

130. Chen SCA, Halliday CL, Meyer W. A review of nucleic acid-based diagnostic tests for systemic mycoses with an emphasis on polymerase chain reaction-based assays. Med Mycol 2002;40(4):333–57.

131. Samson RA, Visagie CM, Houbraken J, et al. Phylogeny, identification and nomenclature of the genus *Aspergillus*. Stud Mycol 2014;78:141–73.

132. Hubka V, Kolarik M. Beta-tubulin paralogue tubC is frequently misidentified as the benA gene in *Aspergillus* section *Nigri* taxonomy: primer specificity testing and taxonomic consequences. Persoonia 2012;29:1–10.

133. Peeters D, Day MJ, Clercx C. An immunohistochemical study of canine nasal aspergillosis. J Comp Pathol 2005;132(4):283–8.

134. Burrow R, McCarroll D, Baker M, et al. Frontal sinus depth at four landmarks in breeds of dog typically affected by sinonasal aspergillosis. Vet Rec 2012; 170(1):20.

135. Belda B, Petrovitch N, Mathews KG. Sinonasal aspergillosis: outcome after topical treatment in dogs with cribriform plate lysis. J Vet Intern Med 2018; 32(4):1353–8.

136. Stanton JA, Miller ML, Johnson P, et al. Treatment of canine sinonasal aspergillosis with clotrimazole infusion in patients with cribriform plate lysis. J Small Anim Pract 2018;59(7):411–4.

137. Vangrinsven E, Girod M, Goossens D, et al. Comparison of two minimally invasive enilconazole perendoscopic infusion protocols for the treatment of canine sinonasal aspergillosis. J Small Anim Pract 2018;59(12):777–82.

138. Burrow R, Baker M, White L, et al. Trephination of the frontal sinuses and instillation of clotrimazole cream: a computed tomographic study in canine cadavers. Vet Surg 2013;42(3):322–8.

139. Schuller S, Clercx C. Long-term outcomes in dogs with sinonasal aspergillosis treated with intranasal infusions of enilconazole. J Am Anim Hosp Assoc 2007;43(1):33–8.

140. Sharman M, Lenard Z, Hosgood G, et al. Clotrimazole and enilconazole distribution within the frontal sinuses and nasal cavity of nine dogs with sinonasal aspergillosis. J Small Anim Pract 2012;53(3):161–7.

141. Montone KT. Pathology of fungal rhinosinusitis: a review. Head Neck Pathol 2016;10(1):40–6.

142. Barr SC, Rishniw M, Lynch M. Questions contents of clotrimazole solution. J Am Vet Med Assoc 2010;236(2):163–4.

143. Lyskova P, Hubka V, Svobodova L, et al. Antifungal susceptibility of the *Aspergillus viridinutans* complex: comparison of two in vitro methods. Antimicrob Agents Chemother 2018;62(4) [pii:e01927-17].

144. Mawby DI, Whittemore JC, Fowler LE, et al. Posaconazole pharmacokinetics in healthy cats after oral and intravenous administration. J Vet Intern Med 2016; 30(5):1703–7.

145. Quimby JM, Hoffman SB, Duke J, et al. Adverse neurologic events associated with voriconazole use in 3 cats. J Vet Intern Med 2010;24(3):647–9.

146. Vishkautsan P, Papich MG, Thompson GR 3rd, et al. Pharmacokinetics of voriconazole after intravenous and oral administration to healthy cats. Am J Vet Res 2016;77(9):931–9.

147. Leshinsky J, McLachlan A, Foster DJR, et al. Pharmacokinetics of caspofungin acetate to guide optimal dosing in cats. PLoS One 2017;12(6):e0178783.

148. Walsh TJ, Anaissie EJ, Denning DW, et al. Treatment of aspergillosis: clinical practice guidelines of the infectious diseases society of America. Clin Infect Dis 2008;46(3):327–60.

149. Mawby DI, Whittemore JC, Fowler LE, et al. Comparison of absorption characteristics of oral reference and compounded itraconazole formulations in healthy cats. J Am Vet Med Assoc 2018;252(2):195–200.

Canine Nasal Disease
An Update

Leah A. Cohn, DVM, PhD

KEYWORDS

- Rhinitis • Nasal discharge • Epistaxis • Sinonasal aspergillosis
- Nasal adenocarcinoma

KEY POINTS

- For dogs with epistaxis unaccompanied by mucoid or mucopurulent nasal discharge, assessment of coagulation status and blood pressure should precede diagnostic investigation aimed at identifying nasal disease.
- Investigation of oral health, including dental probing and dental radiographs as needed, is warranted before more expensive or invasive diagnostics are undertaken in dogs with nasal discharge.
- Primary bacterial rhinitis is uncommon as a cause of nasal disease signs, but antibiotics often result in temporary improvement in signs related to secondary bacterial infections.
- In retrospective studies, nasal neoplasia is often the most common cause of chronic nasal discharge or epistaxis in dogs.
- If the dog's owners are willing to undertake expensive therapies (eg, radiation therapy for nasal carcinoma), should they be indicated, computed tomography or magnetic resonance imaging is indicated early in the disease evaluation.

INTRODUCTION
Nature of the Problem

Canine nasal disease is commonly encountered in small animal practice. Clinical signs are similar regardless of the specific cause of nasal disease (**Box 1**), but some signs are more often associated with specific disease process (eg, facial deformity is more often identified in dogs with nasal neoplasia than other causes of nasal disease). In addition, nasal signs can be identified in dogs with systemic rather than nasal disease (**Box 2**).

A thorough history and physical examination, followed by a stepwise diagnostic evaluation, often identify a specific diagnosis and thus facilitate an accurate prognosis and development of an optimum treatment plan. Several studies have described a specific clinical disease that results in nasal signs[1–10] or have described diagnostic

Department of Veterinary Medicine and Surgery, University of Missouri, 900 East Campus Drive, Columbia, MO 65211, USA
E-mail address: cohnl@missouri.edu

Vet Clin Small Anim 50 (2020) 359–374
https://doi.org/10.1016/j.cvsm.2019.11.002
0195-5616/20/© 2019 Elsevier Inc. All rights reserved.

vetsmall.theclinics.com

Box 1
Clinical signs associated with canine nasal disease

- Nasal discharge
  - Serous
  - Mucoid
  - Mucopurulent
  - Purulent
  - Sanguineus/epistaxis
  - Mixed

- Sneezing

- Pawing or rubbing at muzzle

- Facial deformity, asymmetry, or ulceration

- Facial pain

- Epiphora

- Exophthalmos

- Loss of pigmentation on the ventral portion of the nostril

- Open mouth breathing

- Halitosis

- Stertor

- Coughing

- Seizure (rare)

Modified from Cohn LA. Canine nasal disease. Vet Clin North Am Small Anim Pract. 2014; 44(1): 75-89; with permission.

---

modalities used in dogs with nasal signs.[11–19] Only a few retrospective studies have investigated the frequency with which a specific diagnosis is determined to cause nasal signs in dogs.[10,20–23] Understanding which diagnoses are most likely is helpful not only in prioritizing diagnostic testing but also in informing pet owners as they consider which of many diagnostic options to authorize. Retrospective studies undertaken at referral institutions likely provide a biased representation of the relative importance of some conditions because common disorders (eg, periodontal disease) could be treated by local veterinarians without need for referral. Nonetheless, retrospective

---

Box 2
Systemic diseases processes with nasal manifestations

Coagulopathy
  Primary hemostatic defects (ie, thrombocytopenia/thrombocytopathia)
  Secondary hemostatic defects (eg, vitamin K rodenticide antagonists)

Severe hypertension

Hyperviscosity syndromes (eg, multiple myeloma, ehrlichiosis)

Systemic infection (eg, distemper virus, ehrlichiosis)

Dysautonomia

Vomiting/regurgitation

From Cohn LA. Canine nasal disease. Vet Clin North Am Small Anim Pract. 2014; 44(1): 75-89; with permission.

studies provide useful information regarding the most common causes of nasal disease (**Fig. 1**).

CLINICAL FINDINGS
History and Signalment

Nasal disease occurs most often in dolichocephalic and mesaticephalic dogs.[16,19–22] In particular, dolichocephalic breeds are 2.5 times more likely to develop nasal neoplasia than are mixed breed dogs, and large dogs are more likely to have nasal neoplasia than small breeds.[24–26] Although some studies suggest a slight overrepresentation of male dogs for nasal neoplasia, other studies find no relationship between sex and various causes of nasal disease.[16,20–23,26] There are relationships between the age of the dog and disease. Nasal neoplasia, one of the most common causes of nasal discharge and epistaxis, is more likely in older dogs.[16,21,22,27] Similarly, periodontal disease is more likely in older dogs. Inflammatory rhinitis occurs in dogs of all ages.[1,6,16,23] Fungal rhinitis can also occur in dogs of any age but is most often recognized in young to middle-aged adults.[28]

History provided by the dog's owners can be useful. Key questions include the following:

- Are there signs of illness that are not directly related to the nose, such as anorexia, weight loss, lethargy, bleeding, or bruising?
- What is the duration of nasal signs, and have any therapies been attempted? If so, what was the response?

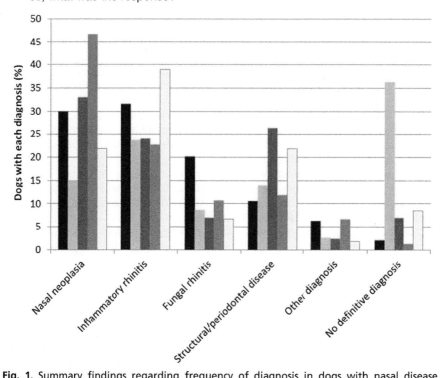

Fig. 1. Summary findings regarding frequency of diagnosis in dogs with nasal disease. Although each study classified disease diagnosis differently, diagnoses have been grouped similarly for summary presentation. (*Data from* Refs.[10,20–23])

- Did the dog's environment change before the clinical signs began (including trips to a boarding facility or a move to a new location)?
- If nasal discharge is present, does it come from 1 nostril (and if so, which one) or both? Has discharge changed from unilateral to bilateral?
- What is the predominant character of nasal discharge, and has it changed over time?
- If nasal signs are long-standing, is there a seasonal change?

Acute nasal signs, nasal signs associated with systemic illness, and epistaxis in the absence of other nasal signs should prompt a thorough consideration of nonnasal disease. For dogs with an acute onset of mucopurulent or purulent discharge, serious consideration should be given to systemic infection (eg distemper, influenza virus) rather than local nasal disease. Although causes of epistaxis directly related to disease of the nose are identified at least 3 times more frequently than are systemic causes of epistaxis, it is still crucial that systemic disorders be ruled out before beginning a search for nasal disease.[29] For dogs presenting with epistaxis in the absence of mucoid/purulent/mucopurulent nasal discharge, coagulation disorders, ehrlichiosis, hypertension, or hyperviscosity syndromes must be ruled out before undertaking nasal imaging or biopsy.

Duration of signs influences the likelihood of various diagnoses. Nasal foreign bodies often result in an acute onset of sneezing and facial pawing, but can remain in place for a long period, resulting in chronic nasal discharge. Signs related to nasal neoplasia or fungal rhinitis can be present for days, weeks, or even months before presentation.[25] However, if signs are present for many months without disease progression, cancer and fungal rhinitis become less likely, whereas structural (eg, nasal stenosis, oronasal fistulae) or inflammatory disease becomes more likely. Seasonal variation in severity of signs is suggestive of inflammatory rather than structural disease.

Laterality of nasal discharge can provide clues to the cause of nasal signs.[10,20,23] Nasal discharge associated with nasal foreign bodies or structural defects is generally unilateral. Discharge associated with either nasal neoplasia or fungal rhinitis often begins as a unilateral problem but progresses to bilateral involvement. Although nasal discharge associated with periodontal disease is often unilateral, dogs with poor oral health can have problems on both sides of the mouth and therefore could show bilateral nasal discharge. Inflammatory rhinitis can present with either bilateral (more common) or unilateral nasal discharge.[1,6,10]

Response to previous therapy with either antihistamines or antibiotics does not necessarily incriminate primary allergic or infectious disease, respectively. Antihistamines can result in minor improvement, regardless of disease causation, through drying of secretions. Similarly, antibiotic therapy can change the quality or quantity of nasal discharge either through elimination of secondary, opportunistic bacterial pathogens or via an anti-inflammatory effect (as seen with doxycycline[30]), regardless of the underlying disease process.

Physical Examination

Physical examination can be useful in establishing and prioritizing differential diagnoses. In addition to an examination of the head, examination of the entire dog is warranted. For animals with epistaxis, look carefully for petechia or ecchymosis, which suggests a coagulopathy. Retinal examination might reveal evidence of either coagulopathy or hypertension. Specific examination should include each of the following:

- Character of nasal discharge, with notation of side or sides
- Facial deformity or ulceration

- Patency of airflow through each nostril
- Condition of the teeth and gums
- Examination of the roof of the mouth to the pharynx (to the degree possible)
- Ability to retro pulse the eyes
- Pain on opening the mouth or manipulating the muzzle
- Epiphora
- Percussion of the frontal sinuses and muzzle
- Pigmentation of the nostrils
- Size and texture of submandibular lymph nodes

A thorough evaluation of the oral cavity includes probing the sulci around the teeth because disease can be present beneath the gum line. Because this examination requires heavy sedation or anesthesia, it is often completed just before, or immediately after, imaging studies or other diagnostic examinations. If probing reveals periodontal disease before advanced imaging is performed, it might obviate that expensive testing. On the other hand, bleeding that can occur as a result of periodontal probing can negatively affect subsequent imaging studies. Therefore, the clinician must use their best judgment in deciding if periodontal probing should precede or follow imaging studies. Tooth root abscess, oronasal fistulae, fractured teeth, osteomyelitis, and intranasal migration of displaced teeth are all potential causes of nasal discharge. Often, dental radiographs are beneficial, especially when disease of a specific tooth is suspected.

Although physical examination rarely provides a definitive diagnosis unless periodontal disease is identified, it often allows for a logical rank order for differential diagnosis. Deformity of the face, epiphora, inability to retro pulse the eyes, or ulceration on the muzzle often suggests space-occupying neoplastic disease.[20] Loss of pigment of the nostril suggests sinonasal aspergillosis,[28] whereas ulcers of the nasal planum can be either fungal or neoplastic in origin. Absence of airflow suggests a space-occupying lesion, although severe mucus accumulation or a foreign body can sometimes produce the same effect.[22]

Nasal discharge can be characterized as either serous, mucoid, purulent, hemorrhagic, or some combination of those types.[10] Although character of the discharge cannot be used to make a diagnosis, certain differential diagnoses are more or less likely to be associated with certain types of discharge (**Box 3**).[10,16,23] Any nasal disease that disrupts the normal protective mechanisms can result in secondary bacterial infection and associated purulent discharge. For this reason, mucopurulent discharge is very common and is perhaps the least useful for ranking differential diagnosis lists.

DIAGNOSTIC MODALITIES

Choice of diagnostic modalities depends on a logically ordered list of differential diagnoses, availability of equipment, and the wishes of the animal's owner (a factor often related to cost). Certain diagnostic techniques can be low yield, but because of simplicity and low cost are still worthwhile. As an example, metastasis of nasal neoplasia to the submandibular lymph nodes at disease diagnosis is uncommon ($\sim$8%), but fine-needle aspirate of those nodes is simple, inexpensive, and minimally invasive and can occasionally provide a definitive disease diagnosis.[27]

Imaging Studies

Imaging studies are useful for the diagnosis of nasal disease in dogs. These studies include the following:

> **Box 3**
> **Characteristics of nasal discharge associated with disease causation**
>
> - Serous discharge
>   Consider: Nasal mites, early viral infection, stress
> - Mucoid or mucopurulent discharge
>   Consider: Systemic disease, oronasal/periodontal disease, nasal neoplasia, inflammatory nasal disease (reactive or primary), fungal rhinitis, chronic foreign body, secondary bacterial infection
> - Epistaxis
>   Consider: Systemic disease, trauma, nasal neoplasia, fungal rhinitis, inflammatory nasal disease, acute foreign body
>
> *Modified from* Cohn LA. Canine nasal disease. Vet Clin North Am Small Anim Pract. 2014; 44(1): 75-89; with permission.

- Dental radiographs (as indicated based on oral examination)
- Skull radiographs
- Thoracic radiographs
- Computed tomography (CT) of the skull with or without contrast enhancement
- Magnetic resonance imaging (MRI) of the skull
- Rhinoscopy, including choanal examination

The usefulness of thoracic radiographs is debatable, because most nasal tumors are locally invasive and unlikely to metastasize to the lungs. However, thoracic imaging is a reasonable diagnostic technique for dogs with suspected nasal neoplasia, because recognition of metastasis likely alters diagnostic and therapeutic plans. When radiographic/CT/MRI imaging of the nose and rhinoscopy are planned, radiographic studies should always precede rhinoscopy, because rhinoscopy results in hemorrhage, which can alter results of radiographic studies.

Numerous studies have described the usefulness of plain film nasal radiographs, CT, and MRI in the diagnosis of nasal disease.[10,13,15–19,27,31,32] Advantages and disadvantages exist with each modality (**Table 1**). Appropriate plain film nasal radiographs require multiple views, including the open mouth view, and thus require general anesthesia.[33] Although either CT or MRI provides significant additional information and increases diagnostic sensitivity in dogs with nasal disease compared with plain radiographs, cost and availability are limitations for some pet owners. However, for pet owners who are likely to consider definitive forms of therapy (eg, radiation for nasal neoplasia or intranasal instillation of antifungal drugs for the treatment of sinonasal aspergillosis), the advantages of advanced imaging are great enough that early referral to an institution with these capabilities is warranted. Although imaging cannot provide a histopathologic diagnosis, advanced imaging can often provide a good degree of confidence in a probable diagnosis.[34] When radiographic/CT/MRI imaging of the nose and rhinoscopy are planned, radiographic studies should always precede rhinoscopy, because rhinoscopy results in hemorrhage, which can alter results of radiographic studies.

Rhinoscopy allows direct visualization of the nasal passages and, via a retroflexed view using a flexible scope, the choanae.[35–37] Rhinoscopy is most useful in combination with, and immediately after, radiographic imaging. Visualization of nasal mites, foreign materials, fungal plaques, or stenosis/atresia can provide a specific diagnosis (**Fig. 2**). Destruction of nasal turbinates in dogs with sinonasal aspergillosis can create a characteristic cavernous appearance with or without visible fungal plaques. Tumors

Table 1
Comparison of imaging techniques for dogs with nasal disease

	Skull Radiographs	CT	MRI
Availability	Readily available	Moderate availability	Least available
General anesthesia	Required	Anesthesia or sedation	Required
Cost	Least expensive	Moderately expensive	Most expensive
Show cribriform plate integrity	Poor	Excellent	Excellent
Ability to discriminate between tissue and mucus	Poor	Excellent (with contrast)	Excellent
Sensitivity to detect soft tissue changes	Poor to moderate	Good	Excellent
Sensitivity to detect bony changes (lysis or hyperostosis)	Moderate	Excellent	Good
Ability to evaluate sinuses	Moderate	Excellent	Good to excellent

From Cohn LA. Canine nasal disease. Vet Clin North Am Small Anim Pract. 2014; 44(1): 75-89; with permission.

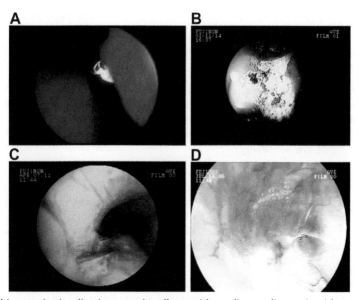

Fig. 2. Rhinoscopic visualization occasionally provides a disease diagnosis without need for additional testing. (*A*) A nasal mite seen in a dog presented for sneezing and pawing at the nose. (*B*) A fungal plaque in a dog with nasal aspergillosis. (*C*) A grass foreign body associated with an acute onset of sneezing. (*D*) Nasopharyngeal stenosis observed on a retro-flexed view to the choanae. (*Courtesy of* [*A*] Dr Carol Reinero, DVM, PhD, DACVIM (SAIM), Columbia, MO; and [*C*] Dr Laura Nafe, DVM, MS, DACVIM (SAIM), Sillwater, OK; and [*B, D*] *From* Cohn LA. Canine nasal disease. Vet Clin North Am Small Anim Pract. 2014; 44(1): 75-89; with permission.)

often block passage of the scope, but malignancy cannot be confirmed by rhinoscopic appearance alone. Hyperemia, mucus, and blood are frequently identified abnormalities but are nonspecific findings. In addition to viewing lesions, rhinoscopy can be used to guide tissue biopsy.[35]

Nonimaging Diagnostic Modalities

Besides diagnostic tests used to rule out systemic causes of nasal signs (eg, blood pressure measurement, coagulation assays), there are a variety of non–imaging-related diagnostic modalities that are useful for animals with nasal disease. Some are applied in nearly all animals with nasal disease (eg, probing of the dental sulci), whereas others are reserved for use in only select cases (eg, fungal serology or culture). Nonimaging diagnostic modalities include the following.

Dental probing under sedation/anesthesia

A simple, noninvasive technique that is applied to essentially all dogs with chronic nasal signs, dental probe examination has a high diagnostic yield when signs are related to oral/periodontal disease.

Serology

Noninvasive blood tests (agar-gel immunodiffusion or immunoglobulin G enzyme-linked immunosorbent assay) provide good sensitivity and excellent specificity for sinonasal aspergillosis, but serum/urine galactomannan assays are of no value.[38,39] The best use of these serologic tests is when aspergillosis is suspected based on clinical findings but either pet owners have declined more expensive diagnostic techniques (ie, advanced imaging studies), or when infection could not be confirmed by other methods. Latex agglutination titers for nasal cryptococcosis provide good sensitivity and specificity, but nasal cryptococcosis is less common in dogs than in cats. Ehrlichiosis is not a common cause of epistaxis but can be ruled out with simple, inexpensive serologic testing.

Fine-needle aspirate of submandibular lymph nodes

The diagnostic yield of this simple, noninvasive technique is low, because metastasis at time of disease diagnosis is uncommon. Submandibular lymph nodes that are enlarged, firm, or ipsilateral to suspected nasal neoplasia warrant aspiration with cytology despite low sensitivity.[25–27]

Nasal cytology

Cytologic assessment of impressions from biopsy specimens, nasal swabs or brush samples (collected with or without visual guidance), or nasal discharge is variably useful for disease diagnosis. Disease diagnosis based on cytologic assessment of nasal discharge is unlikely; however, guided sampling of a visualized lesion can provide higher diagnostic yield if disease is caused by neoplasia or fungal infection.[21,40]

Nasal fungal culture

Fungal cultures require substantial time for pathogen growth and are not inexpensive. The sensitivity of culture for dogs with sinonasal aspergillosis can be as high as 80% if samples are collected from areas containing rhinoscopically visible plaques, but are likely lower from randomly obtained samples.[38] It can be argued that fungal culture is not necessary if fungal plaques are visualized.

Nasal bacterial culture

Because the nasal passages of healthy dogs are not sterile, and because primary bacterial rhinitis is rare, the author finds little use for bacterial culture from dogs with nasal disease. The culture collection method likely influences culture results from dogs as it does for cats.[41] If collected, culture of material (tissue or swab) from deep within the nasal passages is recommended. Light bacterial growth and mixed cultures are typically not reflective of infection.[1]

Nasal biopsy with histopathologic evaluation

Although biopsy is an invasive technique that requires general anesthesia, biopsy is typically required for a definitive diagnosis. It is the only means to make a diagnosis of inflammatory rhinitis, including lymphoplasmacytic rhinitis (LPR).[1,6,42] Histopathologic examination of biopsy tissue can identify fungal pathogens (special stains may be required) or confirm a specific type of nasal neoplasia.[26] Biopsy techniques include rhinoscopically guided biopsy, biopsy guided by radiographic imaging, stereotactic CT-guided biopsy, blind biopsy, or nasal hydropulsion.[37,43–46] Care must be used in obtaining biopsy without visual guidance to avoid injury (**Fig. 3**). Sampling, even with visual guidance, can miss the lesion and obtain only adjacent tissue, thereby providing misleading information.[46] Histologic evidence of inflammation does not prove disease causation without interrogation of all available information. For example, the inflammation characteristic of LPR can be identical to the inflammation associated with nasal aspergillosis. Misdiagnosis could result if only histologic evidence of inflammation is considered without considering the full case, including history and examination as well as other imaging modalities. The same kind of misdiagnosis can happen when a biopsy demonstrates peritumoral inflammation yet misses a nearby neoplastic population of cells.

Nasal lavage

Nasal lavage/hydropulsion can be used as a diagnostic tool in anesthetized dogs. It is most helpful either when used to dislodge tumor tissue for histopathologic examination or when used to dislodge foreign material (eg, plant material).[44] Cytologic evaluation or culture of the lavage solution can occasionally allow identification of fungal hyphae or neoplastic cells.

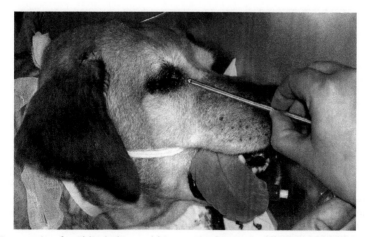

Fig. 3. Preparation for "blinded" nasal biopsy. The biopsy instrument should be measured against the distance from the nares to the medial canthus of the eye before biopsy. (*From* Cohn LA. Canine nasal disease. Vet Clin North Am Small Anim Pract. 2014; 44(1): 75-89; with permission.)

Rhinotomy/sinusotomy/frontal sinus trephination

This most invasive option for diagnosis of nasal disease is usually reserved for those cases that elude diagnosis using other techniques. Although CT or MRI might strongly suggest a diagnosis of sinonasal aspergillosis, confirmation by rhinoscopic visualization of fungal plaques in the nasal cavity or fungal culture is not always possible.[9] In these cases, surgical access to the sinuses can both confirm a diagnosis and facilitate treatment. Similarly, neoplastic disease is sometimes best accessed through a surgical approach when other methods have failed to yield a diagnosis. However, surgical debulking of nasal neoplasia is not curative, with radiation therapy generally the preferred option for treatment with or without surgical exenteration.[47,48]

PATHOLOGY

Confirmation of tumor type depends on histopathologic evaluation of nasal tissue. In dogs, carcinoma accounts for as much as two-thirds of nasal neoplasia, with adenocarcinoma the most common tumor type (**Box 4**).

Pathologic assessment of tissue biopsy is also necessary for diagnosis of inflammatory nasal disease. Diagnosis of inflammatory nasal disease is often frustrating both because of the lack of any specific findings other than histopathologic changes and because these same histopathologic changes can be identified in dogs with other types of nasal disease. Idiopathic lymphoplasmacytic inflammation is the most commonly identified inflammatory rhinitis, but suppurative rhinitis, eosinophilic rhinitis, and granulomatous rhinitis occur as well.[16] Clinicians must keep in mind that inflammation can reflect a response to disease rather than the disease itself. For example, nasal discharge can occur in animals with vomiting or regurgitation as a result of aspiration of materials into the choanae or caudal nasal passage (**Fig. 4**); tissue biopsy from these dogs shows inflammation on microscopic examination, but not disease causation. In addition, biopsy samples can miss the underlying disease and show only surrounding inflammation. When biopsy identifies only inflammation, but neoplastic or fungal rhinitis are suspected based on clinical signs or imaging results, either alternative diagnostic testing (eg, fungal serology) or more aggressive/directed

---

Box 4
Canine nasal neoplasia

Most commonly identified nasal tumor types
- Adenocarcinoma
- Undifferentiated carcinoma
- Chondrosarcoma
- Squamous cell carcinoma

Occasionally identified nasal tumor types
- Fibrosarcoma
- Osteosarcoma
- Undifferentiated sarcoma
- Lymphoma

Rarely identified nasal tumor types (other types are possible)
- Melanoma
- Hemangiosarcoma
- Transmissible venereal tumor
- Neuroendocrine carcinoma
- Mast cell tumors

Data from Refs.[3,16,25–27]

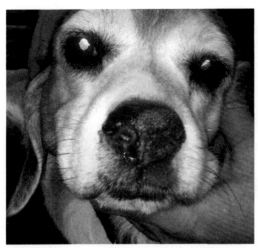

Fig. 4. Severe mucopurulent nasal discharge owing to inflammation induced by severe persistent vomiting in a dog with pancreatitis. (*From* Cohn LA. Canine nasal disease. Vet Clin North Am Small Anim Pract. 2014; 44(1): 75-89; with permission.)

repeat biopsy (eg, rhinotomy, stereotactic CT-guided biopsy) may be warranted. In 1 study, approximately one-third of all histologic diagnoses of nasal neoplasia required 1 or more repeat biopsies.[46]

CASE STUDIES
Case Study 1

A 5-year-old female spayed (FS) Siberian husky presented for an episode of severe epistaxis.

History
Although the dog presented for acute epistaxis, its owners acknowledged that mucopurulent nasal discharge had been present for 2 to 3 weeks; they were unsure as to which side or sides had been affected.

Physical examination
Temperature, pulse, and respiration were normal. Examination (including ocular and conscious oral examination) was unremarkable save for bilateral mucopurulent discharge with some blood, and loss of pigmentation at the ventral portion of the nostril (**Fig. 5**). The dog resented manipulation of the muzzle. Patent airflow was present from both nares.

Diagnostic evaluation
The combination of epistaxis with mucopurulent discharge and the absence of petechia or ecchymosis made systemic disease (eg, coagulopathy, hypertension) less likely than nasal disease. Patent airflow, pain on manipulation of the muzzle, and loss of pigmentation brought nasal aspergillosis to the top of the differential list, which still included periodontal disease, nasal neoplasia, inflammatory nasal disease, or foreign body.

Under general anesthesia, a thorough oral examination with dental probing did not identify important periodontal disease. CT showed cavitary destruction of the turbinates as well as loss of nasal septal bone and mucosal thickening; the cribriform plate

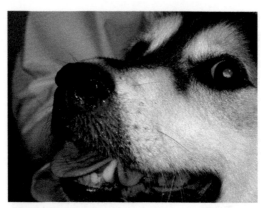

Fig. 5. A 5-year-old FS Siberian husky presented for epistaxis. Notice mucopurulent nasal discharge and loss of pigmentation on nasal planum. The eventual diagnosis was nasal aspergillosis. (*From* Cohn LA. Canine nasal disease. Vet Clin North Am Small Anim Pract. 2014; 44(1): 75-89; with permission.)

was intact. Rhinoscopy, completed after CT examination, showed loss of nasal turbinates, mucoid/sanguinous nasal discharge, and multiple white plaques typical of sinonasal aspergillosis. Fungal culture was not obtained, but samples were submitted for histopathologic examination and confirmed the presence of fungal elements. The combination of clinical and diagnostic findings provided enough confidence in the diagnosis of fungal rhinitis to warrant treatment during the same anesthetic episode as the diagnostic testing. The nasal cavity was debrided and treated with installation of enilconazole.[28] The dog made a complete recovery and did not require subsequent therapy.

Case Study 2

An 11-year-old male castrated (MC) Labrador retriever presented for epistaxis.

History
The dog had a month-long history of sneezing unresponsive to antihistamines, glucocorticoids, or antibiotics and was referred for diagnostic testing after an acute episode of epistaxis from the left nostril. Other than the recent nose bleed, no other discharge had been noticed.

Physical examination
Temperature was 41.1°C (103°F), and the dog was panting on initial examination. Facial asymmetry was present, with swelling under the left eye, elevation of the nictitans on the left, and inability to retro pulse the left eye; the dog acted as if in pain when retropulsion was attempted. Airflow was absent through the left nasal passage. The left submandibular lymph node was slightly firm and enlarged. The remainder of the examination was unremarkable except for 2 movable subcutaneous masses on the flank.

Diagnostic evaluation
The combination of epistaxis with sneezing, facial asymmetry, and obstructed airflow pointed toward nasal rather than systemic disease. Facial asymmetry and absence of airflow on the left side of the face suggested a space-occupying lesion, and nasal neoplasia rose to the top of the differential diagnosis list.

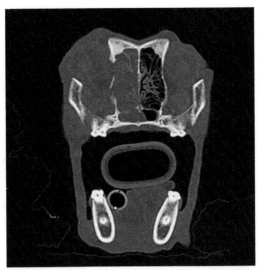

Fig. 6. CT image from an 11-year-old MC Labrador retriever with a 1 month history of sneezing and acute onset epistaxis. Nearly the entire left nasal cavity was filled with contrast-enhancing soft tissue with widespread destruction of the nasal turbinates. Multifocal lysis of the medial aspect of the left orbit with extension of the nasal mass into the medial aspect of the orbit was identified, with mild exophthalmus on the left. Findings were strongly suggestive of nasal neoplasia as was confirmed on biopsy. (*From* Cohn LA. Canine nasal disease. Vet Clin North Am Small Anim Pract. 2014; 44(1): 75-89; with permission.)

The dog's owner was unsure if he would be willing to treat neoplastic disease should that be the final diagnosis. With this in mind, evaluation began with fine-needle aspirate of the left submandibular node; aspirate was nondiagnostic. Thoracic radiographs were offered to check for metastasis, but were declined because of the low likelihood of identifying metastatic nasal disease. The owner did agree to allow blind nasal biopsy. Biopsy revealed only LPR.

One week later, the dog's owner decided to pursue CT imaging (**Fig. 6**). Images were strongly suggestive of nasal neoplasia, with a contrast-enhancing space-occupying mass, substantial bony destruction, and enlargement of the regional lymph node. Repeat biopsies were obtained with guidance provided by the CT images, and the histopathologic diagnosis was nasal adenocarcinoma. The owner opted against radiation therapy.

SUMMARY

Nasal disease is a common problem in dogs, most often manifest as nasal discharge with or without other nasal signs. Attention to signalment, history, and physical examination findings often allows development of a logically ordered list of differential diagnosis. Once systemic and oral/periodontal disease have been ruled out, a combination of imaging techniques and tissue sampling for microscopic examination is usually necessary to achieve a diagnosis. Advanced imaging, such as CT or MRI, offers important advantages over traditional skull radiographs but are less widely available and more costly. Bacterial culture is seldom beneficial, and fungal culture is reserved for select cases likely to have fungal rhinitis. Nasal biopsy is often required to confirm a specific diagnosis and is always required for diagnosis of specific tumor type or for inflammatory rhinitis.

DISCLOSURE

The author has nothing to disclose.

REFERENCES

1. Lobetti R. Idiopathic lymphoplasmacytic rhinitis in 33 dogs. J S Afr Vet Assoc 2014;85(1):01–5.
2. Hazuchova K, Neiger R, Stengel C. Topical treatment of mycotic rhinitis-rhinosinusitis in dogs with meticulous debridement and 1% clotrimazole cream: 64 cases (2007–2014). J Am Vet Med Assoc 2017;250(3):309–15.
3. Madewell BR, Priester WA, Gillette EL, et al. Neoplasms of the nasal passages and paranasal sinuses in domesticated animals as reported by 13 veterinary colleges. Am J Vet Res 1976;37(7):851–6.
4. MacEwen EG, Withrow SJ, Patnaik AK. Nasal tumors in the dog: retrospective evaluation of diagnosis, prognosis, and treatment. J Am Vet Med Assoc 1977; 170(1):45–8.
5. Van Pelt DR, McKiernan BC. Pathogenesis and treatment of canine rhinitis. Vet Clin North Am Small Anim Pract 1994;24(5):789–806.
6. Windsor RC, Johnson LR, Herrgesell EJ, et al. Idiopathic lymphoplasmacytic rhinitis in dogs: 37 cases (1997-2002). J Am Vet Med Assoc 2004;224(12): 1952–7.
7. Windsor RC, Johnson LR, Sykes JE, et al. Molecular detection of microbes in nasal tissue of dogs with idiopathic lymphoplasmacytic rhinitis. J Vet Intern Med 2006;20(2):250–6.
8. Windsor RC, Johnson LR. Canine chronic inflammatory rhinitis. Clin Tech Small Anim Pract 2006;21(2):76–81.
9. Johnson LR, Drazenovich TL, Herrera MA, et al. Results of rhinoscopy alone or in conjunction with sinuscopy in dogs with aspergillosis: 46 cases (2001-2004). J Am Vet Med Assoc 2006;228(5):738–42.
10. Plickert H, Tichy A, Hirt R. Characteristics of canine nasal discharge related to intranasal diseases: a retrospective study of 105 cases. J Small Anim Pract 2014;55(3):145–52.
11. Park RD, Beck ER, LeCouteur RA. Comparison of computed tomography and radiography for detecting changes induced by malignant nasal neoplasia in dogs. J Am Vet Med Assoc 1992;201:1720–4.
12. Burk RL. Computed tomographic imaging of nasal disease in 100 dogs. Vet Radiol Ultrasound 1992;33:177–80.
13. Codner EC, Lurus AG, Miller JB, et al. Comparison of computed tomography with radiography as a noninvasive diagnostic technique for chronic nasal disease in dogs. J Am Vet Med Assoc 1993;202(7):1106–10.
14. Saunders JH, van Bree H, Gielen I, et al. Diagnostic value of computed tomography in dogs with chronic nasal disease. Vet Radiol Ultrasound 2003;44(4): 409–13.
15. Saunders JH, van Bree H. Comparison of radiography and computed tomography for the diagnosis of canine nasal aspergillosis. Vet Radiol Ultrasound 2003; 44(4):414–9.
16. Lefebvre J, Kuehn NF, Wortinger A. Computed tomography as an aid in the diagnosis of chronic nasal disease in dogs. J Small Anim Pract 2005;46(6):280–5.
17. Miles MS, Dhaliwal RS, Moore MP, et al. Association of magnetic resonance imaging findings and histologic diagnosis in dogs with nasal disease: 78 cases (2001-2004). J Am Vet Med Assoc 2008;232(12):1844–9.

18. Furtado A, Caine A, Herrtage M. Diagnostic value of MRI in dogs with inflammatory nasal disease. J Small Anim Pract 2014;55(7):359–63.
19. Auler Fde A, Torres LN, Pinto AC, et al. Tomography, radiography, and rhinoscopy in diagnosis of benign and malignant lesions affecting the nasal cavity and paranasal sinuses in dogs: comparative study. Top Companion Anim Med 2015;30(2):39–42.
20. Lobetti RG. A retrospective study of chronic nasal disease in 75 dogs. J S Afr Vet Assoc 2009;80(4):224–8.
21. Meler E, Dunn M, Lecuyer M. A retrospective study of canine persistent nasal disease: 80 cases (1998-2003). Can Vet J 2008;49(1):71–6.
22. Tasker S, Knottenbelt CM, Munro EA, et al. Aetiology and diagnosis of persistent nasal disease in the dog: a retrospective study of 42 cases. J Small Anim Pract 1999;40(10):473–8.
23. Bondy PJ Jr, Cohn LA. Retrospective review of chronic nasal discharge in the dog. J Vet Intern Med 2003;17:386 (abstract).
24. Reif JS, Bruns C, Lower KS. Cancer of the nasal cavity and paranasal sinuses and exposure to environmental tobacco smoke in pet dogs. Am J Epidemiol 1998;147(5):488–92.
25. LaDue TA, Dodge R, Page RL, et al. Factors influencing survival after radiotherapy of nasal tumors in 130 dogs. Vet Radiol Ultrasound 1999;40(3):312–7.
26. Malinowski C. Canine and feline nasal neoplasia. Clin Tech Small Anim Pract 2006;21(2):89–94.
27. Avner A, Dobson JM, Sales JI, et al. Retrospective review of 50 canine nasal tumours evaluated by low-field magnetic resonance imaging. J Small Anim Pract 2008;49:233–9.
28. Sharman M, Lenard Z, Hosgood G, et al. Clotrimazole and enilconazole distribution within the frontal sinuses and nasal cavity of nine dogs with sinonasal aspergillosis. J Small Anim Pract 2012;53(3):161–7.
29. Bissett SA, Drobatz KJ, McKnight A, et al. Prevalence, clinical features, and causes of epistaxis in dogs: 176 cases (1996-2001). J Am Vet Med Assoc 2007;231(12):1843–50.
30. Leite LM, Carvalho AG, Ferreira PL, et al. Anti-inflammatory properties of doxycycline and minocycline in experimental models: an in vivo and in vitro comparative study. Inflammopharmacology 2011;19(2):99–110.
31. Saunders JH, Clercx C, Snaps FR, et al. Radiographic, magnetic resonance imaging, computed tomographic, and rhinoscopic features of nasal aspergillosis in dogs. J Am Vet Med Assoc 2004;225(11):1703–12.
32. Johnson EG, Wisner ER. Advances in respiratory imaging. Vet Clin North Am Small Anim Pract 2007;37(5):879–900, vi.
33. Finck M, Durand A, Hammond G, et al. Evaluation of the ventro 20° rostral-dorsocaudal oblique radiographic projection for the investigation of canine nasal disease. J Small Anim Pract 2015;56(8):491–8.
34. Kuehn NF. Diagnostic imaging for chronic nasal disease in dogs. J Small Anim Pract 2014;55(7):341–2.
35. Lent SE, Hawkins EC. Evaluation of rhinoscopy and rhinoscopy-assisted mucosal biopsy in diagnosis of nasal disease in dogs: 119 cases (1985-1989). J Am Vet Med Assoc 1992;201(9):1425–9.
36. Willard MD, Radlinsky MA. Endoscopic examination of the choanae in dogs and cats: 118 cases (1988-1998). J Am Vet Med Assoc 1999;215(9):1301–5.
37. Elie M, Sabo M. Basics in canine and feline rhinoscopy. Clin Tech Small Anim Pract 2006;21(2):60–3.

38. Pomrantz JS, Johnson LR, Nelson RW, et al. Comparison of serologic evaluation via agar gel immunodiffusion and fungal culture of tissue for diagnosis of nasal aspergillosis in dogs. J Am Vet Med Assoc 2007;230(9):1319–23.

39. Billen F, Peeters D, Peters IR, et al. Comparison of the value of measurement of serum galactomannan and Aspergillus-specific antibodies in the diagnosis of canine sino-nasal aspergillosis. Vet Microbiol 2009;133(4):358–65.

40. De Lorenzi D, Bonfanti U, Masserdotti C, et al. Diagnosis of canine nasal aspergillosis by cytological examination: a comparison of four different collection techniques. J Small Anim Pract 2006;47(6):316–9.

41. Johnson LR, Kass PH. Effect of sample collection methodology on nasal culture results in cats. J Feline Med Surg 2009;11(8):645–9.

42. Furtado A, Constantino-Casas F. Histopathology inflammation scoring and classification in 34 dogs with inflammatory nasal disease. Vet Rec 2013;173(3):71.

43. Kuhlman GM, Taylor AR, Thieman-Mankin KM, et al. Use of a frameless computed tomography-guided stereotactic biopsy system for nasal biopsy in five dogs. J Am Vet Med Assoc 2016;248(8):929–34.

44. Ashbaugh EA, McKiernan BC, Miller CJ, et al. Nasal hydropulsion: a novel tumor biopsy technique. J Am Anim Hosp Assoc 2011;47(5):312–6.

45. Sapierzynski R, Zmudzka M. Endoscopy and histopathology in the examination of the nasal cavity in dogs. Pol J Vet Sci 2009;12(2):195–201.

46. Harris B, Lourenço B, Dobson J, et al. Diagnostic accuracy of three biopsy techniques in 117 dogs with intra-nasal neoplasia. J Small Anim Pract 2014;55(4): 219–24.

47. Adams WM, Bjorling DE, McAnulty JE, et al. Outcome of accelerated radiotherapy alone or accelerated radiotherapy followed by exenteration of the nasal cavity in dogs with intranasal neoplasia: 53 cases (1990-2002). J Am Vet Med Assoc 2005;227(6):936–41.

48. Tan-Coleman B, Lyons J, Lewis C, et al. Prospective evaluation of a 5 x 4 Gy prescription for palliation of canine nasal tumors. Vet Radiol Ultrasound 2013;54(1): 89–92.

Feline Asthma
Diagnostic and Treatment Update

Julie E. Trzil, DVM, MS

KEYWORDS

- Feline asthma • Feline lower-airway disease • Airway eosinophilia
- Airway hyperresponsiveness

KEY POINTS

- Feline asthma is an important chronic lower-airway disease of cats. Definitive diagnosis is challenging due to overlapping clinicopathologic features with other lower-airway disorders; however, this is necessary due to differences in treatment and prognosis.
- Emerging diagnostics, including thoracic computed tomography and pulmonary function testing, may help differentiate feline asthma from other chronic lower-airway diseases.
- Therapy for feline asthma using glucocorticoids and bronchodilators might be inadequate or contraindicated in some cats. Experimental treatments could be beneficial in refractory cases or as adjuncts for glucocorticoid-sparing effects.

INTRODUCTION

Asthma is a common lower-airway inflammatory disease in cats thought to be allergic in origin.[1] Aeroallergen-induced stimulation of a T-helper 2 response leads to elaboration of a variety of cytokines that cause pathologic changes in the airways. The 3 major hallmarks of asthma include airway inflammation, airway hyperresponsiveness, and airflow limitation (the latter being at least in part reversible).[2] Long term, these changes lead to airway remodeling and fixed airway obstruction.

Feline asthma is estimated to affect approximately 1% to 5% of the feline population.[3] Although the median age at presentation is 4 to 5 years, many cats have a history of chronic signs suggesting that disease onset occurs much earlier in life.[4–6] Asthma is most commonly treated with glucocorticoids and bronchodilators. Although these are effective treatments in many cats, some are unresponsive or minimally responsive. In addition, chronic glucocorticoid therapy might be poorly tolerated or contraindicated in cats with certain disease, such as diabetes mellitus, chronic kidney disease, or congestive heart failure. Finally, these therapies fail to reverse the abnormal immune response and do not ameliorate chronic airway remodeling that results in declining lung function. New therapies capable of restoring immune tolerance or blunting airway remodeling would be desirable. Evaluation of novel therapeutics in clinical trials of pet

IndyVet Emergency and Specialty Hospital, 5425 Victory Drive, Indianapolis, IN 46203, USA
E-mail address: jtrzil@indyvet.com

Vet Clin Small Anim 50 (2020) 375–391
https://doi.org/10.1016/j.cvsm.2019.10.002
0195-5616/20/© 2019 Elsevier Inc. All rights reserved.

cats with asthma is hindered by a lack of consensus on what defines asthma and how it can be discriminated from other lower-airway disorders. Thus, development of additional diagnostic tests in this arena is needed. This article reviews what is currently known regarding the diagnosis and treatment of feline asthma.

DIFFERENTIAL DIAGNOSES

Because there is no single test to definitively diagnose feline asthma, it is important to rule out other diseases that can mimic clinicopathologic features of asthma.

Chronic Bronchitis

Chronic bronchitis is common in cats and shares many clinical features with asthma, such as chronic cough. It is thought to arise secondary to a previous airway insult, such as respiratory infections or inhaled irritants. These previous insults lead to permanent damage to the airways and results in many of the same historical, physical examination, and radiographic features of asthma. Although cats with either asthma or bronchitis can have a bronchial pattern radiographically, cats with asthma typically display bronchoconstriction in response to inhaled aeroallergens or irritants. Bronchoconstriction can result in "air-trapping," visualized on thoracic radiographs as hyperlucent lung fields and displacement of the diaphragm caudally. Bronchoconstriction and air-trapping should be partially reversible with the use of bronchodilators in asthmatic cats. Cats with chronic bronchitis do not have spontaneous bronchoconstriction, although they can have fixed airflow limitation secondary to cellular infiltrates or remodeling changes. Both disorders have differences in cellular infiltrates identified on bronchoalveolar lavage fluid (BALF) cytology with some overlap. Feline asthma is primarily characterized by eosinophilic inflammation ($\geq$17% eosinophils identified in BALF).[7] Chronic bronchitis causes primarily nondegenerate neutrophilic inflammation in BALF.[8] Despite this, there is not always a clear-cut distinction based on BALF because chronic eosinophilic asthma may cause damage to the airways resulting in some neutrophilic inflammation,[9] and mixed inflammation is common in cats with inflammatory airway disease.

Aelurostrongylosis

Several pulmonary parasitic diseases, including *Aelurostrongylus abstrusus*, can result in clinical findings similar to those seen in asthma. *Aelurostrongylus* is a metastrongyloid nematode that infects cats through ingestion of snails, slugs, or paratenic hosts. Radiographically, bronchial to bronchointerstitial lung patterns are typically noted with infection. Although airway eosinophilia is seen with parasitic infection as with allergic asthma, *Aelurostrongylus* infection can sometimes be differentiated by the presence of larvae on BALF cytology or fecal Baermann examination.[10] Parasites are shed intermittently in the feces, and larvae can become trapped in upper-airway secretions; therefore, the lack of larvae in these samples does not exclude a diagnosis of *Aelurostrongylus*. Empirical treatment with fenbendazole is recommended in cats with appropriate clinical signs to more confidently rule out this disorder.

Heartworm-Associated Respiratory Disease

Infection with *Dirofilaria immitis* has been proposed to result in heartworm-associated respiratory disease (HARD). Death of immature L5 larvae in the pulmonary arteries triggers eosinophilic inflammation in the airways and pulmonary parenchyma.[11,12] The presence of adult heartworms is not necessary for this disease to occur because it is primarily mediated by the larval stage.[12] Therefore, heartworm antigen tests and echocardiography to identify adult heartworms are not useful in ruling out HARD. HARD should be considered in any cat in a heartworm-endemic region that displays appropriate clinicopathologic features. A positive heartworm antibody test might increase suspicion of HARD; however, recent studies have demonstrated use of heartworm-preventative medications can cause heartworm antibody tests to be only transiently positive while continued abnormal lung pathologic condition can be identified radiographically.[13] Interestingly, bronchoalveolar lavage cytology was normal in cats that were treated with preventative medications, despite demonstration of these radiographic abnormalities.[13] Cats suspected of having HARD should be treated with an appropriate heartworm-preventative medication and glucocorticoids as previously recommended.[14] Finally, there is evidence to suggest that the heartworm endosymbiont, *Wolbachia*, could contribute to bronchial hyperreactivity in cats with HARD.[15] Thus, it is useful to treat cats suspected of having HARD with doxycycline to eliminate *Wolbachia*. The American Heartworm Society web site should be consulted for the most recent diagnostic and therapeutic recommendations.

Toxocariasis

Toxocara cati infection is relatively common in the pet cat population. Pulmonary and transtracheal migration induced pulmonary and vascular disease in experimentally infected cats.[16,17] Experimental *T cati* infection also induced bronchointerstitial lesions on thoracic radiographs and caused BALF eosinophilia; however, cats with *T cati* were clinically asymptomatic and did not appear to have airway hyperresponsiveness, a defining feature of asthma.[18] The role of *T cati* as a differential for spontaneous feline asthma is unclear because airway lesions may be incidental; however, this deserves further study.[4,5,9,19]

DIAGNOSTICS

Diagnosis of feline asthma is based on a combination of appropriate clinical signs and physical examination findings (**Box 1**) as well as diagnostic testing.

Clinicopathologic Findings

In general, clinicopathologic abnormalities of cats with asthma are nonspecific. Complete blood cell counts have revealed peripheral eosinophilia in 17% to 46% of cases,[4,5,9,19] but this does not correlate with the degree of airway eosinophilia.[5,9,19]

Box 1
Clinical signs and physical examination findings in feline asthma

Clinical signs
- Cough
- Increased respiratory effort
- Open mouth breathing
- Tachypnea
- Vomiting

Physical examination findings
- Inducible cough on tracheal palpation
- Expiratory wheeze
- Tachypnea
- Increased abdominal effort ("push") on expiration

Thoracic Imaging

Common radiographic findings in asthmatic cats include a bronchial or bronchointer-stitial lung pattern.[4,5,9,19,20] Collapse of a lung lobe, particularly the right middle lung lobe, presumably owing to mucus trapping and atelectasis, can also occur in a minority of cats.[4,20] As mentioned previously, air trapping can result in hyperlucent lung fields and caudal displacement of the diaphragm. Lack of radiographic abnormalities does not rule out feline asthma because radiographs can be normal in up to 23% of cases.[4] In addition, other lower respiratory diseases as detailed above and even infectious lower-airway disease can result in similar radiographic findings.

Computed tomography (CT) is used in the evaluation of human asthmatic patients.[21–23] Thoracic CT of cats with lower-airway disease can identify abnormalities, such as bronchial wall thickening, patchy alveolar patterns, and bronchiectasis[24]; however, these findings are not exclusive to asthmatic cats. Thoracic CT can help to identify subtle lesions that otherwise may not be appreciated on survey radiographs (**Fig. 1**). CT can be performed in cats using a Plexiglas chamber, allowing acquisition of images without chemical restraint, eliminating anesthetic risks.[24] Obtaining CT images via a Plexiglas chamber provides an important benefit in cats with respiratory distress unable to tolerate the stress of restraint for radiography. CT abnormalities have been shown to be similar in cats with naturally occurring and experimentally induced asthma and different from healthy cats.[25] Further studies have shown that the bronchial walls are significantly thicker in asthmatic cats compared with healthy cats[26]; however, although CT is useful in evaluating asthmatic cats, it does not discriminate asthma from other lower-airway diseases.

Pulmonary CT findings have been investigated in experimental infections with *A abstrusus*, *T cati*, and *D immitis*. In experimental *Aelurostrongylus* infection, bronchial wall thickening was noted similar to asthmatic cats.[27] However, multiple, variably sized nodules were noted throughout the lung parenchyma, which might help differentiate this disease process from asthma.[27] In *T cati* experimental infections, CT lesions were most often identified in the caudal lung lobes and consisted of random patches of linear densities interspersed among normal lung.[18] Bronchial wall thickening was also noted.[18] In experimental heartworm infection in cats, increased interstitial densities as well as pulmonary arterial enlargement were noted.[28] Although CT findings can be similar to asthma in these diseases, subtle differences may help to differentiate these disorders from asthma. However, the increased sensitivity of CT scans revealing subclinical abnormalities must also be taken into consideration.[29]

Bronchoscopy and Bronchoalveolar Lavage Cytology

Bronchoscopy is useful for visual inspection and collection of samples from cats with lower-airway disease. Lesions include mucus accumulation, mucosal hyperemia, epithelial irregularities, airway collapse, and stenosis, as well as bronchiectasis; however, these abnormalities do not discriminate between asthma and other forms of lower respiratory disease.[30] BALF samples for cytologic examination can be collected using either bronchoscopy or a blind technique. Eosinophilic inflammation is noted on BALF cytology of asthmatic cats; however, what constitutes normal cellular percentages in BALF fluid is controversial. Eosinophil percentages in reportedly "normal" cats have ranged from 0% to 83%.[31–35] In many of these studies, healthy cats have been defined as those free of clinical signs, which is problematic because signs of asthma are often intermittent in nature. In human asthmatics, airway inflammation can be present despite the absence of overt symptoms,[36,37] and subclinical inflammation has also been documented in pet cats.[38] Thus, it is possible that some healthy control

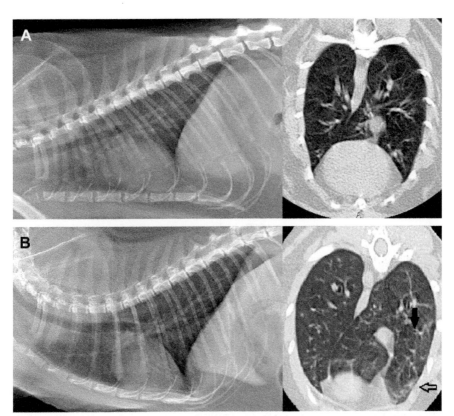

Fig. 1. Representative right lateral thoracic radiographs and thoracic CT images of 2 awake feline cats with naturally occurring asthma. The CT images were obtained with the cats positioned in a restraining device without the use of anesthetics. The lateral thoracic radiograph of both demonstrates a moderate, diffuse bronchointerstitial lung pattern. On the thoracic CT image of cat A, there is minimal bronchial wall thickening. On the thoracic CT image of cat B, there is prominent bronchial wall thickening (*filled arrow*). In addition, there is a ground-glass appearance to the pulmonary parenchyma particularly in the right lateral lung fields (*open arrow*) with a slight haziness of the lung parenchyma and vasculature from motion artifact. Overall, the CT scan of cat B has increased lung attenuation suggestive of more significant pulmonary remodeling, whereas cat A has less opaque lung parenchyma despite the fact that cat A's lung field is less aerated than cat B. This highlights the benefits of CT scans in assessing the severity of structural changes of the pulmonary parenchyma compared with thoracic radiography. (*Courtesy of* Isabelle Masseau, DVM, PhD, DACVR, Columbia, MO.)

cats in studies of BALF cytology were not appropriate, and a cutoff of $\geq$17% BALF eosinophils in pet cats has been proposed as abnormal for some studies.[7,31] Finally, as discussed previously, other parasitic diseases result in airway eosinophilia; thus, eosinophilic inflammation is not specific to feline asthma and should be interpreted in conjunction with clinical signs and other diagnostic testing.

Adjunctive Testing

Culture of BALF, regardless of whether organisms are detected on cytology, is warranted. In addition, if cultures of *Mycoplasma* spp cannot be performed, polymerase chain reaction should be considered because this is one of the more common opportunistic pathogens in feline lower-airway disease.[39] Cats suspected to have asthma with airway eosinophilia should have a heartworm antibody/antigen test to evaluate for HARD in endemic regions and a fecal flotation and Baermann examination for *T cati* and *A abstrusus*, respectively. It is important to realize that negative results do not rule out these diseases completely. Empirical deworming with fenbendazole is often recommended, and if the patient is not yet on a heartworm preventative, this should be considered.

Allergy Testing

Allergy testing by intradermal skin testing (IDST) or serum allergen-specific immunoglobulin E (IgE) can be used to investigate sensitizing allergens, although these are not commonly performed in pet cats with asthma because tests are not completely reliable. With appropriate identification, allergen avoidance or, in the future, allergen-specific immunotherapy (ASIT) might be used to reduce or eliminate clinical signs in affected cats (see later discussion in the Treatment section).

Pulmonary Function Testing

An important clinical feature of asthma is airflow limitation, which is partially or completely reversible with bronchodilators. In humans, spirometry is used to gauge lung function, but this requires patient compliance to exhale maximally through a mouthpiece, making it unsuitable for use in cats. Alternative pulmonary function testing in cats includes tidal breathing flow-volume loops using a tight-fitting face mask, forced expiratory flow-volume curves using a thoracic compression technique, barometric whole body plethysmography (BWBP), and ventilator-acquired lung mechanics.[40–44] The use of pulmonary function testing is reviewed elsewhere,[45] and in this issue.

There has been growing interest in using BWBP as a noninvasive test to differentiate between feline asthma and chronic bronchitis. In a study, bronchoprovocation using BWBP discriminated normal cats from cats with lower-airway disease,[46] although it is important to understand that BWBP is influenced by the respiratory cycle and does not directly measure airway resistance.[47] Cats with asthma were more likely to demonstrate airflow limitation in response to challenge with an indirect bronchoprovocant than cats with chronic bronchitis.[46] Another study showed a correlation between the degree and type of airway inflammation and airflow limitation measured by BWBP in spontaneous feline bronchial disease.[48] Namely, cats with airway eosinophilia demonstrated airway hyperresponsiveness at lower doses of the bronchoprovocant than cats with airway neutrophilia. The varying degree of airway hyperresponsiveness suggests that BWBP could be useful in differentiating asthma from chronic bronchitis.

The gold-standard technique to measure airway resistance is direct pulmonary mechanics. In experimental feline asthma, ventilator-acquired pulmonary mechanics allow direct and specific calculations of airway resistance and have particular value in assessing effects of therapy on airflow limitation.[43,49,50] Although there is value in assessing pulmonary mechanics, its use in clinical practice is limited due to the need for anesthesia and specialized equipment.

Biomarkers

There are several biomarkers that have been evaluated to try to differentiate feline asthma from other respiratory diseases; however, little progress has been made. The proinflammatory mediator, endothelin-1, has been associated with the pathogenesis of asthma,[51] and endothelin-1 concentrations were higher in BALF of cats with experimentally induced asthma compared with healthy control cats.[52] However, endothelin-1 has not been investigated in naturally occurring airway disease or other airway diseases of cats, so it is uncertain if this will be helpful in differentiating cats with similar clinical signs.

Exhaled breath biomarkers have been evaluated in human[53–58] and cats with experimentally induced asthma[59,60] Exhaled breath condensates (EBC) can be obtained by placing the cat in an acrylic chamber attached to tubing immersed in an ice bath and collecting the volume of breath condensate over 30 minutes.[61] Hydrogen peroxide (H_2O_2) is a marker of oxidative stress[54] and correlated with BALF eosinophilia in allergen-sensitized cats.[60] A more recent study demonstrated that acetone was increased in the EBC of 74% of cats with experimentally induced asthma.[59] More study is needed at this time to determine if measurement of metabolites in EBC will become a clinically useful biomarker for asthma in a clinical setting.

TREATMENT

The mainstay of therapy for feline asthma consists of lifelong steroids with or without bronchodilators. Unfortunately, these medications are not effective in all cats, can be associated with adverse effects, and are contraindicated with some concurrent diseases. Therapies that might help reverse the underlying immunopathology of asthma or could be used as adjuncts in refractory asthma are being investigated in experimental feline asthma models. Although these models are important in identifying therapies that may be effective in asthma, they might not accurately reflect all aspects of naturally occurring asthma. Thus, it is critical that future studies are performed in pet cats with asthma.

Traditional therapies

Glucocorticoids
Steroids are potent anti-inflammatories that have long been used for the treatment of feline asthma. They are most often administered orally in the form of prednisolone; however, inhaled therapy using modified spacing devices (Aerokat; Trudell Medical International, Ontario, Canada) is widely accepted. There are no prospective, controlled studies evaluating the use of oral glucocorticoids in cats with spontaneous asthma; however, many retrospective studies have reported a beneficial response to steroids.[4,5,19,20] Unfortunately, therapeutic response in these studies is often based on improvement in clinical signs without documenting improvement in airway inflammation or hyperresponsiveness. Given the waxing and waning nature of the clinical signs of asthma, it is difficult to assess the true effectiveness of therapy based on clinical signs alone.

In experimental feline asthma, both oral prednisone (10 mg/d) and inhaled flunisolide (500 μg/d) significantly decreased airway eosinophilia compared with placebo.[62] Using a different experimental feline asthma model, fluticasone propionate with salmeterol (500 μg fluticasone/50 μg salmeterol twice daily) was as effective as oral prednisolone (2 mg/kg/d) at reducing airway inflammation in acute asthma.[63] In a follow-up study by the same group, oral prednisolone (2 mg/kg/d) was compared with inhaled salmeterol (50 μg twice daily) over a 4-day period.[64] Only oral prednisolone was capable of eliminating the late-phase asthmatic reaction in response to inhaled allergen.[64] Although an effective dose in pet cats has not been established, comparison of varying doses of inhaled fluticasone (44, 110, or 220 μg twice daily) suggested that all are equipotent in controlling airway eosinophilia in cats with experimentally induced asthma.[65] In naturally occurring asthma, inhaled budesonide improved clinical signs in pet cats and also resulted in improvement in BWBP parameters compared with pretreatment values.[66]

Bronchodilators

Bronchodilators reduce bronchoconstriction in acute asthma attacks. However, they should not be used for monotherapy because they fail to control the airway inflammation that exacerbates airway hyperresponsiveness.[2] Several different types of bronchodilators have been assessed, mostly in experimentally induced asthma in cats, including methylxanthines,[67,68] short-acting and long-acting beta-2 agonists (SABA[19,69–71] and LABA,[64,69,70] respectively), and anticholinergics.[67,69,70] When using a compound that directly constricts smooth muscle (ie, carbachol), inhalation of several of these drugs via a metered dose inhaler and nebulization were equally effective in blunting airway hyperresponsiveness.[69] Also, SABA were more potent than LABA, and with combination SABA/anticholinergic bronchodilator therapy, synergism was noted.[69] Interestingly, after specific allergen bronchoprovocation, inhaled bronchodilators did not improve time to recovery compared with no treatment.[67] For this reason, the author prefers use of the injectable bronchodilator, terbutaline, in pet cats with life-threatening status asthmaticus. Although SABA are critical in treating life-threatening bronchoconstriction, overuse by inhalation has been associated with increased risk of death in human asthmatics.[72] Inhalant albuterol is a racemic mixture consisting of the R-enantiomer, which possesses bronchodilatory properties, and the S-enantiomer, which promotes bronchospasm and inflammation.[73] With repeated use, the S-enantiomer preferentially accumulates in the lung because of slower metabolism/clearance, enhancing bronchoconstrictive and proinflammatory effects.[74] Chronic use (twice daily for 2 weeks) in healthy cats induced de novo neutrophilic airway inflammation; in experimentally asthmatic cats, eosinophilic airway inflammation was exacerbated.[73] Thus, inhaled albuterol can be an important therapy for acute bronchoconstriction (especially as at-home treatment), it should not be used in the daily management of asthmatic cats. A single-isomer form of R-albuterol (levalbuterol) is available, is not associated with negative adverse effects, and could be considered an option for chronic therapy.

Experimental Therapies

Allergen-specific immunotherapy

No therapy to date reverses the underlying immunopathology associated with spontaneous feline allergic asthma. ASIT is proposed to reverse the T helper 2–mediated allergic response by inducing immunologic tolerance to allergen. Several different protocols have been investigated in an experimental model of feline asthma using an abbreviated administration (rush immunotherapy, RIT) and have successfully diminished airway eosinophilia.[75–77] Before pet cats with asthma can be treated, allergens implicated in airway sensitization must be identified. Using cats experimentally sensitized to Bermuda grass or house dust mite, the sensitivity and specificity of IDST and 2 different forms of serum allergen testing using either an FcεR1α-based enzyme-linked immunosorbent assay (ELISA) or an enzymoimmunometric assay were investigated.[78] The sensitivity of the IDST was greater than the FcεR1α-based ELISA (ie, better screening test); however, both were specific (ie, suitable for allergen selection for RIT). Disappointingly, the enzymoimmunometric assay produced unreliable results, including failure to detect allergen-specific IgE and identification of allergens to which the cats had not been sensitized. Future studies should be performed to more rigorously evaluate the accuracy of diagnostic laboratories offering allergen-specific IgE testing for ASIT. To determine the importance of closely matched allergens for use in RIT, an additional study was performed in experimentally asthmatic cats.[79] Use of allergens not implicated in sensitization or use of only 1 of 2 sensitizing allergens in RIT still led to reductions in airway eosinophilia. However, only closely matched allergens had the potential to induce an immunologic cure by induction of tolerance, potentially allowing for eventual discontinuation of therapy with permanent benefit. With RIT, time is required to result in improvement in clinical signs. Thus, many cats are likely to be concurrently treated with glucocorticoids. In 1 study, oral glucocorticoids blunted the effectiveness of immunotherapy.[80] Thus, inhaled glucocorticoids or other therapies that do not affect the immune system may be better for use in conjunction with RIT.

Omega-3 fatty acids/nutraceuticals

Omega-3 polyunsaturated fatty acids (ω3 PUFAs) act as anti-inflammatory agents through reduction in the availability of arachidonic acid in cell membranes for production of inflammatory eicosanoids.[81] The use of dietary ω3 PUFAs in combination with the antioxidant, luteolin, has been evaluated in experimental feline asthma.[82] This treatment failed to resolve airway eosinophilia, but diminished airway hyperresponsiveness as assessed by BWBP. Although clearly unsuitable as monotherapy, additional studies in pet cats with asthma might help determine if ω3 PUFAs could be used as adjunctive therapy.

Inhaled lidocaine

Lidocaine has received interest in human medicine as a potential treatment of severe asthma[83–85] and has been investigated in an experimental feline asthma model.[86] In the latter study, nebulized lidocaine (2 mg/kg every 8 hours) was administered to healthy and experimentally asthmatic cats for 2 weeks. Lidocaine decreased airway hyperresponsiveness without decreasing airway eosinophilia. Importantly, no adverse effects were noted in the cats despite the known sensitivity of cats to injectable lidocaine. Further study is needed to determine if lidocaine might be useful to treat airflow limitation in spontaneous feline asthma.

Tyrosine kinase inhibitors

Blockade of key cell signaling pathways involved in the immunopathogenesis of asthma could lead to novel avenues of treatment. Both receptor and nonreceptor tyrosine kinase inhibitors (TKIs) have potential in this regard. For example, stem cell factor, the growth factor for the c-kit receptor, is associated with proliferation and activation of both mast cells and eosinophils,[87] and in experimental feline asthma, these can be inhibited with TKIs, such as masitinib.[43] Cats with experimental disease receiving (50 mg/d orally) masitinib had decreased BALF eosinophilia and lung compliance as measured by ventilator-acquired pulmonary mechanics; however, side effects were dose limiting. A preliminary study using inhibition of the janus kinase cytokine signaling pathway by a nonreceptor TKI was also evaluated in experimental feline asthma[88] and suggested a reduction of airway eosinophilia without a significant effect on airway hyperresponsiveness. Further research is needed before TKIs can be routinely recommended for treatment.

Stem cells

Stem cells have been studied for the treatment of a variety of respiratory disorders, including asthma. In murine asthma models, stem cells can reduce airway eosinophilia, airway hyperresponsiveness, and airway remodeling.[89–92] In a pilot study that delivered adipose-derived stem cells shortly after experimental induction of asthma, airway eosinophil percentages decreased to within normal reference ranges by 9 months after treatment.[93] In addition, airway hyperresponsiveness and CT evidence of bronchial wall thickening were improved. When adipose-derived stem cells were administered to cats with chronically established experimentally induced asthma, there was no difference in airway eosinophilia and hyperresponsiveness compared with control cats,[94] although there was some reduction in bronchial wall thickening as assessed by CT. Stem cells used in these studies are *not* the same as the current commercially available products, and further research is needed before they can be recommended for use in cats with naturally occurring asthma.

Ineffective Therapies

Leukotriene antagonists are used for treatment of human asthmatics. Unfortunately, cysteinyl-leukotrienes do not appear to be important mediators of feline asthma,[95,96] and a clinical trial with the leukotriene antagonist, zafirlukast, failed to reduce airway eosinophilia or hyperresponsiveness in experimental feline asthma.[62]

Serotonin is a preformed mediator in mast cells and is thought to be important in mediating bronchoconstriction in response to allergen exposure.[96,97] Cyproheptadine, a nonspecific serotonin antagonist, at a low dose (2 mg every 12 hours orally) failed to reduce airway reactivity and airway inflammation in experimentally asthmatic cats.[62] A subsequent study[98] evaluated a higher dose of cyproheptadine (8 mg every 12 hours orally) based on a pharmacokinetic study, suggesting cats may require substantially higher doses than what has been traditionally recommended to reach therapeutic concentrations.[99] Even at this dose, cyproheptadine was ineffective at reducing airway eosinophilia. Because hyperresponsiveness was not evaluated in this study, it is uncertain if the higher dose could alleviate airflow limitation. Although not advocated for monotherapy, the higher dose deserves further study to evaluate possible bronchodilatory properties.

Histamine, like serotonin, is present in the granules of mast cells and could have similar effects on airway reactivity.[97,100–103] A study investigating the second-generation antihistamine, cetirizine (5 mg every 12 hours orally), found that airway eosinophilia was not significantly diminished.[98] The effect of cetirizine on airway hyperresponsiveness is currently not known, and further study is needed before this therapy can be recommended.

A salivary tripeptide (feG-COOH) identified as a modulator of the immune response reduced allergen-induced airway inflammation in other animal models of asthma.[104,105] Chronic administration of feG-COOH (1 mg/kg/d for 2 weeks) did not blunt airway eosinophilia compared with placebo in experimental feline asthma and cannot be advocated.[106]

N-acetylcysteine is a mucolytic with antioxidant properties that could have a benefit in asthma; however, nebulized delivery in humans is known to induce bronchospasm. Similarly, in experimentally asthmatic cats, nebulization of N-acetylcysteine increased baseline airway resistance by an average of approximately 150% and should not be administered by this route.[50]

Oral doxycycline (5 mg/kg/d) failed to blunt airway eosinophilia or hyperresponsiveness.[64] Finally, a neurokinin-1 antagonist failed to ameliorate clinical symptoms, airway eosinophilia, or airway hyperresponsiveness in either acute[107] or chronic[108] manifestations of experimental asthma.

SUMMARY

Much work has been done in experimental models to better define feline asthma and discriminate it from other lower-airway diseases. Importantly, accurately identifying asthmatics will help more appropriately select candidates for targeted therapies acting along the allergic cascade. Although some experimental therapies have shown promise in models of feline asthma, work is needed to determine if these will be beneficial in the pet cat population.

ACKNOWLEDGMENTS

The author thanks Dr Carol Reinero for her contributions to the first version of this article.

DISCLOSURE

The author has nothing to disclose.

REFERENCES

1. Reinero CR. Advances in the understanding of pathogenesis, and diagnostics and therapeutics for feline allergic asthma. Vet J 2011;190(1):28–33.
2. Busse W, Camargo C Jr, Boushey H, et al. Expert panel report 3: guidelines for the diagnosis and management of asthma. Bethesda (MD): National Heart, Lung, and Blood Institute; 2007. Available at: http://www.nhlbi.nih.gov/guidelines/asthma/asthgdln.htm. Accessed June 24, 2013.
3. Padrid P. Chronic bronchitis and asthma in cats. Philadelphia: WB Saunders; 2009.
4. Adamama-Moraitou KK, Patsikas MN, Koutinas AF. Feline lower airway disease: a retrospective study of 22 naturally occurring cases from Greece. J Feline Med Surg 2004;6(4):227–33.
5. Corcoran BM, Foster DJ, Fuentes VL. Feline asthma syndrome: a retrospective study of the clinical presentation in 29 cats. J Small Anim Pract 1995;36(11): 481–8.
6. Dye JA. Feline bronchopulmonary disease. Vet Clin North Am Small Anim Pract 1992;22(5):1187–201.
7. Nafe LA, DeClue AE, Lee-Fowler TM, et al. Evaluation of biomarkers in bronchoalveolar lavage fluid for discrimination between asthma and chronic bronchitis in cats. Am J Vet Res 2010;71(5):583–91.
8. Dear JD, Johnson LR. Lower respiratory tract endoscopy in the cat: diagnostic approach to bronchial disease. J Feline Med Surg 2013;15(11):1019–27.
9. Moise NS, Wiedenkeller D, Yeager AE, et al. Clinical, radiographic, and bronchial cytologic features of cats with bronchial disease: 65 cases (1980-1986). J Am Vet Med Assoc 1989;194(10):1467–73.
10. Lacorcia L, Gasser RB, Anderson GA, et al. Comparison of bronchoalveolar lavage fluid examination and other diagnostic techniques with the Baermann technique for detection of naturally occurring Aelurostrongylus abstrusus infection in cats. J Am Vet Med Assoc 2009;235(1):43–9.
11. Dillon AR, Blagburn BL, Tillson D, et al. Immature heartworm infection produces pulmonary parenchymal, airway, and vascular disease in cats. [abstract] J Vet Intern Med 2007;21(3):608–9.
12. Dillon AR, Blagburn BL, Tillson M, et al. Heartworm-associated respiratory disease (HARD) induced by immature adult Dirofilaria immitis in cats. Parasit Vectors 2017;10(Suppl 2):514.
13. Dillon AR, Blagburn BL, Tillson M, et al. The progression of heartworm associated respiratory disease (HARD) in SPF cats 18 months after Dirofilaria immitis infection. Parasit Vectors 2017;10(Suppl 2):533.

14. Nelson CT, McCall JW, Jones S, et al. Current feline guidelines for the prevention, diagnosis, and management of heartworm infection (Dirofilaria immitis) in cats. Wilmington (DE): American Heartworm Society; 2014. Available at: https://www.heartwormsociety.org/veterinary-resources/american-heartworm-society-guidelines. Accessed July 20, 2019.

15. Garcia-Guasch L, Caro-Vadillo A, Manubens-Grau J, et al. Is Wolbachia participating in the bronchial reactivity of cats with heartworm associated respiratory disease? Vet Parasitol 2013;196(1–2):130–5.

16. Sprent JF. The life history and development of Toxocara cati (Schrank 1788) in the domestic cat. Parasitology 1956;46(1–2):54–78.

17. Swerczek TW, Nielsen SW, Helmboldt CF. Ascariasis causing pulmonary arterial hyperplasia in cats. Res Vet Sci 1970;11(1):103–4.

18. Dillon AR, Tillson DM, Hathcock J, et al. Lung histopathology, radiography, high-resolution computed tomography, and bronchio-alveolar lavage cytology are altered by Toxocara cati infection in cats and is independent of development of adult intestinal parasites. Vet Parasitol 2013;193(4):413–26.

19. Dye JA, McKiernan BC, Rozanski EA, et al. Bronchopulmonary disease in the cat: historical, physical, radiographic, clinicopathologic, and pulmonary functional evaluation of 24 affected and 15 healthy cats. J Vet Intern Med 1996; 10(6):385–400.

20. Foster SF, Allan GS, Martin P, et al. Twenty-five cases of feline bronchial disease (1995-2000). J Feline Med Surg 2004;6(3):181–8.

21. Mitsunobu F, Tanizaki Y. The use of computed tomography to assess asthma severity. Curr Opin Allergy Clin Immunol 2005;5(1):85–90.

22. Niimi A, Matsumoto H, Amitani R, et al. Airway wall thickness in asthma assessed by computed tomography. Relation to clinical indices. Am J Respir Crit Care Med 2000;162(4 Pt 1):1518–23.

23. Niimi A, Matsumoto H, Takemura M, et al. Clinical assessment of airway remodeling in asthma: utility of computed tomography. Clin Rev Allergy Immunol 2004; 27(1):45–58.

24. Oliveira CR, Mitchell MA, O'Brien RT. Thoracic computed tomography in feline patients without use of chemical restraint. Vet Radiol Ultrasound 2011;52(4): 368–76.

25. Masseau I, Banuelos A, Dodam J, et al. Comparison of lung attenuation and heterogeneity between cats with experimentally induced allergic asthma, naturally occurring asthma and normal cats. Vet Radiol Ultrasound 2015;56(6):595–601.

26. Won S, Yun S, Lee J, et al. High resolution computed tomographic evaluation of bronchial wall thickness in healthy and clinically asthmatic cats. J Vet Med Sci 2017;79(3):567–71.

27. Dennler M, Bass DA, Gutierrez-Crespo B, et al. Thoracic computed tomography, angiographic computed tomography, and pathology findings in six cats experimentally infected with Aelurostrongylus abstrusus. Vet Radiol Ultrasound 2013; 54(5):459–69.

28. Ray Dillon A, Tillson DM, Wooldridge A, et al. Effect of pre-cardiac and adult stages of Dirofilaria immitis in pulmonary disease of cats: CBC, bronchial lavage cytology, serology, radiographs, CT images, bronchial reactivity, and histopathology. Vet Parasitol 2014;206(1–2):24–37.

29. Lamb CR, Jones ID. Associations between respiratory signs and abnormalities reported in thoracic CT scans of cats. J Small Anim Pract 2016;57(10):561–7.

30. Johnson LR, Vernau W. Bronchoscopic findings in 48 cats with spontaneous lower respiratory tract disease (2002-2009). J Vet Intern Med 2011;25(2):236–43.

31. Hawkins EC, DeNicola DB, Kuehn NF. Bronchoalveolar lavage in the evaluation of pulmonary disease in the dog and cat. State of the art. J Vet Intern Med 1990;4(5):267–74.

32. McCarthy GM, Quinn PJ. Bronchoalveolar lavage in the cat: cytological findings. Can J Vet Res 1989;53(3):259–63.

33. McCarthy GM, Quinn PJ. Age-related changes in protein concentrations in serum and respiratory tract lavage fluid obtained from cats. Am J Vet Res 1991;52(2):254–60.

34. Padrid PA, Feldman BF, Funk K, et al. Cytologic, microbiologic, and biochemical analysis of bronchoalveolar lavage fluid obtained from 24 healthy cats. Am J Vet Res 1991;52(8):1300–7.

35. Shibly S, Klang A, Galler A, et al. Architecture and inflammatory cell composition of the feline lung with special consideration of eosinophil counts. J Comp Pathol 2014;150(4):408–15.

36. Laprise C, Laviolette M, Boutet M, et al. Asymptomatic airway hyperresponsiveness: relationships with airway inflammation and remodelling. Eur Respir J 1999;14(1):63–73.

37. Obase Y, Shimoda T, Kawano T, et al. Bronchial hyperresponsiveness and airway inflammation in adolescents with asymptomatic childhood asthma. Allergy 2003;58(3):213–20.

38. Cocayne CG, Reinero CR, DeClue AE. Subclinical airway inflammation despite high-dose oral corticosteroid therapy in cats with lower airway disease. J Feline Med Surg 2011;13(8):558–63.

39. Foster SF, Martin P, Braddock JA, et al. A retrospective analysis of feline bronchoalveolar lavage cytology and microbiology (1995-2000). J Feline Med Surg 2004;6(3):189–98.

40. Bark H, Epstein A, Bar-Yishay E, et al. Non-invasive forced expiratory flow-volume curves to measure lung function in cats. Respir Physiol Neurobiol 2007;155(1):49–54.

41. Hoffman AM, Dhupa N, Cimetti L. Airway reactivity measured by barometric whole-body plethysmography in healthy cats. Am J Vet Res 1999;60(12):1487–92.

42. Kirschvink N, Leemans J, Delvaux F, et al. Non-invasive assessment of airway responsiveness in healthy and allergen-sensitised cats by use of barometric whole body plethysmography. Vet J 2007;173(2):343–52.

43. Lee-Fowler TM, Guntur V, Dodam J, et al. The tyrosine kinase inhibitor masitinib blunts airway inflammation and improves associated lung mechanics in a feline model of chronic allergic asthma. Int Arch Allergy Immunol 2012;158(4):369–74.

44. McKiernan BC, Johnson LR. Clinical pulmonary function testing in dogs and cats. Vet Clin North Am Small Anim Pract 1992;22(5):1087–99.

45. Balakrishnan A, King LG. Updates on pulmonary function testing in small animals. Vet Clin North Am Small Anim Pract 2014;44(1):1–18.

46. Hirt RA, Galler A, Shibly S, et al. Airway hyperresponsiveness to adenosine 5'-monophosphate in feline chronic inflammatory lower airway disease. Vet J 2011;187(1):54–9.

47. Bates J, Irvin C, Brusasco V, et al. The use and misuse of Penh in animal models of lung disease. Am J Respir Cell Mol Biol 2004;31:373–4.

48. Allerton FJ, Leemans J, Tual C, et al. Correlation of bronchoalveolar eosinophilic percentage with airway responsiveness in cats with chronic bronchial disease. J Small Anim Pract 2013;54(5):258–64.

49. Masseau I, Chang CH, LeFloch M, et al. Assessment of airway hyperresponsiveness in tandem with remodeling using pulmonary mechanics and computed tomography in experimental feline asthma [Abstract R-3]. J Vet Intern Med 2013;27(3):754.

50. Reinero CR, Lee-Fowler TM, Dodam JR, et al. Endotracheal nebulization of N-acetylcysteine increases airway resistance in cats with experimental asthma. J Feline Med Surg 2011;13(2):69–73.

51. Xu J, Zhong NS. Mechanisms of bronchial hyperresponsiveness: the interaction of endothelin-1 and other cytokines. Respirology 1999;4(4):413–7.

52. Sharp CR, Lee-Fowler TM, Reinero CR. Endothelin-1 concentrations in bronchoalveolar lavage fluid of cats with experimentally induced asthma. J Vet Intern Med 2013;27(4):982–4.

53. Accordino R, Visentin A, Bordin A, et al. Long-term repeatability of exhaled breath condensate pH in asthma. Respir Med 2008;102(3):377–81.

54. Aldakheel FM, Thomas PS, Bourke JE, et al. Relationships between adult asthma and oxidative stress markers and pH in exhaled breath condensate: a systematic review. Allergy 2016;71(6):741–57.

55. Antczak A, Nowak D, Shariati B, et al. Increased hydrogen peroxide and thiobarbituric acid-reactive products in expired breath condensate of asthmatic patients. Eur Respir J 1997;10(6):1235–41.

56. Hanazawa T, Kharitonov SA, Barnes PJ. Increased nitrotyrosine in exhaled breath condensate of patients with asthma. Am J Respir Crit Care Med 2000;162(4 Pt 1):1273–6.

57. Kostikas K, Papatheodorou G, Ganas K, et al. pH in expired breath condensate of patients with inflammatory airway diseases. Am J Respir Crit Care Med 2002;165(10):1364–70.

58. Loukides S, Bouros D, Papatheodorou G, et al. The relationships among hydrogen peroxide in expired breath condensate, airway inflammation, and asthma severity. Chest 2002;121(2):338–46.

59. Fulcher YG, Fotso M, Chang CH, et al. Noninvasive recognition and biomarkers of early allergic asthma in cats using multivariate statistical analysis of NMR spectra of exhaled breath condensate. PLoS One 2016;11(10):e0164394.

60. Kirschvink N, Marlin D, Delvaux F, et al. Collection of exhaled breath condensate and analysis of hydrogen peroxide as a potential marker of lower airway inflammation in cats. Vet J 2005;169(3):385–96.

61. Sparkes AH, Mardell EJ, Deaton C, et al. Exhaled breath condensate (EBC) collection in cats–description of a non-invasive technique to investigate airway disease. J Feline Med Surg 2004;6(5):335–8.

62. Reinero CR, Decile KC, Byerly JR, et al. Effects of drug treatment on inflammation and hyperreactivity of airways and on immune variables in cats with experimentally induced asthma. Am J Vet Res 2005;66(7):1121–7.

63. Leemans J, Kirschvink N, Clercx C, et al. Effect of short-term oral and inhaled corticosteroids on airway inflammation and responsiveness in a feline acute asthma model. Vet J 2012;192(1):41–8.

64. Leemans J, Kirschvink N, Bernaerts F, et al. Salmeterol or doxycycline do not inhibit acute bronchospasm and airway inflammation in cats with experimentally-induced asthma. Vet J 2012;192(1):49–56.

65. Cohn LA, DeClue AE, Cohen RL, et al. Effects of fluticasone propionate dosage in an experimental model of feline asthma. J Feline Med Surg 2010;12(2):91–6.

66. Galler A, Shibly S, Bilek A, et al. Inhaled budesonide therapy in cats with naturally occurring chronic bronchial disease (feline asthma and chronic bronchitis). J Small Anim Pract 2013;54(10):531–6.

67. Leemans J, Kirschvink N, Clercx C, et al. Functional response to inhaled salbutamol and/or ipratropium bromide in Ascaris suum-sensitised cats with allergen-induced bronchospasms. Vet J 2010;186(1):76–83.

68. Stursberg U, Zenker I, Hecht S, et al. Use of propentofylline in feline bronchial disease: prospective, randomized, positive-controlled study. J Am Anim Hosp Assoc 2010;46(5):318–26.

69. Leemans J, Kirschvink N, Bernaerts F, et al. A pilot study comparing the antispasmodic effects of inhaled salmeterol, salbutamol and ipratropium bromide using different aerosol devices on muscarinic bronchoconstriction in healthy cats. Vet J 2009;180(2):236–45.

70. Leemans J, Kirschvink N, Gustin P. A comparison of in vitro relaxant responses to ipratropium bromide, beta-adrenoceptor agonists and theophylline in feline bronchial smooth muscle. Vet J 2012;193(1):228–33.

71. Rozanski EA, Hoffman AM. Pulmonary function testing in small animals. Clin Tech Small Anim Pract 1999;14(4):237–41.

72. Spitzer WO, Suissa S, Ernst P, et al. The use of beta-agonists and the risk of death and near death from asthma. N Engl J Med 1992;326(8):501–6.

73. Reinero CR, Delgado C, Spinka C, et al. Enantiomer-specific effects of albuterol on airway inflammation in healthy and asthmatic cats. Int Arch Allergy Immunol 2009;150(1):43–50.

74. Dhand R, Goode M, Reid R, et al. Preferential pulmonary retention of (S)-albuterol after inhalation of racemic albuterol. Am J Respir Crit Care Med 1999; 160(4):1136–41.

75. Lee-Fowler TM, Cohn LA, DeClue AE, et al. Evaluation of subcutaneous versus mucosal (intranasal) allergen-specific rush immunotherapy in experimental feline asthma. Vet Immunol Immunopathol 2009;129(1–2):49–56.

76. Reinero CR, Byerly JR, Berghaus RD, et al. Rush immunotherapy in an experimental model of feline allergic asthma. Vet Immunol Immunopathol 2006; 110(1–2):141–53.

77. Reinero CR, Cohn LA, Delgado C, et al. Adjuvanted rush immunotherapy using CpG oligodeoxynucleotides in experimental feline allergic asthma. Vet Immunol Immunopathol 2008;121(3–4):241–50.

78. Lee-Fowler TM, Cohn LA, DeClue AE, et al. Comparison of intradermal skin testing (IDST) and serum allergen-specific IgE determination in an experimental model of feline asthma. Vet Immunol Immunopathol 2009;132(1):46–52.

79. Reinero C, Lee-Fowler T, Chang CH, et al. Beneficial cross-protection of allergen-specific immunotherapy on airway eosinophilia using unrelated or a partial repertoire of allergen(s) implicated in experimental feline asthma. Vet J 2012;192(3):412–6.

80. Chang CH, Cohn LA, Declue AE, et al. Oral glucocorticoids diminish the efficacy of allergen-specific immunotherapy in experimental feline asthma. Vet J 2013; 197(2):268–72.

81. Calder PC. Polyunsaturated fatty acids and inflammation. Biochem Soc Trans 2005;33(Pt 2):423–7.

82. Leemans J, Cambier C, Chandler T, et al. Prophylactic effects of omega-3 poly-unsaturated fatty acids and luteolin on airway hyperresponsiveness and inflammation in cats with experimentally-induced asthma. Vet J 2010;184(1):111–4.

83. Decco ML, Neeno TA, Hunt LW, et al. Nebulized lidocaine in the treatment of severe asthma in children: a pilot study. Ann Allergy Asthma Immunol 1999;82(1):29–32.

84. Hunt LW, Swedlund HA, Gleich GJ. Effect of nebulized lidocaine on severe glucocorticoid-dependent asthma. Mayo Clin Proc 1996;71(4):361–8.

85. Hunt LW, Frigas E, Butterfield JH, et al. Treatment of asthma with nebulized lidocaine: a randomized, placebo-controlled study. J Allergy Clin Immunol 2004;113(5):853–9.

86. Nafe LA, Guntur VP, Dodam JR, et al. Nebulized lidocaine blunts airway hyper-responsiveness in experimental feline asthma. J Feline Med Surg 2013;15(8):712–6.

87. Guntur VP, Reinero CR. The potential use of tyrosine kinase inhibitors in severe asthma. Curr Opin Allergy Clin Immunol 2012;12(1):68–75.

88. Chang CH, Dodam JR, Cohn LA. An experimental janus kinase (JAK) inhibitor suppresses eosinophilic airway inflammation in feline asthma. ACVIM Forum Proceedings. Available at: http://www.vin.com/Members/Proceedings/Proceedings. Published 2013. Accessed June 24, 2013.

89. Bonfield TL, Koloze M, Lennon DP, et al. Human mesenchymal stem cells suppress chronic airway inflammation in the murine ovalbumin asthma model. Am J Physiol Lung Cell Mol Physiol 2010;299(6):L760–70.

90. Firinci F, Karaman M, Baran Y, et al. Mesenchymal stem cells ameliorate the histopathological changes in a murine model of chronic asthma. Int Immunopharmacol 2011;11(8):1120–6.

91. Goodwin M, Sueblinvong V, Eisenhauer P, et al. Bone marrow-derived mesenchymal stromal cells inhibit Th2-mediated allergic airways inflammation in mice. Stem Cells 2011;29(7):1137–48.

92. Ou-Yang HF, Huang Y, Hu XB, et al. Suppression of allergic airway inflammation in a mouse model of asthma by exogenous mesenchymal stem cells. Exp Biol Med (Maywood) 2011;236(12):1461–7.

93. Trzil JE, Masseau I, Webb TL, et al. Intravenous adipose-derived mesenchymal stem cell therapy for the treatment of feline asthma: a pilot study. J Feline Med Surg 2016;18(12):981–90.

94. Trzil JE, Masseau I, Webb TL, et al. Long-term evaluation of mesenchymal stem cell therapy in a feline model of chronic allergic asthma. Clin Exp Allergy 2014;44(12):1546–57.

95. Norris CR, Decile KC, Berghaus LJ, et al. Concentrations of cysteinyl leukotrienes in urine and bronchoalveolar lavage fluid of cats with experimentally induced asthma. Am J Vet Res 2003;64(11):1449–53.

96. Padrid PA, Mitchell RW, Ndukwu IM, et al. Cyproheptadine-induced attenuation of type-I immediate-hypersensitivity reactions of airway smooth muscle from immune-sensitized cats. Am J Vet Res 1995;56(1):109–15.

97. Mitchell RW, Cozzi P, Ndukwu IM, et al. Differential effects of cyclosporine A after acute antigen challenge in sensitized cats in vivo and ex vivo. Br J Pharmacol 1998;123(6):1198–204.

98. Schooley EK, McGee Turner JB, Jiji RD, et al. Effects of cyproheptadine and cetirizine on eosinophilic airway inflammation in cats with experimentally induced asthma. Am J Vet Res 2007;68(11):1265–71.

99. Norris CR, Boothe DM, Esparza T, et al. Disposition of cyproheptadine in cats after intravenous or oral administration of a single dose. Am J Vet Res 1998; 59(1):79–81.
100. Banovcin P, Visnovsky P, Korpas J. Pharmacological analysis of reactivity changes in airways due to acute inflammation in cats. Acta Physiol Hung 1987;70(2–3):181–7.
101. Barnes PJ. Histamine and serotonin. Pulm Pharmacol Ther 2001;14(5):329–39.
102. Wenzel SE, Fowler AA 3rd, Schwartz LB. Activation of pulmonary mast cells by bronchoalveolar allergen challenge. In vivo release of histamine and tryptase in atopic subjects with and without asthma. Am Rev Respir Dis 1988;137(5): 1002–8.
103. Wilson AM. The role of antihistamines in asthma management. Treat Respir Med 2006;5(3):149–58.
104. Dery RE, Mathison R, Davison J, et al. Inhibition of allergic inflammation by C-terminal peptides of the prohormone submandibular rat 1 (SMR-1). Int Arch Allergy Immunol 2001;124(1–3):201–4.
105. Dery RE, Ulanova M, Puttagunta L, et al. Frontline: inhibition of allergen-induced pulmonary inflammation by the tripeptide feG: a mimetic of a neuro-endocrine pathway. Eur J Immunol 2004;34(12):3315–25.
106. Eberhardt JM, DeClue AE, Reinero CR. Chronic use of the immunomodulating tripeptide feG-COOH in experimental feline asthma. Vet Immunol Immunopathol 2009;132(2–4):175–80.
107. Grobman M, Krumme S, Outi H, et al. Acute neurokinin-1 receptor antagonism fails to dampen airflow limitation or airway eosinophilia in an experimental model of feline asthma. J Feline Med Surg 2016;18(2):176–81.
108. Grobman M, Graham A, Outi H, et al. Chronic neurokinin-1 receptor antagonism fails to ameliorate clinical signs, airway hyper-responsiveness or airway eosinophilia in an experimental model of feline asthma. J Feline Med Surg 2016;18(4): 273–9.

Canine Chronic Bronchitis

An Update

Elizabeth Rozanski, DVM

KEYWORDS

- Cough • Inflammatory • Pulmonary pharmacology • Cough suppressant

KEY POINTS

- Chronic cough is a syndrome not a final diagnosis.
- Evaluation of potential underlying causes is important to exclude more treatable and curable disease.
- Chronic bronchitis is an inflammatory disease, and glucocorticoids tapered to the lowest possible dose to control signs are most commonly required.
- Owners should be advised that some cough may always exist, and goals of therapy are focused on improving quality of life.

Canine chronic bronchitis is an inflammatory pulmonary disease that results in cough and can lead to exercise intolerance and respiratory distress.[1] Clinical signs vary from mild to severe, with the most severe cases resulting in death or euthanasia from relentless cough. This variation can be particularly frustrating for clinicians and clients alike, because dogs often feel well when not coughing, and, when inflammation has been managed, cough suppression might successfully suppress cough but result in a heavily sedated pet.

This article (1) reviews an overall approach to diagnosis and management of chronic bronchitis; (2) reviews pathophysiology associated with chronic bronchitis; and (3) highlights emerging areas and concepts, specifically providing an update on advances in this topic since 2014, when the last review article was published.

OVERVIEW

Cough is defined as a sudden noisy expulsion of air, associated with efforts to clear the airway. Both acute and chronic cough are common presenting complaints for dogs in small animal practice. Other airway sounds can be confused with cough, including so-called reverse sneezing, stridor, and stertor. Dogs with tracheal collapse honk, which is usually associated with airway obstruction and is commonly mislabeled

Section of Critical Care, Cummings School of Veterinary Medicine, 200 Westboro Road, North Grafton, MA 01536, USA
E-mail address: elizabeth.rozanski@tufts.edu

Vet Clin Small Anim 50 (2020) 393–404
https://doi.org/10.1016/j.cvsm.2019.10.003
0195-5616/20/© 2019 Elsevier Inc. All rights reserved.
vetsmall.theclinics.com

as a cough. Smartphone recording of suspect sounds is particularly useful in further clarifying the type of sound, particularly if it is transient.

In some dogs, particularly small breed dogs, cough is accepted as normal by many clients, and, unfortunately, further evaluation is not pursued until signs are advanced.

There are many possible causes for cough and identification and therapy for the specific cause of cough is more likely to result in an amelioration of clinical signs than simple supportive care. Canine chronic bronchitis (CCB) is defined as cough on most days of the preceding 2 months, without any other cause identified. Therefore, it is important to exclude other causes of cough, particularly infection, before making a diagnosis of chronic bronchitis. Chronic bronchitis can also coexist with other cardiopulmonary conditions, such as mitral regurgitation, tracheal collapse, and bronchomalacia, and/or it can lead to pulmonary hypertension. However, panel members on the American College of Veterinary Internal Medicine consensus statement on pulmonary hypertension, due to be published in 2020, debated whether or not dogs with chronic bronchitis develop pulmonary hypertension or whether pulmonary hypertension is associated with an alternate cause in affected dogs.

Common causes of cough in dogs include infectious causes, as well as lung tumors, pleural effusion, upper airway dysfunction with gastroesophageal reflux, interstitial lung disease, and congestive heart failure. Although infectious disease is most common in puppies and in dogs exposed to other dogs through activities such as boarding or grooming, it is also a common cause of an exacerbation of signs in older dogs with preexisting pulmonary disease. Dogs that have decompensated after a period of stability should always be evaluated for infection.

Lung tumors are often bronchial adenocarcinomas, and, as such, they grow around a bronchus. Pleural effusion is a less common cause of cough but is thought to cause cough by diaphragmatic irritation or because of airway compression associated with lung collapse. Upper airway dysfunction (eg, laryngeal paralysis) causes cough by intermittent aspiration of food, liquids, or oropharyngeal contents. In geriatric dogs, laryngeal paralysis can be associated with pharyngeal dysfunction, which also can lead to cough.[2] One report described reversible laryngeal dysfunction associated with gastroesophageal reflux in a St. Bernard dog.[3] Although not widely appreciated in veterinary medicine, in people, gastroesophageal reflex disease is a common cause of cough.[4] In brachycephalic dogs, a relationship has been observed between gastrointestinal and respiratory signs of obstruction,[5] providing support for a link between the respiratory and digestive systems.

Interstitial lung disease most often causes tachypnea and exercise intolerance, although cough also can be present in some dogs. Congestive heart failure is expected to result in tachypnea and increased respiratory rate and should not cause cough, although dogs with heart failure can have a dry cough. Cough has classically been associated with marked left atrial enlargement causing compression of the mainstem bronchi, although 1 study suggested that these dogs likely have airway collapse and consequent inflammation causing cough.[6] Importantly, because dogs with mitral valve disease and CCB are often similar in breed and age, it is crucial to establish that an apparent exacerbation of CCB is not congestive heart failure. Detection of tachypnea and tachycardia, and radiographic evidence of pulmonary edema and pulmonary venous engorgement, would support congestive heart failure as an cause of cough.

Tracheal and airway collapse are increasingly being promoted to represent 2 separate entities, namely an obstructive airway disease associated with tracheal malformation in the most severe form of tracheal collapse (grade IV), and less severe forms of tracheal collapse (grades I–III, tracheomalacia) with or without more widespread bronchomalacia. Cough is more commonly associated with malacia, and honk is more commonly associated with airway obstruction. Importantly, both of these syndromes can coexist with CCB.

CLINICAL APPROACH

Evaluation of a dog with cough starts with review of the recent history and environmental exposures, and a complete physical examination. Signalment is helpful in establishing a suspicion of chronic bronchitis, because it is most common in older dogs. Cocker spaniels have been identified with an increased risk of bronchiectasis,[7] which can occur as a sequela to poorly controlled bronchitis in some cases, whereas all breeds have been reported to develop bronchitis. Pertinent historical considerations include exposure, even if limited, to other dogs/puppies in which infectious disease could be a consideration, and evidence of systemic disease, such as exercise intolerance. Exposure to passive (secondhand) smoking or excessive environmental odors/perfumes anecdotally seems to contribute to cough, although this has not been scientifically established.[8] In addition, the nature of cough should be explored, including dry or productive, paroxysmal, constant, or intermittent, and its relation to eating and activity. Voice change or reluctance to bark can support an upper airway disease such as laryngeal paralysis or hemiparalysis and indicates that microaspiration should be considered as a cause of cough. The role of this in development or exacerbation of CCB is unclear. Prior use of prescription or home remedies and the perceived effect on the cough should be explored.

A complete physical examination should focus on the cardiopulmonary system as well as identifying signs of systemic disease, including recent weight loss or gain, loss of appetite, and weakness or lethargy. Auscultation of the lungs can provide clues of lower airway disease, although a variety of findings should be anticipated, ranging from normal to harsh lung sounds, crackles, or expiratory wheezes. The presence or absence of a murmur should be noted, although, even when a mitral murmur is detected, chronic cough is more likely of pulmonary rather than cardiac origin. A respiratory arrhythmia is a common auscultatory finding in dogs with chronic bronchitis thought to be associated with increased vagal tone. A cough can often be induced by palpation of the trachea; this is useful to better characterize the cough and to exclude other conditions that could be mistaken for cough, such as reverse sneezing. Most dogs with chronic bronchitis are systemically well geriatric dogs, with only persistent productive cough as the major complaint.

Some dogs have syncope associated with cough, or the so-called cough-drop syndrome, which is most likely associated with high vagal tone. This condition must be differentiated from syncope associated with pulmonary hypertension or an intermittent arrhythmia.

Diagnostic testing should be tailored to the individual patient; however, the tests that are typically performed include baseline laboratory testing, such as a complete blood count, chemistry profile, and urinalysis. These laboratory tests are useful in establishing general health and are anticipated to be largely normal in dogs with chronic bronchitis. Peripheral eosinophilia is of particular interest in baseline laboratory results, because circulating eosinophilia can be associated with pulmonary eosinophilia or parasite infection. Other laboratory tests that should be considered include heartworm antigen testing and fecal analysis for both eggs and lungworm larva. Consideration should be given to evaluation of N-terminal pro–brain natriuretic peptide (NT-proBNP), a biomarker that is at increased levels in the presence of left atrial enlargement/congestive heart failure as well as in pulmonary hypertension. An increased NT-proBNP level suggests potential complicating diseases and should prompt further evaluation by echocardiography.[9]

Lung Function Testing

Pulmonary function testing is widely used in human medicine to better characterize the specific defects in airflow associated with chronic bronchitis. Although difficult to evaluate routinely in clinical veterinary cases, lung function is markedly affected by chronic bronchitis. As a review, lung function is a combination of (1) adequate gas exchange, which can be evaluated by arterial blood gas analysis, pulse oximetry, or end-tidal CO_2 analysis; and (2) work of breathing, as indicated by lung mechanics. Lung mechanics are mathematical descriptions of the relationships between gas flow rates, air volume/tidal volume, and airway pressure changes during breathing. See Anusha Balakrishnan and Carissa W. Tong's article, "Clinical Application of Pulmonary Function Testing in Small Animals," in this issue for further details.

In chronic bronchitis, airway lumen narrowing develops from a combination of airway thickening and excessive mucus production and accumulation, which result in increased airway resistance. This resistance is especially pronounced during expiration. In addition, there can be expiratory flow limitation caused by airway collapse and narrowing, which leads to air trapping or dynamic hyperinflation. Hyperinflation subsequently increases the work of breathing and perpetuates lung dysfunction. Importantly, in contrast with asthmatic people, cats, and horses, dogs have little to no naturally occurring bronchoconstriction with chronic bronchitis.

Although pulmonary function testing is simple to perform in dogs, lack of readily available standardized equipment limits its utility at this time. In addition, subtle deficits in people are most effectively revealed with testing designed to evaluate maximal effort, such as the forced expiratory volume in 1 second (FEV_1), and these are impossible to perform in patients that cannot provide voluntary cooperation. Tidal breathing flow-volume loops have been described in dogs with CCB and show expiratory flow abnormalities.[10] However, there are 2 forms of pulmonary function testing that are more practical for clinical evaluation and can be used in dogs, specifically collection of an arterial blood gas sample and use of the 6-minute walk test (6MWT). Arterial blood gas analysis can document mild hypoxemia or an increased alveolar-arterial gradient to support pulmonary dysfunction. Small breed dogs most commonly affected by CCB can be difficult to collect arterial samples from, either because of size or because of challenges with restraint. The 6MWT is easily performed in animals of any size by measuring the distance that a dog can walk over 6 minutes. An example is available on YouTube (https://www.youtube.com/watch?v=rzkLDEyDfy4).

Distances of less than 400 m are supportive of significant lung disease.[11] Owners are able to perform a 6MWT at home as well and can use this assessment to determine response to therapy.

Diagnostic Imaging

Chest radiographs are helpful in evaluating dogs with cough. If diagnostic testing is limited for an individual patient, chest radiographs will be the most useful test. Chest radiographs should be evaluated for evidence of bronchial thickening, as shown by visualization of "donuts" (airway walls in cross section) and tramlines (longitudinal airways in parallel) (**Fig. 1**). Additional signs consistent with chronic bronchitis include obesity, bronchiectasis, and less commonly hyperinflation. Chest radiographs are also useful to exclude other conditions that can cause cough, such as pneumonia, congestive heart failure, lung masses, pleural effusion, and interstitial lung disease.

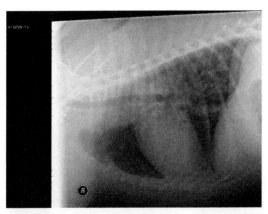

Fig. 1. Right lateral radiograph of dog with a marked bronchointerstitial pattern consistent with chronic bronchitis. (*From* Rozanski E. Canine chronic bronchitis. Vet Clin North Am Small Anim Pract. 2014;44(1):107-116; with permission.)

Fluoroscopy can be useful to evaluate the tracheal and larger airway for collapse, but are less helpful for evaluation of chronic cough unless concurrent tracheobroncho-malacia is suspected. Ultrasonography is useful if an isolated peripheral lesion is found on radiographs or in the presence of pleural effusion but is not useful in bronchitis.

Computed tomography (CT), which is widely used in people with airway diseases, is growing in popularity for identification of canine bronchial disease as well. CT scanning usually requires brief general anesthesia, so is commonly combined with evaluation of laryngeal function, bronchoscopy, and collection of airway cytology samples in dogs suspected of having CCB. The airway detail shown by CT scanning is much improved compared with routine thoracic radiographs.

Bronchoscopy, if available, is the preferred technique to evaluate and visualize the airway (**Fig. 2**). In a study of chronic bronchitis, all dogs showed irregular mucosal surfaces with a loss of the glistening appearance seen in healthy airways.[10] Often the mucosa was noted as being thickened and granular with a roughened appearance. Most dogs in the same study had hyperemia of mucosal vessels and showed partial collapse of bronchi during expiration, suggesting concurrent bronchomalacia. The presence of excessive mucus in the airways is also consistent with chronic bronchitis.[10,12] In people, bronchoscopy is not required for the diagnosis of chronic bronchitis, with more focus on lung function testing. However, it is the author's opinion that bronchoscopy provides useful information in dogs with chronic bronchitis and should be pursued if practical.

Airway Sampling

Collection of airway samples for cytology and bacterial culture is useful in further characterizing chronic bronchitis and excluding other causes of cough. Cytology samples can be collected by tracheal wash, blind bronchoalveolar lavage, or with a bronchoscope.[13] The technique chosen reflects clinician preference and the availability of supplies and equipment.

Airway samples for cytologic assessment should be placed in tubes containing ethylenediaminetetraacetic acid (EDTA) or can be submitted in syringes or suction traps. They should be processed promptly to avoid changes in the cell counts and cytologic appearance. If analysis will be delayed, a small aliquot of the sample should be

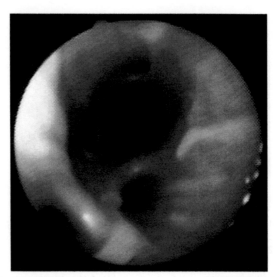

Fig. 2. Endoscopic view of a dog with severe chronic bronchitis. The epithelium is hyperemic and irregular. Copious mucus accumulation is apparent. (*Courtesy of* Lynelle Johnson, DVM, MS, PhD, DACVIM, Davis, CA.)

centrifuged and a direct smear made of the pellet. Respiratory cytology from a dog with chronic bronchitis typically reveals a predominantly neutrophilic infiltrate with excessive mucus (**Fig. 3**). Small numbers of lymphocytes, eosinophils, goblet cells, ciliated cells, and epithelial cells, and variable numbers of alveolar macrophages, are also commonly observed. If a sample shows marked eosinophilia, eosinophilic bronchopneumopathy or parasitic infection (heartworm/lung worm) should be considered. In Europe, the French heartworm (*Angiostrongylus vasorum*) is a concern when airway eosinophilia is detected, and this infection has the potential to extend across North America in the future.[14]

Bacterial culture is commonly performed in association with airway cytology to rule out an infectious cause of cough. Detection of low numbers of bacteria is common, but does not reflect true infection because the lower airways are not sterile. Positive bacterial cultures should be evaluated in light of the clinical appearance of the dog and in conjunction with observed cytology. For example, if cytology contains nondegenerate neutrophils and no intracellular bacteria, but microbiology isolates 1+ growth (or light growth) of a highly sensitive strain of *Escherichia coli*, it is unlikely that bacteria are playing a role in the clinical syndrome. In contrast, if cytology documents multiple degenerate neutrophils with intracellular bacteria, a positive bacterial culture provides useful information for treating that dog for pneumonia.

In people with chronic bronchitis, exacerbations associated with secondary bacterial infection are common, although they are not the primary cause of bronchitis. It is unclear whether this occurs in dogs with chronic bronchitis. *Mycoplasma* spp are incriminated as a respiratory pathogen, although this can be a fastidious organism to isolate using conventional bacteriologic techniques.[15] Polymerase chain reaction can be useful in identifying the offending pathogen when appropriate primers are used. Pneumonia is a reasonable differential for cough; however, in contrast with dogs with chronic bronchitis, dogs with pneumonia are more commonly systemically

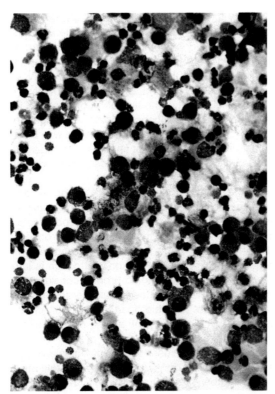

Fig. 3. Airway cytology from a dog with chronic bronchitis reveals increased neutrophils (53%, normal 5%–8%) as well as evidence of hemorrhage, mucin accumulation, and extra-cellular bacteria suggestive of contamination. (Wright-Giemsa, original magnification ×40) (*Courtesy of* Lynelle Johnson, DVM, MS, PhD, DACVIM, Davis, CA.)

unwell with fever and lethargy, have a shorter duration of clinical signs, and more often display an alveolar infiltrate on thoracic radiographs.

PATHOPHYSIOLOGY

Chronic bronchitis results in inflammatory changes within the lower airways, including neutrophilic inflammation and evidence of increased mucus production. Bronchial wall thickening and malacia contribute to airflow obstruction and worsen development of inflammation. The inflammatory response also perpetuates coughing and contributes to progressive decline in lung function. Although exposure to tobacco smoke is by far the most common cause for the development of chronic bronchitis in people, the specific factors that are responsible for disease in dogs remain unknown.

TREATMENT

Following diagnostic testing, if the clinical impression remains that the dog has chronic bronchitis, it is important to initiate therapy. Treatment goals for dogs with chronic bronchitis include reducing inflammation, limiting cough, and improving exercise stamina. Treatment also ideally prevents or slows disease progression and the associated airway remodeling.

Any environmental pollutants should be eliminated. Owners should be advised not to smoke indoors and to limit exposure of the dog to any airborne irritants, including air fresheners and heavily scented cleaning products. Exposure to potentially sick puppies should be avoided and trips to dog parks, grooming parlors, and boarding kennels should be limited to avoid the complication of infectious disease.

Obesity should be aggressively treated, because it markedly worsens cough and lung function and also limits activity. The author recognizes the frustration of this in a dog that must also be treated with glucocorticoids, and diligent efforts are required along with strict instructions for weight loss. Consultation with a veterinary nutritionist can be helpful, and use of a weight loss diet should be considered. A harness should be used in place of a collar, and episodes of excessive barking should be curtailed with appropriate behavioral modification.

Glucocorticoids are the mainstay of treatment of CCB because they reduce inflammation and this reduces cough. Glucocorticoids can be administered orally or via inhalation. Prednisone is the most commonly used glucocorticoid and is dosed at 1 to 2 mg/kg/d initially and then tapered to the lowest effective dose that controls clinical signs. For example, a 10-kg dog with severe chronic bronchitis might be started on 10 mg of prednisone twice daily for 7 days, or until cough is improved by 85% to 90%. Failure of the cough to improve should prompt consideration of an alternative diagnosis. Following improvement, the dose could be decrease by 25% every 2 to 3 weeks until ideally the lowest possible dose is reached. Alternate-day therapy is preferred to allow normalization of the hypothalamic-pituitary axis and to limit clinical signs associated with use of exogenous glucocorticoids.

Inhaled glucocorticoids have been used widely in people and are used with growing frequency in dogs with CCB. Most dogs can be trained to tolerate the facemask fairly easily, and 1 study showed benefits of therapy with fluticasone (125 μg twice daily).[16] Inhaled steroids are delivered via a spacer chamber and face mask designed especially for dogs (AeroDawg, Trudell Medical). Inhaled glucocorticoids are currently much more expensive than oral glucocorticoids, although the systemic steroid-sparing effect can be worthwhile in improving quality of life. In the United States, fluticasone is available as 44 μg/puff; 110 μg/puff, and 220 μg/puff. The dosing approach is less clear in animals than in humans, because a substantial portion of the inhaled medication may not make it to the lungs/lower airways. A reasonable starting point is 10 to 20 μg/kg twice a day, rounded up to the available dose.

Bronchodilators are commonly prescribed for dogs with chronic bronchitis, although there is limited evidence of efficacy in dogs.

Antibiotics are warranted in dogs with an acute exacerbation of chronic bronchitis and a reasonable suspicion of infection. Pending bacterial culture results, doxycycline is a good choice for dogs with chronic bronchitis, as is azithromycin, because these drugs have antiinflammatory properties as well as antimicrobial effects. Fluoroquinolones also have good respiratory penetration and could be useful in chronic bronchitis, although overuse of this class of drug leads to increased bacterial resistance.

Cough suppressants are helpful in CCB for improving the quality of life for dogs as well as for the families, and should be instituted when inflammation has been reasonably controlled. Also, on-going cough promotes inflammation, which results in more cough. Over-the-counter cough suppressants are rarely effective in dogs, and narcotic cough suppressants are most effective, with hydrocodone being the most widely used (**Table 1**). A study in human medicine has just reported on the efficacy of gabapentin for control of cough in people, and this deserves investigation in dogs as well.[17]

Table 1
Cough suppressants used in canine chronic bronchitis

Drug	Dose	Comments
Opioids (Most Effective)		
Butorphanol	0.25–1.1 mg/kg every 8–12 h	Expensive; titrate up
Hydrocodone	0.2–0.3 mg/kg every 6–12 h	—
Tramadol	2–5 mg/kg by mouth every 8–12 h	Less effective, inexpensive
Nonopioids (Less Effective)		
Gabapentin	2-5 mg/kg by mouth every 8 h	Unestablished efficacy
Methocarbamol	15–30 mg/kg every 12	Unestablished efficacy

Opioids may be titrated up as needed, although tolerance can result. Side effects are primarily excessive sedation.

From Rozanski E. Canine chronic bronchitis. Vet Clin North Am Small Anim Pract. 2014;44(1):107-116; with permission.

PROGNOSIS

The clinical course of chronic bronchitis is variable. In most dogs, there are permanent changes in the airways at the time of diagnosis, and the disease cannot be cured. Proper medical management can typically ameliorate clinical signs, and stop or slow progression of bronchial damage. Periodic relapses of cough are common and require adjustments in the treatment protocol, such as a temporary increase in the dose of glucocorticoids, or addition of antibiotics or cough suppressants until improvement in clinical signs. Quality of life may be affected in the dogs and in their owners, particularly when cough is frequent, nocturnal, or unrelenting.

WHAT IS NEW SINCE 2014?

Although CCB is a common and at times a frustrating disease, there have been only a limited number of peer-reviewed publications in the last 5 years.

Pharmacologic Therapy

Major developments include difficulty in sourcing extended-release theophylline and the current opioid crisis that is facing much of the United States. Theophylline is no longer available for use in people, and therefore needs to be compounded for use in dogs. Efficacy and bioavailability of these products are unknown. Opioid dependency and abuse is at an all-time high in people, which has led to challenges both with pharmacies stocking controlled drugs and with the need for monthly, signed, hard-copy, tamper-proof prescriptions, even for dogs on chronic therapy. Some clinicians have exchanged diphenoxylate (Lomotil) for opioids because it is sometimes easier to obtain, but this is also a scheduled drug.

Another challenge is determining drug efficacy. As all clinicians are aware, some clients tolerate very little cough and others are much more tolerant. Thus it can be hard to evaluate the degree of efficacy of a specific medication objectively. In people, it is possible to use cough counters, as well as diaries to better determine the efficacy of a medication.

The only chronic bronchitis/chronic cough pharmaceutical study in the last 5 years evaluated the use of maropitant in chronic bronchitis in a small group of dogs.[18] Results of this non–placebo-controlled trial suggested that maropitant has some antitussive properties but was not effective at reducing airway inflammation.[18]

Other laboratory investigations into chronic bronchitis have evaluated C-reactive protein levels in affected dogs and found them lower than in dogs with acute pneumonia. It might be possible that an increase in C-reactive protein levels could signal an infectious exacerbation of CCB.[19] In addition, 1 study of dogs with chronic rhinitis and chronic bronchitis documented an allergic phenotype, compared with normal dogs, with increased proportion of CC chemokine receptor 4 (CCR4)–positive cells.[20]

In addition, from an imaging standpoint, 1 study evaluated the utility of CT in confirming the diagnosis of chronic bronchitis, but found limited additional value.[21] However, another study identified a predictable increase in the ratio of the bronchial wall to the pulmonary artery and suggested using this as a CT marker of bronchitis.[22] It is unclear whether this would reliably distinguish neutrophilic chronic bronchitis from eosinophilic lung disease.

WHAT TO DO WHEN THE DOG IS STILL COUGHING?

Persistent or poorly responsive cough is frustrating for clients, veterinarians, and likely dogs. In dogs with a confirmed diagnosis of chronic bronchitis that are presenting with recurrent or worsening cough, it is worthwhile to confirm that the dog and owner have been compliant with the prescribed medications, because small dogs in particular are often difficult to medicate. In addition, it is prudent to reevaluate the diagnosis via auscultation and thoracic radiographs. Congestive heart failure could develop in a dog with progressive mitral valve disease, and other diseases, such as pneumonia, pulmonary neoplasia, and pulmonary fibrosis, can develop. In dogs without apparent confounding disease, one option to control cough is increasing the dose and frequency of administration of a cough suppressant until the dog is heavily sedated at least for 12 to 24 hours to limit inflammation that perpetuates cough. In addition, in people, and likely in dogs with exacerbations, antibiotics are often helpful in reducing bacterial colonization of diseased airways. In addition, increasing the prednisone dose or administering parenteral glucocorticoids is often useful. When clinical signs abate, the dose is tapered back to a lower amount that controls clinical signs. In some cases, hospitalizing the dog for supplemental oxygen and rest can permit the dog's signs to improve and additionally allow the owners a night of uninterrupted sleep, which can increase their enthusiasm and tolerance for treating the dog.

SUMMARY

CCB is a common cause of chronic cough and is a condition that is frequently treated by practicing clinicians. A sound understanding of the pathophysiology, diagnosis, and treatment of the condition allows prolonged quality of life for the patient. Owner education of dogs with chronic bronchitis is essential because CCB is a progressive, chronic disease. Treatment can ameliorate clinical signs, but on-going airway disease and some form of cough will likely persist. Frequent checkups and tailoring of the therapeutic plan to the individual dog provide the best outcome. Advancement in methods for early detection of chronic bronchitis and more effective treatments will improve the understanding of this disease and allow clinicians to limit the long-term effects it has on dogs.

DISCLOSURE

The author has nothing to disclose.

REFERENCES

1. Johnson LR, Queen EV, Vernau W, et al. Microbiologic and cytologic assessment of bronchoalveolar lavage fluid from dogs with lower respiratory tract infection: 105 cases (2001-2011). J Vet Intern Med 2013;27:259–67.

2. Stanley BJ, Hauptman JG, Fritz MC, et al. Esophageal dysfunction in dogs with idiopathic laryngeal paralysis: a controlled cohort study. Vet Surg 2010;39(2):139–49.

3. Lux CN, Archer TM, Lunsford KV. Gastroesophageal reflux and laryngeal dysfunction in a dog. J Am Vet Med Assoc 2012;240:1100–3.

4. Madanick RD. Management of GERD-related chronic cough. Gastroenterol Hepatol (N Y) 2013;9:311–3.

5. Poncet CM, Dupre GP, Freiche VG, et al. Prevalence of gastrointestinal tract lesions in 73 brachycephalic dogs with upper respiratory syndrome. J Small Anim Pract 2005;46:273–9.

6. Singh MK, Johnson LR, Kittleson MD, et al. Bronchomalacia in dogs with myxomatous mitral valve degeneration. J Vet Intern Med 2012;26:312–9.

7. Hawkins EC, Basseches J, Berry CR, et al. Demographic, clinical, and radiographic features of bronchiectasis in dogs: 316 cases (1988-2000). J Am Vet Med Assoc 2003;223:1628–35.

8. Hawkins EC, Clay LD, Bradley JM, et al. Demographic and historical findings, including exposure to environmental tobacco smoke, in dogs with chronic cough. J Vet Intern Med 2010;24:825–31.

9. Oyama MA, Rush JE, Rozanski EA. Assessment of serum N-terminal pro-B-type natriuretic peptide concentration for differentiation of congestive heart failure from primary respiratory tract disease as the cause of respiratory signs in dogs. J Am Vet Med Assoc 2009;235(11):1319–25.

10. Padrid PA, Hornof WJ, Kurpershoek CJ, et al. Canine chronic bronchitis: a pathophysiologic evaluation of 18 cases. J Vet Intern Med 1990;4:172–80.

11. Swimmer RA, Rozanski EA. Evaluation of the 6-minute walk test in pet dogs. J Vet Intern Med 2011;25:405–6.

12. Brownlie SEJ. A retrospective study of diagnosis in 109 cases of canine lower respiratory disease. J Small Anim Pract 1990;31:371–6.

13. Creevy KE. Airway evaluation and flexible endoscopic procedures in dogs and cats: laryngoscopy, transtracheal wash, tracheobronchoscopy, and bronchoalveolar lavage. Vet Clin North Am Small Anim Pract 2009;39:869–80.

14. Conboy GA. Canine angiostrongylosis: the French heartworm: an emerging threat in North America. Vet Parasitol 2011;176:382–9.

15. Chandler JC, Lappin MR. Mycoplasmal respiratory infections in small animals: 17 cases (1988-1999). J Am Anim Hosp Assoc 2002;38:111–9.

16. Bexfield NH, Foale RD, Davison LJ, et al. Management of 13 cases of canine respiratory disease using inhaled corticosteroids. J Small Anim Pract 2006;47:377–82.

17. Ryan NM, Birring SS, Gibson PG. Gabapentin for refractory chronic cough: a randomised, double-blind, placebo-controlled trial. Lancet 2012;380(9853):1583–9.

18. Grobman M, Reinero C. Investigation of neurokinin-1 receptor antagonism as a novel treatment for chronic bronchitis in dogs. J Vet Intern Med 2016;30(3):847–52.

19. Viitanen SJ, Laurila HP, Lilja-Maual LI, et al. Serum C-reactive protein as a diagnostic biomarker in dogs with bacterial respiratory disease. J Vet Intern Med 2014;28(1):84–91.
20. Yamaya Y, Watari T. Increased proportions of CCR4(+) cells among peripheral blood CD4(+) cells and serum levels of allergen-specific IgE antibody in canine chronic rhinitis and bronchitis. J Vet Med Sci 2015;77(4):421–5.
21. Mortier JR, Mesquita L, Ferrandis I, et al. Accuracy of and interobserver agreement regarding thoracic computed tomography for the diagnosis of chronic bronchitis in dogs. J Am Vet Med Assoc 2018;253(6):757–62.
22. Szabo D, Sutherland-Smith J, Barton B, et al. Accuracy of a computed tomography bronchial wall thickness to pulmonary artery diameter ratio for assessing bronchial wall thickening in dogs. Vet Radiol Ultrasound 2015;56(3):264–71.

Canine Infectious Respiratory Disease

Krystle L. Reagan, DVM, PhD*, Jane E. Sykes, BVSc (Hons), PhD

KEYWORDS

• CIRD • Kennel cough • *Bordetella* • Parainfluenza virus • Pneumonia

KEY POINTS

- Multiple bacterial and viral pathogens can result in clinical signs of canine infectious respiratory disease complex (CIRDC), with coinfection by multiple pathogens commonly identified.
- A clinical diagnosis of CIRDC can typically be made with a history and physical examination; however, an etiologic diagnosis should be pursued in dogs with severe or prolonged clinical signs or in disease outbreak situations.
- Clinical signs of CIRDC are typically mild and self-limiting, resolving after approximately 1 week.
- Antimicrobial treatment is warranted in dogs suspected to have bacterial pneumonia and optimally should be directed based on bacterial culture and susceptibility results. The development of pneumonia should raise concern for underlying canine distemper virus infection or other underlying immunosuppressive disease.
- Vaccinations do not induce sterilizing immunity; therefore, more comprehensive prevention strategies are necessary, especially in group-housing situations.

Canine infectious respiratory disease complex (CIRDC), commonly referred to as "kennel cough," refers to a syndrome characterized by acute onset of contagious respiratory disease in dogs that can be caused by a wide range of etiologic agents.[1] These infections are of particular concern when large numbers of dogs are housed together, such as in animal shelters, boarding facilities, or day-care facilities.[2] Outbreaks associated with CIRDC are reported worldwide,[2–4] and dogs are more likely to develop clinical signs of CIRDC the longer they are in a group-housing environment.[5]

Historically, the most common pathogens associated with CIRDC have been canine parainfluenza virus (CPIV), canine adenovirus type 2 (CAV-2), and *Bordetella bronchiseptica* (**Table 1**).[6] In the past 2 decades, outbreaks of novel pathogens, including

Veterinary Medical Teaching Hospital, University of California, Davis, 1 Garrod Drive, Davis, CA 95616, USA
* Corresponding author.
E-mail address: kreagan@ucdavis.edu

Vet Clin Small Anim 50 (2020) 405–418
https://doi.org/10.1016/j.cvsm.2019.10.009
0195-5616/20/© 2019 Elsevier Inc. All rights reserved.
vetsmall.theclinics.com

Table 1
Summary of the primary pathogens associated with canine infectious respiratory disease complex

Organism	Incubation Period (d)	Clinical Presentation	Vaccination
B bronchiseptica	2–6	Variable ranging from commensal to mild upper-respiratory signs to severe bronchopneumonia	Parenteral inactivated; attenuated live intranasal, mucosal vaccine
Mycoplasma cynos	3–10	Clinical syndrome not completely described. Isolated as a single agent from dogs with pneumonia	None available
Streptococcus equi subsp zooepidemicus	Probably days	Although has been associated with severe, rapidly progressing hemorrhagic pneumonia in overcrowded environments, can also cause mild upper-respiratory signs or subclinical infections	None available
Canine adenovirus 2	3–6	Mild upper-respiratory signs and harsh cough of 2-wk duration	Attenuated live parenteral and mucosal vaccines; cross-protection for CAV-1
Canine distemper virus	3–6	Respiratory signs in combination with lethargy, ocular discharge, fever; rapidly progressive and can include GI and central nervous system signs	Parenteral attenuated live and recombinant vaccines; core vaccines
Canine herpesvirus-1	6–10	Subclinical or mild respiratory signs in adults; moderate to severe ocular changes; severe disease in neonates	None available
Canine influenza virus	2–4	Variable, ranging from subclinical to severe clinical disease with secondary bacterial infection	Parenteral inactivated vaccines for H3N2, H3N8, or both
Canine parainfluenza virus	3–10	Highly contagious; upper-respiratory signs lasting up to 10 d	Attenuated live parenteral and mucosal vaccines
Canine respiratory coronavirus	Probably days	Variable; subclinical to mild upper-respiratory signs	None available; no cross-protection afforded by the CCoV vaccine

Data from Sykes JE. Canine Viral Respiratory Infections. In: Sykes JE, ed. Canine and Feline Infectious Diseases. Saint Louis: W.B. Saunders; 2014:170-181.

canine herpesvirus-1 (CHV-1) and canine influenza virus (CIV), have been reported, and advances in molecular identification methods have identified other potential pathogens that may be playing a role in this disease complex.[3,7–13]

The agents associated with CIRDC are transmitted via the aerosol route and frequently cause subclinical or mild upper-respiratory signs that last on average 1 to

2 weeks. More severe clinical signs can be noted in dogs that have coinfections with multiple CIRDC pathogens or secondary bacterial pneumonia.[14–17] Here, potential pathogens involved in CIRDC are discussed, including both viral and bacterial pathogens (see **Table 1**), preventative measures to limit the spread of these infections, available diagnostics, and treatment options.

BACTERIAL ORGANISMS ASSOCIATED WITH CANINE INFECTIOUS RESPIRATORY DISEASE COMPLEX
Bordetella bronchiseptica

B bronchiseptica is a worldwide cause of respiratory disease in dogs and also causes disease in other species, including cats, pigs, rabbits, and people. Different strains of this gram-negative coccobacilli likely vary in their host range and ability to cause disease,[18–20] and isolation of B bronchiseptica from apparently healthy dogs can occur.[21–24]

Transmission of B bronchiseptica is via the airborne route, and it is highly contagious. Once inhaled, the organisms adhere to the respiratory cilia by way of adhesion molecules (fimbrial adhesions, filamentous hemagglutinin, pertactin, and lipopolysaccharides).[6] The organisms can evade the host defenses using virulence factors, such as the outer capsule, or the O antigen, which protects the bacteria from phagocytosis and complement mediated attacks.[25] Other virulence factors have also been described, including type III secretion systems that allow for bacterial colonization,[26–28] adenylate cyclase toxin with anti-inflammatory and immune evasion properties,[29,30] and exotoxins that cause necrosis of epithelial cells.[31] Once colonization has been established, altered respiratory epithelial cell function leads to excessive mucus secretion and further impairment of the local innate immune defenses, predisposing the host to infection by opportunistic secondary pathogens. The incubation period of B bronchiseptica ranges from 2 to 10 days. Clinical signs can vary dramatically. Mild upper-respiratory tract disease can lead to mucopurulent nasal discharge, sneezing, and a cough. In more severe disease cases that involve the lower-respiratory tract, signs of systemic illness can be present, including lethargy, decreased appetite, fever, and a productive cough. The organism can be shed for at least 1 month, and in some cases, for several months.[32,33]

Mycoplasma cynos

Many Mycoplasma spp are commensal organisms that colonize the mucous membranes of the respiratory tract, and their role in canine infectious respiratory disease is not clear. Mycoplasma spp are fastidious organisms that lack a cell wall, are the smallest known free-living organisms, and can be isolated from the lungs or trachea of about 25% of healthy adult dogs.[34] M cynos is the only Mycoplasma spp significantly associated with respiratory disease in dogs,[35] most commonly pneumonia.[36,37] It is still unclear if M cynos is a primary or secondary pathogen in dogs, because it can be cultured from the lungs of dogs both with[34,35] and without[35,36] other identifiable infectious respiratory disease. Recently it was associated with lethal bronchopneumonia in a litter of golden retriever puppies[38] and a colony of laboratory beagles.[39]

Experimental infection of dogs, by either endobronchial infection or exposure to infected dogs, results in development of clinical pneumonia, destruction and loss of respiratory cilia, and influx of neutrophils and macrophages into the alveolus.[37,40] Younger dogs are more likely to be infected with this organism as compared with older dogs, and dogs become infected within the first 2 to 3 weeks upon entering an animal shelter.[35] M cynos can persist in the lung for up to 3 weeks following infection and be transmitted via aerosols.[40] It is unknown how long the organism can persist in the environment. However, other *Mycoplasma* spp can survive for several weeks outside of the host; therefore, it should be assumed that *M cynos* can also persist in the environment.

Streptococcus equi Subspecies zooepidemicus

Streptococcus equi subsp *zooepidemicus*, a β-hemolytic, Lancefield group C streptococcus, has emerged as a cause of acute, severe bronchopneumonia in dogs. It is a commensal organism of the upper-respiratory tract of horses, but also can cause opportunistic infections, such as abscesses, and endometritis and can result in abortion.[41] Outbreaks of severe hemorrhagic pneumonia have been described in several populations of group-housed dogs in which *S equi* subsp *zooepidemicus* was identified as the causative agent.[42–44] A history of contact with horses has been identified in some, but not all infected dogs.[45] Rarely, *S equi* subsp *zooepidemicus* can be isolated from dogs without clinical signs.[42–44]

Dogs initially have mild clinical signs, including a cough and nasal discharge; however, their clinical signs can rapidly progress within 24 to 48 hours of onset, resulting in development of severe acute fibrinosuppurative, necrotizing, and hemorrhagic bronchopneumonia.[46] The pathogenesis is not fully elucidated; however, bacterial exotoxin genes have been identified in *S equi* subsp *zooepidemicus*, and the course of clinical disease in dogs is similar to that of streptococcal exotoxin-induced toxic shock syndrome in people, in which an overzealous host immune response induces significant pathologic condition.[46,47] Coinfection with other pathogens has been noted in some, but not all cases. In experimental models, coinfection of *S equi* subsp *zooepidemicus* with CIV (H3N8) resulted in severe clinical signs, whereas infection with *S equi* subsp *zooepidemicus* alone did not induce disease.[16]

Miscellaneous Bacteria

Other bacterial species have been isolated from dogs with CIRDC, including *Streptococcus canis*, *Pasteurella* spp, *Pseudomonas* spp, *Staphylococcus* spp, and coliforms, such as *Escherichia coli* and *Klebsiella pneumoniae*[48,49]; however, they are likely to represent secondary opportunistic infections as opposed to primary pathogens.

VIRUSES ASSOCIATED WITH CANINE INFECTIOUS RESPIRATORY DISEASE COMPLEX
Canine Adenovirus 2

Canine adenovirus-2, genus *Mastadenovirus* of the family Adenoviridae, is a nonenveloped double-stranded DNA virus that is a worldwide cause of infectious respiratory disease in dogs.[50] CAV-2 infects the nonciliated bronchiolar epithelial cells; epithelial cells of the nasal mucosa, pharynx, and tonsillar crypts; mucous cells in the trachea and bronchi; and type 2 alveolar epithelial cells.[51] Clinical signs are most often mild and consist of sneezing, nasal discharge, and a dry cough; however, more severe clinical signs are observed when coinfections with other CIRDC pathogens are present.[52] Viral shedding typically wanes 1 to 2 weeks after infection; however, the virus can survive in the environment for weeks to months.[53]

Canine Distemper Virus

Canine distemper virus (CDV) is in the genus *Morbillivirus* and family Paramyxoviridae. CDV is an enveloped RNA virus that can cause a myriad of clinical signs, primarily respiratory, with variable gastrointestinal (GI) and neurologic signs.[54] CDV is highly contagious and spread through aerosol secretions. Viral particles initially infect monocytes within the lymphoid and tonsillar tissues of the upper-respiratory tract and then disseminate throughout the body via the lymphatics.[55] CDV also infects lymphocytes, in particular, CD4[+] T lymphocytes, and causes widespread lymphocyte destruction, leading to lymphopenia in the first few days after infection; then widespread dissemination to multiple organ systems occurs.[56]

Clinical signs associated with CDV infection can vary from subclinical infection to death. Dogs that present with respiratory signs consistent with CIRD that also have GI signs, ocular discharge, neurologic signs, and/or an unknown vaccination history should be considered at high risk of having distemper. CDV is shed from all bodily secretions starting at 5 days after infection, and shedding can continue for up to 4 months.[54] Because of the viral envelope, environmental survival is only several hours, and routine disinfectants will inactivate the virus.

Canine Herpesvirus

Canine herpesvirus-1 (Canid alphaherpesvirus-1) is an enveloped doubled-stranded DNA virus belonging to the family Herpesviridae. The major clinical syndrome associated with CHV-1 is reproductive failure in bitches and severe illness in neonates.[52,57] CHV-1 also has been isolated from lung and tracheal specimens from dogs with rhinitis and pharyngitis, and a high seroprevalence has been noted in dogs housed in kennel situations, implicating it as a CIRDC pathogen.[58–62] Experimental infections of dogs with CHV-1 can lead to rhinitis, tracheobronchitis, and ocular signs, including keratitis and conjunctivitis.[63]

CHV-1 infects the epithelial cells of the upper-respiratory mucosa, and the incubation period is 6 to 10 days.[53] CHV-1, like other herpesviruses, becomes latent in neurologic tissue, and reactivation of latent infections can occur after considerable stress or pharmacologic immunosuppression, with intermittent shedding in respiratory secretions throughout the life of the patient.[52]

Canine Influenza Virus

Influenza viruses have segmented, negative-sense RNA genomes and are enveloped. CIV belongs to the family Orthomyxoviridae and genus *Alphainfluenzavirus* (influenza A) and is further subtyped based on its hemagglutinin (H) and neuraminidase (N) genes. Influenza viruses infect a wide variety of animals, including birds and mammals, and significant genetic reassortment can occur when multiple subtypes infect a single host.

CIV is caused by 2 subtypes of influenza that have adapted to spread throughout the dog population. The first was documented in a population of racing greyhounds in Florida in 2004. The virus is closely related to equine influenza virus subtype H3N8.[64,65] Serosurveys of greyhounds indicate that the virus first emerged in the canine population between 1999 and 2000.[3] The virus then spread throughout the country, mostly being reported in kennels and shelters, and sporadically within the pet population.[10] The overall prevalence of this infection has been declining, and extinction in the US dog population has been suspected. In 2015, an outbreak of CIV was noted in Chicago, Illinois caused by an H3N2 influenza subtype that is genetically similar to a strain previously reported in South East Asia, suspected to be the result of a mutated avian influenza virus that has now adapted to the dog.[66] Since 2015, this strain of CIV has spread throughout the United States,[66] and reintroductions from Asia have resulted in the appearance of additional outbreaks.

CIV typically causes mild clinical respiratory signs, including lethargy, cough, nasal and ocular discharge, and occasionally more severe clinical signs associated with pneumonia. Clinical signs may be more severe with H3N2 than H3N8 infections. After experimental infection, H3N8 CIV induced necrotizing and hyperplastic tracheitis and bronchitis in all dogs, and mild bronchiolitis and pneumonia in some dogs.[8] Many dogs also developed secondary bacterial pneumonia.[8] Viral shedding decreases dramatically 1 week after infection; however, H3N2 has been isolated from dogs up to 3 weeks after infection.[8,67]

Canine Parainfluenza Virus

CPIV is an enveloped single-stranded negative-sense RNA virus belonging to the family Paramyxoviridae and genus *Rubulavirus* and is closely related to simian virus 5. CPIV is a highly contagious cause of respiratory disease in dogs worldwide. Before introduction of vaccines, CPIV could be isolated from up to 50% of dogs with respiratory disease in a kennel situation.[68]

CPIV is spread via respiratory droplets, and infection occurs within the respiratory epithelial cells. Dogs can exhibit no clinical signs or mild clinical signs of a dry, harsh cough for 2 to 6 days with or without pyrexia and nasal discharge. Clinical signs appear more severe when coinfections occur. In experimental infections, clinical signs of respiratory disease are absent or very mild.[69] Histologic examination shows rhinitis with mixed inflammatory cell infiltration, tracheobronchitis, and bronchiolitis with loss of ciliated respiratory cells, and epithelial hyperplasia.[69] Viral shedding decreases 1 to 2 weeks after infection. The envelope of CPIV renders it susceptible to inactivation by most commercial disinfectants.

Canine Respiratory Coronavirus

Canine respiratory coronavirus (CRCoV) is a group 2a coronavirus in the family Coronaviridae and is an enveloped RNA virus. This virus was first described in a group of shelter dogs with respiratory disease in 2003 in the United Kingdom and has now been identified in dogs worldwide.[12] It can be found in dogs with and without clinical signs of respiratory disease.

Infection with CRCoV is associated with mild clinical signs, including nasal discharge, cough, and sneezing.[70] Experimental CRCoV infection of dogs resulted in mild respiratory disease, with virus infecting most respiratory tissue and respiratory associated lymphoid tissue, such as the tonsils and local lymph nodes. Infection of lymphoid tissue is associated with histopathologic changes that include damage to or loss of respiratory cilia.[53,70] Although respiratory tissue appears to be the primary site of viral replication, CRCoV has also been detected in the stool or intestines of dogs that presented with primary respiratory disease in the absence of GI signs and in 2 dogs with coinfections with other enteric viral pathogens in the absence of respiratory signs.[71] Viral shedding has been detected up to 10 days after infection.

Other Viruses Potentially Associated with Canine Infectious Respiratory Disease Complex

Molecular techniques have identified other viruses in dogs afflicted with CIRDC. Pantropic canine coronavirus, a group 1a coronavirus, is a strain of canine enteric coronavirus (CCoV) that was isolated from a group of dogs in Italy with severe respiratory disease. This strain of pantropic CCoV has been associated with severe clinical disease in puppies less than 3 months of age, as compared with those 6 months and older. Outbreaks have been reported throughout Europe, and coinfection with canine parvovirus has also been reported.[72]

Canine pneumovirus is a member of the family Paramyxoviridae. Infections have been reported in dogs from 2 animal shelters in the United States that had respiratory disease with no other causative agents discovered.[73] Other viruses that have been identified in dogs with respiratory disease include canine reovirus, canine bocavirus, and canine hepacivirus.[13] The role of these viruses in the induction of respiratory disease is unclear, and further investigation is warranted to elucidate their individual roles in CIRDC.

DIAGNOSIS

Diagnosis of disease associated with CIRDC starts with collection of a history and thorough physical examination. Most causative agents of CIRDC have short incubation periods ranging from a few days up to 2 weeks. A history of exposure to other dogs is often present because most agents are transmitted by inhalation of respiratory droplets, although fomite transmission can take place with some pathogens. Most dogs will exhibit mild clinical signs of a paroxysmal, harsh cough; serous ocular discharge; nasal discharge; and/or sneezing. Typically, energy and appetite will remain normal. Dogs that are exhibiting pyrexia, lethargy, decreased appetite, or other more severe clinical signs likely have secondary bacterial infections.

Complete blood count, serum biochemistry, and urinalysis are usually normal or show evidence of inflammation, including mild to moderate neutrophilia, presence of band neutrophils, and lymphopenia. Thoracic radiographs are often normal or have mild abnormalities ranging from an interstitial to a bronchointerstitial pulmonary pattern. Dogs with more severe clinical signs or secondary bacterial infection can have an alveolar pulmonary pattern.

Findings on the history, physical examination, blood work, and radiographs can raise suspicion for disease caused by a pathogen within the CIRDC; however, an etiologic diagnosis cannot be elucidated without pathogen-specific diagnostic assays. For dogs that (1) have severe or rapidly progressive clinical signs, (2) have clinical signs that last for more than 7 to 10 days, or (3) exist in an outbreak setting, an attempt to obtain an etiologic diagnosis is recommended.

Bacterial cultures can be performed from specimens obtained from nasal swab, oropharyngeal swab, tracheal wash, or bronchoalveolar lavage. Cultures of the upper-respiratory tract should be interpreted with caution because they can yield growth of normal flora, and many CIRDC pathogens, such as *B bronchiseptica*, can be isolated from healthy animals. Isolation of the same pathogen from multiple animals within an outbreak setting would likely be more meaningful. Collection of a tracheal wash or bronchoalveolar lavage specimen is indicated in dogs with more severe clinical signs or evidence of pneumonia. Growth of a CIRDC pathogen such a *B bronchiseptica* or *M cynos* in a dog with consistent clinical signs can provide some support for their involvement; however, coinfection with other pathogens should still be considered, and negative test results do not rule out the presence of other pathogens (such as CDV). Growth of multiple bacterial species may represent opportunistic secondary infection or contamination. False negatives can occur with low bacterial burden or if antimicrobials have been administered.

Molecular diagnostic assays, such as those based on the polymerase chain reaction (PCR), have become widely available from commercial laboratories. Respiratory panels have been developed using real-time PCR that detect the nucleic acid from pathogens, including CPIV, CAV-2, CDV, CRCoV, CHV, CIV, *B bronchiseptica*, and *Mycoplasma* spp.[15,74–76] Swabs of the nasal cavity, oropharyngeal cavity, or specimens collected from the lower-respiratory tract can be submitted for PCR. False negative results can be common because of transient or low-level shedding or sample degradation during transit to the laboratory. Vaccination within the previous few weeks with live-attenuated vaccines can lead to false positive results.[77]

Virus isolation is increasingly being replaced with PCR assays, but is still offered by specialized virology laboratories (eg, the Animal Health Diagnostic Laboratory at

Cornell University, Ithaca, NY, USA). Swabs from the upper-respiratory tract or specimens collected from the lower-respiratory tract can be submitted. Virus isolation suffers from some of the same pitfalls as PCR with false negatives because of low or intermittent viral shedding or degradation of virus particles during transit. If possible, the laboratory should be contacted in advance of specimen collection to provide instruction on storage and transport conditions for collected specimens.

Serologic assays for measurement of antibodies to CIRDC viral pathogens are available; however, their clinical use is limited because antibodies occurring in response to vaccination cannot be distinguished from those produced owing to infection or to subclinical infection.

TREATMENT

Treatment of dogs with uncomplicated signs of CIRDC typically involves supportive care. Clinical signs in most dogs will resolve without treatment, so if clinical signs have been present for less than 1 week and the dog is bright with a good appetite, no specific therapy is recommended under current guidelines.[78] Expectorant medications, such as guaifenesin, have not been shown to be beneficial in reducing clinical signs of CIRDC and therefore are not recommended.[6] Use of a cough suppressant can be considered in order to provide relief for affected dogs and their owners, especially as the cough can persist for weeks and can occur throughout the night. Over-the-counter antitussive medications might be somewhat effective in dogs with mild clinical signs. Narcotic antitussives, such as hydrocodone, are more effective at reducing clinical signs; however, administration is contraindicated in animals with productive cough because there can be diminished clearance of bacteria when they are administered, predisposing to secondary infections.[79] There are currently no labeled antiviral therapies for dogs with CIRDC and no published recommendations for administration of commercially available influenza antivirals used in human medicine; therefore, antiviral therapy is not recommended.

Dogs that have clinical signs persisting beyond 1 week or any signs of bacterial pneumonia, such as pyrexia, lethargy, decreased appetite, or an alveolar pulmonary pattern on thoracic radiographs, should be treated with antimicrobials. Ideally, treatment of bacterial pathogens, *B bronchiseptica*, or opportunistic secondary pathogens should be guided by culture and susceptibility testing, because antimicrobial resistance is increasingly being recognized, especially among *Bordetella* isolates.

Empiric antimicrobial therapy should be based on the most likely agent to be present. Doxycycline is recommended for dogs with suspected *B bronchiseptica* or *M cynos* infection. If a bacterial infection is suspected to be secondary to an underlying viral infection, broad-spectrum antimicrobials are more appropriate. In severe cases, a parenteral antimicrobial combination that includes a fluoroquinolone and penicillin or clindamycin is recommended.[78]

Additional supportive care is advised and should be tailored to the patient's need. This additional supportive care can include hydration and/or nutritional support, oxygen therapy, nebulization, and coupage. Care should be taken to prevent further irritation to the trachea by avoiding a neck lead and removing barking triggers.

PREVENTION OF CANINE INFECTIOUS RESPIRATORY DISEASE

Vaccines are available for many common CIRDC pathogens (see **Table 1**): CAV-2, CDV, CPIV, CIV H3N8, and H3N2, and *B bronchiseptica*. With the exception of CDV, these vaccines do not produce sterilizing immunity but rather decrease the severity of clinical signs and magnitude of pathogen shedding.[5] The CDV vaccine is a core vaccine that should be administered to all dogs. The remaining vaccinations are recommended in dogs that have risk of exposure.

Both mucosally administered (intranasal or transoral) and parenteral vaccines are available for CPIV, CAV-2, and *B bronchiseptica*. The route of vaccine delivery for these pathogens and its impact on the immune response have been debated in the literature. Intranasal or intraoral vaccination has been recommended to improve mucosal immune responses and permit rapid onset of protection in overcrowded environments, such as shelters. However, mucosal vaccination can sometimes result in vaccine-induced disease, and it can be difficult to know whether disease in a shelter environment is secondary to the vaccine or natural infection. Concern has also been raised that intranasal vaccine strains of *B bronchiseptica* might be capable of causing human disease in the immunosuppressed, although molecular evidence of this is lacking. Vaccination with intranasal vaccines is followed by the development of low titers of serum immunoglobulin G (IgG), whereas serum IgG responses are higher after parenteral vaccination.[80] A recent study suggested that intranasal vaccination may provide greater clinical protection against challenge than oral vaccination.[81] Additional studies are warranted to further assess the optimal vaccine type for dogs. Parenteral vaccines are available for reduction of clinical signs owing to CIVs, including individual H3N8 or H3N2 vaccines and combination (bivalent) vaccines.[82,83] No commercially available vaccines are available for reduction of clinical signs caused by CRCoV and CHV.

Although vaccination is a major prevention strategy, other precautions must be taken because immunization does not protect against all infections. In group-housing situations, precautionary measures should include an isolation period for dogs entering the population, rigorous daily monitoring for development of clinical signs within the group, and quarantine protocols for dogs with clinical signs associated with CIRDC. Care should be taken to prevent overcrowding and stress within the population. If an outbreak does occur, facilities should have an infectious disease protocol in place to limit exposure to other dogs in the facility, isolating ill animals from the population at large and applying proper disinfection protocols. An attempt should be made to determine the etiologic agent so targeted prevention and treatment protocols can be instituted.

SUMMARY

Contagious respiratory disease is a pervasive problem in group-housed dogs and pets that comingle with other dogs. Molecular techniques have led to discoveries of CIRDC pathogens that were not previously associated with the disease complex and highlighted the importance of coinfections in disease severity. With increased travel of dogs around the world, it is likely that novel pathogens will continue to emerge as CIV variants have in the past 2 decades. Because there are no specific therapies available for viral CIRDC pathogens, and available vaccines do not convey sterilizing immunity, prevention of infection is vital in group-housed dogs.

DISCLOSURE

Dr J.E. Sykes receives honoraria and research funding from Boehringer Ingelheim, Zoetis, Elanco, Merck, and IDEXX Laboratories.

REFERENCES

1. Buonavoglia C, Martella V. Canine respiratory viruses. Vet Res 2007;38:355–73.

2. Mitchell JA, Cardwell JM, Leach H, et al. European surveillance of emerging pathogens associated with canine infectious respiratory disease. Vet Microbiol 2017;212:31–8.

3. Anderson TC, Bromfield CR, Crawford PC, et al. Serological evidence of H3N8 canine influenza-like virus circulation in USA dogs prior to 2004. Vet J 2012; 191:312–6.

4. Barrell EA, Pecoraro HL, Torres-Henderson C, et al. Seroprevalence and risk factors for canine H3N8 influenza virus exposure in household dogs in Colorado. J Vet Intern Med 2010;24:1524–7.

5. Edinboro CH, Ward MP, Glickman LT. A placebo-controlled trial of two intranasal vaccines to prevent tracheobronchitis (kennel cough) in dogs entering a humane shelter. Prev Vet Med 2004;62:89–99.

6. Ford RB. Canine infectious respiratory disease. In: Greene CE, editor. Infectious diseases of the dog and cat. 4th edition. St. Louis (MO): Saunders Elsevier; 2013. p. 55–65.

7. Buonavoglia C, Decaro N, Martella V, et al. Canine coronavirus highly pathogenic for dogs. Emerg Infect Dis 2006;12:492–4.

8. Castleman W, Powe J, Crawford P, et al. Canine H3N8 influenza virus infection in dogs and mice. Vet Pathol 2010;47:507–17.

9. Decaro N, Buonavoglia C. An update on canine coronaviruses: viral evolution and pathobiology. Vet Microbiol 2008;132:221–34.

10. Dubovi EJ, Njaa BL. Canine influenza. Vet Clin North Am Small Anim Pract 2008; 38:827–35.

11. Erles K, Shiu K-B, Brownlie J. Isolation and sequence analysis of canine respiratory coronavirus. Virus Res 2007;124:78–87.

12. Erles K, Toomey C, Brooks HW, et al. Detection of a group 2 coronavirus in dogs with canine infectious respiratory disease. Virology 2003;310:216–23.

13. Priestnall SL, Mitchell JA, Walker CA, et al. New and emerging pathogens in canine infectious respiratory disease. Vet Pathol 2014;51:492–504.

14. Damián M, Morales E, Salas G, et al. Immunohistochemical detection of antigens of distemper, adenovirus and parainfluenza viruses in domestic dogs with pneumonia. J Comp Pathol 2005;133:289–93.

15. Erles K, Dubovi EJ, Brooks HW, et al. Longitudinal study of viruses associated with canine infectious respiratory disease. J Clin Microbiol 2004;42:4524–9.

16. Larson LJ, Henningson J, Sharp P, et al. Efficacy of the canine influenza virus H3N8 vaccine to decrease severity of clinical disease after cochallenge with canine influenza virus and Streptococcus equi subsp. zooepidemicus. Clin Vaccine Immunol 2011;18:559–64.

17. Maboni G, Seguel M, Lorton A, et al. Canine infectious respiratory disease: new insights into the etiology and epidemiology of associated pathogens. PLoS One 2019;14:e0215817.

18. Binns SH, Speakman AJ, Dawson S, et al. The use of pulsed-field gel electrophoresis to examine the epidemiology of *Bordetella bronchiseptica* isolated from cats and other species. Epidemiol Infect 1998;120:201–8.

19. Dawson S, Jones D, McCracken CM, et al. *Bordetella bronchiseptica* infection in cats following contact with infected dogs. Vet Rec 2000;146:46–8.

20. Foley JE, Rand C, Bannasch MJ, et al. Molecular epidemiology of feline bordetellosis in two animal shelters in California, USA. Prev Vet Med 2002;54:141–56.

21. Chalker VJ, Toomey C, Opperman S, et al. Respiratory disease in kennelled dogs: serological responses to *Bordetella bronchiseptica* lipopolysaccharide

do not correlate with bacterial isolation or clinical respiratory symptoms. Clin Diagn Lab Immunol 2003;10:352–6.

22. Decaro N, Mari V, Larocca V, et al. Molecular surveillance of traditional and emerging pathogens associated with canine infectious respiratory disease. Vet Microbiol 2016;192:21–5.

23. Schulz BS, Kurz S, Weber K, et al. Detection of respiratory viruses and *Bordetella bronchiseptica* in dogs with acute respiratory tract infections. Vet J 2014;201:365–9.

24. Lavan R, Knesl O. Prevalence of canine infectious respiratory pathogens in asymptomatic dogs presented at US animal shelters. J Small Anim Pract 2015;56:572–6.

25. Inatsuka CS, Xu Q, Vujkovic-Cvijin I, et al. Pertactin is required for *Bordetella* species to resist neutrophil-mediated clearance. Infect Immun 2010;78:2901–9.

26. Pilione MR, Harvill ET. The *Bordetella bronchiseptica* type III secretion system inhibits gamma interferon production that is required for efficient antibody-mediated bacterial clearance. Infect Immun 2006;74:1043–9.

27. Jacob-Dubuisson F, Reveneau N, Willery E, et al. Molecular characterization of *Bordetella bronchiseptica* filamentous haemagglutinin and its secretion machinery. Microbiology 2000;146:1211–21.

28. Weyrich LS, Rolin OY, Muse SJ, et al. A type VI secretion system encoding locus is required for *Bordetella bronchiseptica* immunomodulation and persistence in vivo. PLoS One 2012;7:e45892.

29. Vojtova J, Kamanova J, Sebo P. *Bordetella* adenylate cyclase toxin: a swift saboteur of host defense. Curr Opin Microbiol 2006;9:69–75.

30. Shrivastava R, Miller JF. Virulence factor secretion and translocation by *Bordetella* species. Curr Opin Microbiol 2009;12:88–93.

31. Mattoo S, Foreman-Wykert AK, Cotter PA, et al. Mechanisms of *Bordetella* pathogenesis. Front Biosci 2001;6:168–86.

32. Bemis DA, Greisen HA, Appel MJG. Pathogenesis of canine bordetellosis. J Infect Dis 1977;135:753–62.

33. Ellis JA. How well do vaccines for *Bordetella bronchiseptica* work in dogs? A critical review of the literature 1977–2014. Vet J 2015;204:5–16.

34. Randolph JF, Moise NS, Scarlett JM, et al. Prevalence of mycoplasmal and ureaplasmal recovery from tracheobronchial lavages and prevalence of mycoplasmal recovery from pharyngeal swab specimens in dogs with or without pulmonary disease. Am J Vet Res 1993;54:387–91.

35. Chalker VJ, Owen WM, Paterson C, et al. Mycoplasmas associated with canine infectious respiratory disease. Microbiology 2004;150:3491–7.

36. Chandler JC, Lappin MR. Mycoplasmal respiratory infections in small animals: 17 cases (1988–1999). J Am Anim Hosp Assoc 2002;38:111–9.

37. Rosendal S. Mycoplasmas as a possible cause of enzootic pneumonia in dogs. Acta Vet Scand 1972;13:137.

38. Zeugswetter F, Weissenbock H, Shibly S, et al. Lethal bronchopneumonia caused by *Mycoplasma cynos* in a litter of golden retriever puppies. Vet Rec 2007;161:626–7.

39. Hong S, Kim O. Molecular identification of *Mycoplasma cynos* from laboratory beagle dogs with respiratory disease. Lab Anim Res 2012;28:61–6.

40. Rosendal S, Vinther O. Experimental mycoplasmal pneumonia in dogs: electron microscopy of infected tissue. Acta Pathol Microbiol Scand B 1977;85B:462–5.

41. Timoney JF. The pathogenic equine streptococci. Vet Res 2004;35:397–409.

42. Chalker VJ, Brooks HW, Brownlie J. The association of *Streptococcus equi* subsp. *zooepidemicus* with canine infectious respiratory disease. Vet Microbiol 2003;95: 149–56.

43. Kim MK, Jee H, Shin SW, et al. Outbreak and control of haemorrhagic pneumonia due to *Streptococcus equi* subspecies *zooepidemicus* in dogs. Vet Rec 2007; 161:528–9.

44. Pesavento PA, Hurley KF, Bannasch MJ, et al. A clonal outbreak of acute fatal hemorrhagic pneumonia in intensively housed (shelter) dogs caused by *Streptococcus equi* subsp. *zooepidemicus*. Vet Pathol 2008;45:51–3.

45. Acke E, Abbott Y, Pinilla M, et al. Isolation of *Streptococcus zooepidemicus* from three dogs in close contact with horses. Vet Rec 2010;167:102–3.

46. Priestnall SL, Erles K, Brooks HW, et al. Characterization of pneumonia due to *Streptococcus equi* subsp. *zooepidemicus* in dogs. Clin Vaccine Immunol 2010;17:1790–6.

47. Paillot R, Darby AC, Robinson C, et al. Identification of three novel superantigen-encoding genes in *Streptococcus equi* subsp. *zooepidemicus*, szeF, szeN, and szeP. Infect Immun 2010;78:4817–27.

48. Radhakrishnan A, Drobatz KJ, Culp WT, et al. Community-acquired infectious pneumonia in puppies: 65 cases (1993–2002). J Am Vet Med Assoc 2007;230: 1493–7.

49. Thrusfield M, Aitken C, Muirhead R. A field investigation of kennel cough: incubation period and clinical signs. J Small Anim Pract 1991;32:215–20.

50. Ditchfield J, Macpherson LW, Zbitnew A. Association of a canine adenovirus (Toronto A26/61) with an outbreak of laryngotracheitis (kennel cough). A preliminary report. Can Vet J 1962;3:238–47.

51. Appel M, Bistner S, Menegus M, et al. Pathogenicity of low-virulence strains of two canine adenovirus types. Am J Vet Res 1973;34(4):543–50.

52. Decaro N, Martella V, Buonavoglia C. Canine adenoviruses and herpesvirus. Vet Clin North Am Small Anim Pract 2008;38:799–814.

53. Sykes JE. Chapter 17–Canine viral respiratory infections. In: Sykes JE, editor. Canine and feline infectious diseases. Saint Louis (MO): W.B. Saunders; 2014. p. 170–81.

54. Martella V, Elia G, Buonavoglia C. Canine distemper virus. Vet Clin North Am Small Anim Pract 2008;38:787–97.

55. Appel M, Shek W, Summers B. Lymphocyte-mediated immune cytotoxicity in dogs infected with virulent canine distemper virus. Infect Immun 1982;37: 592–600.

56. Iwatsuki K, Okita M, Ochikubo F, et al. Immunohistochemical analysis of the lymphoid organs of dogs naturally infected with canine distemper virus. J Comp Pathol 1995;113:185–90.

57. Appel MJ, Menegus M, Parsonson IM, et al. Pathogenesis of canine herpesvirus in specific-pathogen-free dogs: 5- to 12-week-old pups. Am J Vet Res 1969;30: 2067–73.

58. Erles K, Brownlie J. Investigation into the causes of canine infectious respiratory disease: antibody responses to canine respiratory coronavirus and canine herpesvirus in two kennelled dog populations. Arch Virol 2005;150:1493–504.

59. Gadsden BJ, Maes RK, Wise AG, et al. Fatal canid herpesvirus 1 infection in an adult dog. J Vet Diagn Invest 2012;24:604–7.

60. Karpas A, Garcia FG, Calvo F, et al. Experimental production of canine tracheobronchitis (kennel cough) with canine herpesvirus isolated from naturally infected dogs. Am J Vet Res 1968;29:1251–7.

61. Kawakami K, Ogawa H, Maeda K, et al. Nosocomial outbreak of serious canine infectious tracheobronchitis (kennel cough) caused by canine herpesvirus infection. J Clin Microbiol 2010;48:1176–81.
62. Ledbetter EC, Kim SG, Dubovi EJ. Outbreak of ocular disease associated with naturally-acquired canine herpesvirus-1 infection in a closed domestic dog colony. Vet Ophthalmol 2009;12:242–7.
63. Ledbetter EC, Kim SG, Dubovi EJ, et al. Experimental reactivation of latent canine herpesvirus-1 and induction of recurrent ocular disease in adult dogs. Vet Microbiol 2009;138:98–105.
64. Payungporn S, Crawford PC, Kouo TS, et al. Influenza A virus (H3N8) in dogs with respiratory disease, Florida. Emerg Infect Dis 2008;14:902–8.
65. Rivailler P, Perry IA, Jang Y, et al. Evolution of canine and equine influenza (H3N8) viruses co-circulating between 2005 and 2008. Virology 2010;408:71–9.
66. Voorhees IEH, Glaser AL, Toohey-Kurth K, et al. Spread of canine influenza A(H3N2) virus, United States. Emerg Infect Dis 2017;23:1950–7.
67. Newbury S, Godhardt-Cooper J, Poulsen KP, et al. Prolonged intermittent virus shedding during an outbreak of canine influenza A H3N2 virus infection in dogs in three Chicago area shelters: 16 cases (March to May 2015). J Am Vet Med Assoc 2016;248:1022–6.
68. McCandlish I, Thompson H, Cornwell H, et al. A study of dogs with kennel cough. Vet Rec 1978;102:293–301.
69. Ellis JA, Krakowka GS. A review of canine parainfluenza virus infection in dogs. J Am Vet Med Assoc 2012;240:273–84.
70. Erles K, Brownlie J. Canine respiratory coronavirus: an emerging pathogen in the canine infectious respiratory disease complex. Vet Clin North Am Small Anim Pract 2008;38:815–25.
71. Yachi A, Mochizuki M. Survey of dogs in Japan for group 2 canine coronavirus infection. J Clin Microbiol 2006;44:2615–8.
72. Zicola A, Jolly S, Mathijs E, et al. Fatal outbreaks in dogs associated with pantropic canine coronavirus in France and Belgium. J Small Anim Pract 2012; 53:297–300.
73. Renshaw RW, Zylich NC, Laverack MA, et al. Pneumovirus in dogs with acute respiratory disease. Emerg Infect Dis 2010;16:993–5.
74. Bellau-Pujol S, Vabret A, Legrand L, et al. Development of three multiplex RT-PCR assays for the detection of 12 respiratory RNA viruses. J Virol Methods 2005;126: 53–63.
75. Jeoung H-Y, Song D-S, Jeong W, et al. Simultaneous detection of canine respiratory disease associated viruses by a multiplex reverse transcription-polymerase chain reaction assay. J Vet Med Sci 2012;75(1):12–0287.
76. Payungporn S, Chutinimitkul S, Chaisingh A, et al. Single step multiplex real-time RT-PCR for H5N1 influenza A virus detection. J Virol Methods 2006;131:143–7.
77. Ruch-Gallie R, Moroff S, Lappin MR. Adenovirus 2, *Bordetella bronchiseptica*, and parainfluenza molecular diagnostic assay results in puppies after vaccination with modified live vaccines. J Vet Intern Med 2016;30:164–6.
78. Lappin MR, Blondeau J, Boothe D, et al. Antimicrobial use guidelines for treatment of respiratory tract disease in dogs and cats: antimicrobial guidelines working group of the International Society for Companion Animal Infectious Diseases. J Vet Intern Med 2017;31:279–94.
79. Thrusfield MV, Aitken CGG, Muirhead RH. A field investigation of kennel cough: efficacy of different treatments. J Small Anim Pract 1991;32:455–9.

80. Ellis JA, Krakowka GS, Dayton AD, et al. Comparative efficacy of an injectable vaccine and an intranasal vaccine in stimulating Bordetella bronchiseptica-reactive antibody responses in seropositive dogs. J Am Vet Med Assoc 2002; 220:43–8.

81. Ellis JA, Gow SP, Waldner CL, et al. Comparative efficacy of intranasal and oral vaccines against *Bordetella bronchiseptica* in dogs. Vet J 2016;212:71–7.

82. Rodriguez L, Nogales A, Murcia PR, et al. A bivalent live-attenuated influenza vaccine for the control and prevention of H3N8 and H3N2 canine influenza viruses. Vaccine 2017;35:4374–81.

83. Rodriguez L, Nogales A, Reilly EC, et al. A live-attenuated influenza vaccine for H3N2 canine influenza virus. Virology 2017;504:96–106.

An Update on Tracheal and Airway Collapse in Dogs

Ann Della Maggiore, DVM

KEYWORDS

- Tracheal collapse • Airway collapse • Bronchomalacia • Chronic cough
- Tracheal stent

KEY POINTS

- Tracheal collapse is characterized by dorsoventral flattening of tracheal rings.
- Tracheal collapse affects the cervical and/or intrathoracic trachea and is seen most commonly in middle-aged to older toy and miniature-breed dogs.
- Airway collapse or bronchomalacia affects large bronchi that contain cartilage and could be associated with similar cartilage defects to those seen with tracheal collapse. This condition is seen in any size of breed of dog.
- Medical management can include reduction of stress, weight loss, antitussives, bronchodilators, and possibly glucocorticoids (when concurrent bronchitis is present) and antibiotics (when infection is discovered).
- Surgical and minimally invasive treatment options are available when medical management fails.

INTRODUCTION

Tracheal or airway collapse is a common cause of cough in dogs and can affect the cervical trachea, intrathoracic trachea, or bronchial walls in isolation, or multiple regions can be affected concurrently. Tracheal collapse most likely results from softening of the tracheal cartilage that results in dorsoventral flattening of the tracheal rings and prolapse of the tracheal membrane into the lumen. This process leads to narrowing of the trachea whenever extraluminal pressure exceeds intraluminal pressure, causing airway collapse and impeding the passage of air. In some dogs with the most severe form of tracheal collapse (grade 4 out of 4), the cartilage rings are sometimes rigid but deviate dorsally into the trachea in a W shape. Clinically, tracheal narrowing results in a persistent dry, paroxysmal goose-honk cough; tracheal sensitivity; and varying degrees of respiratory difficulty. When the principal bronchi are also involved, the condition is termed tracheobronchomalacia. Bronchomalacia,

MarQueen Pet Emergency and Specialty Group, 9205 Sierra College Boulevard #120, Roseville, CA 95661, USA
E-mail address: adellamaggiore@yahoo.com

Vet Clin Small Anim 50 (2020) 419–430
https://doi.org/10.1016/j.cvsm.2019.11.003
0195-5616/20/© 2019 Elsevier Inc. All rights reserved.
vetsmall.theclinics.com

which is recognized in people and in dogs, is a defect of the principal bronchi and other smaller airways supported by cartilage that causes narrowing and loss of luminal dimensions in intrathoracic airways and a reduction in ability to clear secretions. These changes result in bronchial collapse, causing chronic cough, wheezing, and intermittent or chronic respiratory difficulty.[1,2]

CAUSE/PATHOPHYSIOLOGY

The cause of malacic airway disease is complex, incompletely understood, and likely multifactorial. In people, proposed causes include congenital conditions, endotracheal intubation, long-term ventilation, closed-chest trauma, chronic airway irritation and inflammation, malignancy, asthma, mechanical anatomic factors, and thyroid disease, but a definitive cause is unknown.[3–12] The cause of tracheobronchomalacia in dogs is also unknown and could be primary (congenital) or secondary to chronic inflammation (acquired). Given the common occurrence of tracheal collapse in small-breed dogs, there could be a primary or congenital abnormality of cartilage with secondary factors playing a role in progression and development of clinical signs.

Tracheal collapse is often associated with softening of cartilage rings caused by a reduction of glycosaminoglycan and chondroitin sulfate, which leads to a weakness and flattening of the tracheal rings. Changes to the tracheal matrix and inability to retain water lead to a decreased ability to maintain functional rigidity.[13,14] Extrinsic compression, chronic inflammation, and alteration in elastic fibers in the dorsal tracheal membrane and annular ligaments have also been considered as possible causes or factors that contribute to collapse.[15,16] Secondary factors that can initiate clinical signs include airway irritants, chronic bronchitis, laryngeal paralysis, respiratory infection, obesity, and tracheal intubation. It is critical to identify these factors for appropriate medical management.

Dynamic collapse of the airway perpetuates additional inflammation, tracheal edema, alterations or failure in the mucociliary apparatus, increased mucus secretion, and mucus trapping within the airways. The cervical trachea collapses during inspiration and the thoracic trachea collapses during expiration because of the pressures developed during the respiratory cycle. Tracheal collapse occurs almost exclusively in small-breed dogs, whereas bronchial collapse occurs in both large-breed and small-breed dogs and most commonly involves the right middle and the left cranial bronchi.[1] In some dogs only bronchial collapse (bronchomalacia) is noted.

PATIENT HISTORY

Tracheal or airway collapse is commonly seen in middle-aged to older miniature, toy, and small-breed dogs. Age at presentation typically ranges from 1 to 15 years and signs have been present for years, although about 25% of affected dogs show clinical signs by the age of 6 months.[17] Breeds over-represented include Yorkshire terriers, Pomeranian, pugs, miniature poodle, Maltese, and Chihuahuas.[18] No sex predilection has been appreciated. Cats and large-breed dogs are rarely diagnosed with tracheal collapse.

Bronchomalacia is reported in 45% to 83% of dogs with tracheal collapse[1,19] and has also been reported in dogs with eosinophilic bronchopneumopathy[20] or bronchitis. Bronchomalacia, unlike tracheal collapse, can affect any canine breed and can be seen in medium-breed and large-breed dogs,[1,2] suggesting that the underlying cause could be different from that of tracheal collapse, although histologic investigations are lacking. Within a population of coughing dogs, dogs with airway collapse are often older, lower in body weight, and have a significantly higher body condition than dogs without airway collapse.[1] Bronchomalacia, and specifically collapse of the left cranial lobar bronchus, has been recognized in a large percentage (87%) of dogs with brachycephalic airway syndrome. In 1 report, pugs were the most common brachycephalic breed affected with this type of collapse, followed by English bulldogs and French bulldogs.[21]

Dogs with tracheal or airway collapse usually present to the veterinarian for evaluation of cough that is initiated by excitement, drinking or eating, or pulling on a leash with a neck lead. Prolonged clinical history is common and ranges from weeks to years, although some dogs present at a very young age with respiratory distress caused by fixed airway narrowing and obstruction. These dogs often have grade 4, or the W shape, to the trachea. Other dogs have paroxysmal or waxing and waning respiratory signs, most often described as a dry, harsh, or honking cough. Worsening tachypnea, exercise intolerance, and respiratory distress tend to occur during physical exertion, heat stress, or in humid conditions. Respiratory compromise can progress and become refractory to treatment. Cyanosis and syncope can also occur because of complete airway obstruction, vagally mediated syncope, or pulmonary hypertension.[22] Occasionally animals present with acute respiratory distress from airway obstruction, often exacerbated by stress, excitement, heat, and/or concurrent respiratory disease.

PHYSICAL EXAMINATION

Dogs presenting for airway collapse are usually systemically healthy and are often overweight. Respiratory pattern is often normal or the dog can show increased respiratory effort caused by airway collapse. Cervical tracheal collapse typically causes respiratory difficulty on inspiration, whereas intrathoracic collapse and bronchomalacia result in increased expiratory effort. Close observation or palpation at the thoracic inlet can sometimes reveal cranial lung herniation through the inlet during expiration in some dogs with intrathoracic airway collapse. Palpation of the trachea frequently initiates cough in affected dogs, indicating nonspecific tracheal sensitivity. This palpation should be performed cautiously because some animals become cyanotic, develop syncope, or go into a life-threatening respiratory crisis because of paroxysmal cough. Collapse of the cervical tracheal can sometimes be appreciated as a flattening of the tracheal rings on cervical palpation.

Auscultation over the trachea can reveal stridorous sounds on both inspiration and expiration caused by the fixed narrowing of the extrathoracic tracheal diameter. This narrowing must be differentiated from laryngeal paralysis, which has been reported in up to 60% of dogs with tracheal collapse,[22] emphasizing the importance of a thorough upper airway examination if the animal is anesthetized. Stertor or stridor could also indicate laryngeal collapse in brachycephalic breeds, with 1 study reporting some degree of laryngeal collapse in almost all brachycephalic dogs as well as an association between laryngeal collapse and collapse of the left cranial lobar bronchus.[21] During thoracic auscultation, referred upper airway sounds are often noted and can compromise assessment of lung sounds. Crackles on both inspiration and expiration are sometimes appreciated in dogs with bronchomalacia and small airway collapse, or this can suggest mucus accumulation in the airways associated with concurrent bronchitis.

A thorough cardiac auscultation is recommended, and a heart murmur associated with mitral regurgitation was found significantly more often in dogs with airway collapse (17%) compared with animals presenting with cough without airway collapse (2%).[1] This finding most likely is related to the commonality of myxomatous mitral valve disease and airway disease in small-breed dogs. The role of cardiomegaly and specifically left atrial enlargement in airway collapse remains unclear. A recent study showed similar severity and location of airway collapse in dogs with and without left atrial enlargement and reported airway inflammation as the likely cause of cough in dogs that had both left atrial enlargement and airway collapse.[23]

Hepatomegaly is common in dogs with tracheal collapse and could be a reflection of obesity, although hepatic dysfunction (as indicated by increases in levels of bile acids) has been reported in dogs with tracheal collapse.[24]

DIAGNOSTIC EVALUATION
Hematologic, Biochemical Evaluation, and Heartworm Screening

The diagnosis of tracheal collapse is strongly suspected based on signalment, history of cough, and physical examination findings. Additional diagnostic evaluation should be performed to rule out concurrent disorders and determine appropriate therapy.

A complete blood count, chemistry panel, and heartworm screening is recommended in any coughing dog before additional diagnostic evaluation. These tests are typically unremarkable in dogs with airway collapse, although evaluation of dogs with severe tracheal collapse showed that 12 out of 26 dogs had increases in the levels of 2 or more liver enzymes, and stimulated bile acid levels were increased in 25 out of 26 dogs.[24] Following stent placement for management of severe, refractory airway obstruction, bile acid concentrations decreased but plasma liver enzyme activity was not significantly influenced.[24] The cause of these changes remains unknown, although hypoxia and development of a centrilobular liver cell necrosis was suggested as a possible cause of liver dysfunction, similar to what has been reported in humans with acute exacerbation of chronic respiratory disease.

Thoracic and Cervical Radiographs

Detection and grading of tracheal collapse is used to identify the location and severity of collapse and to monitor progression of the disease. Because tracheal and airway collapse are considered dynamic processes, it is ideal to perform diagnostic imaging in multiple stages of the respiratory cycle. Collapse of the cervical trachea should be evident on inspiration and the intrathoracic trachea will collapse on expiration. It is

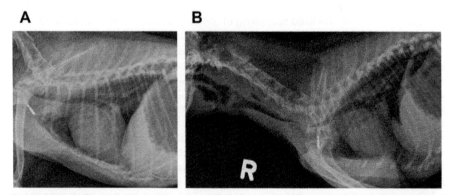

Fig. 1. Lateral thoracic (*A*) and cervical (*B*) radiographs of a dog with cervical tracheal collapse at the thoracic inlet. Note that the additional view (*B*) improves the ability to identify cervical tracheal collapse. Retraction of the larynx in (*B*) likely reflects upper airway obstruction. (*Courtesy of* Lynelle Johnson, DVM, MS, PhD, DACVIM, Davis, CA.)

recommended to evaluate a lateral radiograph of the thorax and cervical region (**Fig. 1**) in both the inspiratory and expiratory phases, although this only slightly improves accuracy in detection of collapse.[18] False-positives and false-negatives are common with plain radiography. Radiographs often underestimate the frequency and severity of tracheal collapse and often fail to detect collapse at the carina, which is reportedly more severe than cervical collapse.[18] Radiographs also underestimate the tracheal diameter compared with computed tomography, making them inadequate for selecting tracheal stent size.[25] However, radiographs are useful in evaluation of concurrent respiratory or cardiac disease.

Fluoroscopy

A fluoroscopic study can be used to evaluate a coughing dog for the presence and location of airway collapse but this technique is only available at universities and large referral hospitals. When radiography was compared with fluoroscopy, assuming the fluoroscopy was correct, radiographic evidence of collapse was at the incorrect location in 44% of dogs and it was not detected in 8% of dogs with radiographs alone.[18] Fluoroscopic identification of lower airway collapse versus tracheal collapse can be important in determining therapy (discussed later) (**Fig. 2**). Importantly, radiography, fluoroscopy, and bronchoscopy might be required to allow complete evaluation of the type of airway collapse present in a dog.[26]

Bronchoscopy

Bronchoscopy is considered the gold standard for diagnosis of bronchomalacia in humans because it allows visualization of the trachea and the principal, lobar, and sublobar bronchi to assess for bronchomalacia.[27] In addition to bronchoscopy, laryngoscopy and bronchoalveolar lavage are recommended in coughing dogs to detect concurrent disease that affects treatment. Bronchoscopy does require anesthesia, which can be associated with complications in animals with severe airway obstruction,

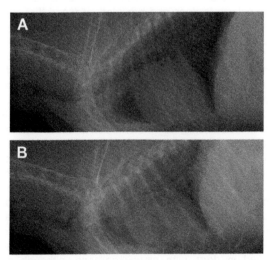

Fig. 2. Images captured from a fluoroscopic study on inspiration (*A*) and expiration (*B*) from a dog with intrathoracic tracheal collapse clearly show the change in luminal diameter of the intrathoracic airway during expiration. (*Courtesy of* Lynelle Johnson, DVM, MS, PhD, DACVIM, Davis, CA.)

marked tracheal sensitivity, dramatic expiratory effort, or those that are obese or overly excitable.

Laryngeal collapse and paralysis can be seen concurrently with tracheal collapse and bronchomalacia, so a thorough upper airway evaluation is recommended and should be performed before intubation at anesthetic induction. Laryngeal collapse is graded in 3 stages based on severity.[28] Stage I is characterized by eversion of the laryngeal saccules, stage 2 by medial displacement of the cuneiform process of the arytenoid cartilages, and stage 3 by collapse of the corniculate processes of the arytenoid cartilages with the loss of the dorsal arch of the rima glottis. Further details are provided in Catriona M. MacPhail's article, "Laryngeal Disease in Dogs and Cats: An Update," elsewhere in this issue. As mentioned previously, in 1 report, laryngeal collapse was significantly correlated with severe bronchial collapse in brachycephalic dogs.[21]

Bronchoscopic examination should be performed in a standardized fashion with the use of tracheal bronchial anatomy and nomenclature as proposed by Amis and McKiernan[29] for proper identification. Grading of tracheal collapse is based on a scheme determined by Tagner and Hobson[30] related to the reduction in luminal dimension (**Fig. 3, Table 1**).

Bronchoscopy also allows evaluation of the principal and lobar bronchi for evidence of bronchomalacia and identifies specific segments of bronchial collapse. Bronchial collapse in both brachycephalic and nonbrachycephalic dogs most commonly involves the left cranial and right middle bronchi.[2,3,21,23] In 1 study, 48% of dogs diagnosed with bronchomalacia had concurrent tracheal collapse,[3] whereas, in another,[1] 41% had tracheal collapse in conjunction with bronchial collapse. In dogs with collapse of sublobar airways, focal airway collapse was identified in 48% and diffuse airway collapse was present in 52% of dogs.[1] Bronchomalacia commonly goes underdiagnosed because it is not visible radiographically and endoscopy is required for definitive diagnosis.

In humans bronchomalacia and dynamic airway collapse are defined as 2 separate entities, and until recently this had not been investigated in dogs. Normal airways are recognized as round or ovoid with minimal luminal variation (subjectively <20%) during the respiratory cycle.[1] One study examined clinical evaluation and endoscopic classification of bronchomalacia in dogs and provided evidence that static and dynamic bronchomalacia seem to occur both independently and concurrently. Dynamic bronchial collapse was found alone in 59% of cases or with static bronchial collapse in 37% of dogs, and most animals (71%) had dynamic bronchial collapse and tracheal collapse.[3] Bronchial collapse in that study was defined as static if a stable airway diameter was seen or dynamic if changes in luminal diameter were noted during respiration (**Fig. 4**). A grading system was developed with grade I collapse defined as static or dynamic collapse with reduction in diameter less than or equal to 50%, grade 2 collapse as diameter reduction greater than 50% and less than or equal to 75%, and grade 3 collapse as greater than 75%, with contact between the dorsal and ventral mucosa of the collapsed bronchus.[3] If use of this grading system becomes widespread, prospective studies could be designed to assess progression of disease and better establish prognosis, as well as guidelines for therapeutic intervention.

Common bronchoscopic findings in some dogs with airway collapse include gross evidence of airway inflammation, hyperemia, and mucus accumulation. Bronchoalveolar lavage cytology is used to document infectious or inflammatory conditions, and culture is used to rule out concurrent infection. Varying types of inflammation have been identified in dogs with airway collapse, although a previous study comparing dogs with airway collapse and dogs without airway collapse showed no clear differences in airway inflammation between groups.[1] In animals with bronchomalacia that have had bronchoalveolar lavage performed, neutrophilic inflammation was

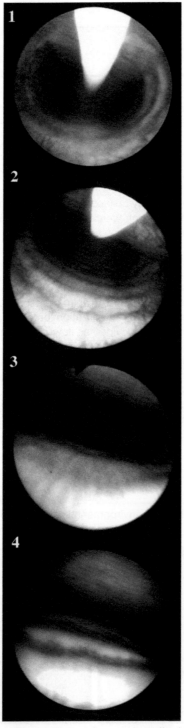

Fig. 3. Grades of tracheal collapse. (*From* Johnson LR, Pollard RE. Tracheal collapse and bronchomalacia in dogs: 58 cases (7/2001-1/2008). J Vet Intern Med 2010;24:298-305; with permission.)

Table 1	
Grading of tracheal collapse	
Grade	**Reduction in Luminal Diameter (%)**
1	25
2	50
3	75
4	90–100 obstruction of lumen or a double lumen (W shaped) trachea

Modified from Maggiore AD. Tracheal and Airway Collapse in Dogs. Vet Clin North Am Small Animal Pract. 2014; 44(1):111-27; with permission.

found in 51%.[3] In dogs with airway collapse and left atrial enlargement, both neutrophilic and lymphocytic inflammation were commonly identified.[21] It remains unclear whether inflammation precedes or follows airway collapse.

TREATMENT

The approach to treatment of airway collapse varies with the location of collapse and the severity of the animal's clinical signs. An animal presenting in respiratory distress is a medical emergency and requires stabilization before diagnostic testing. Stress should be minimized and oxygen provided as flow-by or in an oxygen cage. Acepromazine (0.01–0.1 mg/kg subcutaneously every 4–6 hours) and butorphanol (0.05–0.1 mg/kg subcutaneously every 4–6 hours) can be synergistic in providing sedation and cough suppression, but caution should be used because oversedation could make intubation necessary. Dogs should be maintained in a cool environment because patients with upper airway obstructions are predisposed to hyperthermia. Glucocorticoids are sometimes necessary to decrease laryngeal inflammation or edema. Once the dog is stabilized, additional diagnostics and treatment options can be considered.

MEDICAL MANAGEMENT
Environmental Factors

As an adjunct to medical therapy, environmental changes should be instituted to maintain the animal in a cool environment with minimal humidity. The owner's ability to

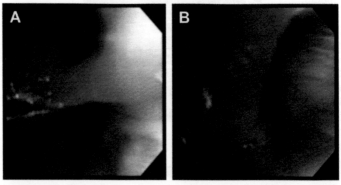

Fig. 4. Inspiratory (*A*) and expiratory (*B*) endoscopic images of the left cranial lobar bronchus in a dog with bronchomalacia. (*Courtesy of* Lynelle Johnson, DVM, MS, PhD, DACVIM, Davis, CA.)

recognize and reduce specific environmental factors that increase barking, anxiety, and excitement can help decrease the stimulus to cough. Using a harness instead of a neck collar reduces direct stimulation and compression of the trachea.

Encouraging weight loss is one of the single most important strategies for reducing clinical signs in dogs with airway collapse. By increasing thoracic wall compliance and reducing extrathoracic and intra-abdominal adipose tissue, cough and respiratory difficulty can be substantially reduced. However, weight loss is typically challenging because many of these dogs cannot effectively exercise. Careful diet planning is essential. Current caloric intake from all sources should be determined and resting energy requirement (RER) calculated through the formula: $RER = 70 \times (body\ weight)^{0.75}$. It is important that owners are given realistic expectations for weight loss, and ideally, a dog should lose 1% to 2% of its weight per week. Caloric restriction alone is used initially with weekly monitoring of weight. If this is unsuccessful, a prescription low-calorie, high-fiber diet should be used. Identification and treatment of secondary medical conditions is also important for appropriate management.

Antitussive Agents

When infection and inflammation have been adequately treated, cough suppressants are recommended to reduce chronic irritation and control cough. These cough suppressants are often the sole therapy used for cough associated with cervical tracheal collapse. Cough suppressants regularly used include hydrocodone (0.22 mg/kg by mouth 2–4 times a day) and butorphanol (0.55 mg/kg by mouth 2–4 times a day). When treating an animal with cough suppressants, it is recommended to start at a frequent dosing interval and gradually prolong the time between dose administration until the lowest effective dose is used at the longest interval. Side effects of these drugs include sedation, constipation, and development of tolerance.

Glucocorticoids

Glucocorticoids are often used short term to reduce laryngeal, tracheal, and bronchial inflammation, unless a concurrent infectious condition is suspected. Initial treatment typically involves an antiinflammatory dose of prednisone (0.5 mg/kg by mouth twice a day) for 5 to 7 days or inhaled steroids (fluticasone propionate, 110 μg/puff, administered via face mask and spacing chamber). A short course of therapy is advised to avoid secondary effects such as panting, which puts added stress on the respiratory system, and weight gain. Use of inhaled in place of systemic corticosteroids can minimize side effects.

Bronchodilators

Bronchodilators are sometimes used when small airway disease is suspected to contribute to intrathoracic airway collapse. Use is based on the theory that any increase in diameter of small (<300 μm) airways improves expiratory airflow, alters pressure dynamics, and reduces the tendency for intrathoracic airways to collapse. Bronchodilators have no effect on the larger airways that are visible during endoscopy and are not indicated for treatment of cervical tracheal collapse. Bronchodilators can play an important role when lower airway collapse/bronchomalacia is suspected or documented on bronchoscopic evaluation, although response is variable. Methylxanthine bronchodilators are most commonly used and extended-release theophylline is recommended at 10 mg/kg by mouth every 12 hours. This drug is no longer available commercially because it is not used in human medicine, and compounding pharmacies must be used to obtain this medication. The efficacy of these extended-release products is unknown and cautious dosing must be used to avoid toxicity, along with clinical assessment of efficacy. β_2-Agonists are more effective as true bronchodilators but do not seem to be as useful in management of airway collapse.

Antibiotics

Infection rarely contributes to clinical signs in airway collapse, but antibiotics can play an important role in treating secondary infections that act as an inciting cause to airway irritation. Doxycycline can be considered pending culture results for treatment of mycoplasma infection as well as for antiinflammatory effects.

Surgical Interventions

When medical management fails to control clinical signs, surgical intervention or placement of an intraluminal stent should be considered. Extraluminal tracheal rings are indicated for cervical tracheal collapse and excellent outcomes have been reported in dogs managed by skilled surgeons.[31] Postoperative laryngeal paralysis can be anticipated as a potential problem caused by impingement or praxis of the recurrent laryngeal nerve, and, if stridor or inspiratory respiratory distress occurs after placement of extraluminal rings, laryngeal lateralization is generally needed. Tracheal necrosis can also be encountered long term if blood supply is damaged.[32–34]

If intrathoracic tracheal collapse is diagnosed and cannot be managed medically, placement of an intraluminal stent can be considered. Complications include bacterial tracheitis, stent fracture/migration, stent collapse/deformation, tracheal perforation during placement, and development of obstructive granulation tissue. Patient selection is important in obtaining good outcomes. Grade 4 W-shaped tracheal malformation and the tapering diameter of the trachea from the cervical to the intrathoracic region could be associated with an increase in the risk of stent fracture and obstructive granulation tissue.[35] Intraluminal stents or surgical management can be lifesaving and excellent short-term and long-term outcomes have been reported.[19,36] Extensive medical management is often required to control cough, infection, and inflammation after stent placement.

Prognosis

Little has been published about overall prognosis in dogs with airway collapse that are medically managed. There is concern that disease will gradually progress over time and dogs will become refractory to treatment. However, most dogs can be successfully managed with diligent attention to weight control, identification and control of infection and inflammation, and appropriate use of interventional therapy.

DISCLOSURE

None.

REFERENCES

1. Johnson LR, Pollard RE. Tracheal collapse and bronchomalacia in dogs: 58 cases (7/2001-1/2008). J Vet Intern Med 2010;24:298–305.
2. Adamama-Moraitou KK, Pardali D, Day MJ, et al. Canine bronchomalacia: a clinicopathological study of 18 cases diagnosed by endoscopy. Vet J 2012;191(2): 261–6.
3. Bottero E, Bellino C, De Lorenzi D, et al. Clinical evaluation and endoscopic classification of bronchomalacia in dogs. J Vet Intern Med 2013;27(4):840–6.
4. Mair E, Parsons DS. Pediatric tracheomalacia and major airway collapse. Ann Otol Rhino Laryngol 1992;101:300–9.

5. Feist JH, Johnson TH, Wilson RJ. Acquired tracheomalacia: etiology and differential diagnosis. Chest 1975;68:340–5.

6. Burden RJ, Shann F, Butt W, et al. Tracheobronchial malacia and stenosis in children in intensive care: bronchograms help to predict outcome. Thorax 1999;54:511–7.

7. Tsugawa C, Nishijima E, Muraji T, et al. A shape memory airway stent for tracheomalacia in children: an experimental and clinical study. J Pediatr Surg 1997;32:50–3.

8. Johnson TH, Mikita J, Wilson RJ, et al. Acquired tracheomalacia. Radiology 1973;109:576–80.

9. Tillie-Lebold I, Wallaert B, Leblond D, et al. Respiratory involvement in relapsing polychondritis. Clinical, functional, endoscopic, and radiographic evaluations. Medicine 1998;77:168–76.

10. Miyazawa T, Miyazu Y, Iwamoto Y, et al. Stenting at the flow-limiting segment in tracheobronchial stenosis due to lung cancer. Am J Respir Crit Care Med 2004;169:1096–102.

11. Nuutinen J. Acquired tracheobronchomalacia. Eur J Respir Dis 1982;63:380–7.

12. McHenry CR, Pitrowski JJ. Thyroidectomy in patients with marked thyroid enlargement: airway management, morbidity, and outcome. Am Surg 1994;60:586–91.

13. Dallman MJ, McClure RC, Brown EM. Normal and collapsed trachea in the dog. Scanning electron microscopy study. Am J Vet Res 1985;46(10):2110–5.

14. Dallman MJ, McClure RC, Brown EM. Histochemical study of normal and collapsed tracheas in dogs. Am J Vet Res 1988;49(12):2117–25.

15. Jokinen K, Palva T, Sutinen S, et al. Acquired tracheobronchomalacia. Ann Clin Res 1977;9:52–7.

16. Kamanta S, Usui N, Sawai T, et al. Pexi of the great vessels for patients with tracheobronchomalacia in infancy. J Pediatr Surg 2000;35:454–7.

17. Herrtage MJ. Medical management of tracheal collapse. In: Bonagura J, Twedt D, editors. Kirks current veterinary therapy XIV. St Louis (MO): Saunders Elsevier; 2009. p. 630–5.

18. Macready DM, Johnson LR, Pollard RE. Fluoroscopic and radiographic evaluation of tracheal collapse in 62 dogs. J Am Vet Med Assoc 2007;230:1870–6.

19. Moritz A, Schneider M, Bauer N. Management of advanced tracheal collapse in dogs using intraluminal self-expanding biliary wall stents. J Vet Intern Med 2004;18:31–42.

20. Clercx C, Peeters D, Snaps F, et al. Eosinophilic bronchopneumopathy in dogs. J Vet Intern Med 2000;14:282–91.

21. De Lorenzi D, Bertoncello D, Drigo M. Bronchial abnormalities found in a consecutive series of forty brachycephalic dogs. J Am Vet Med Assoc 2009;235:835–40.

22. Johnson LR. Diseases of airways. In: Johnson LR, editor. Clinical canine and feline respiratory medicine. Ames (IA): Wiley-Blackwell publishing; 2010. p. 97–103.

23. Singh MK, Johnson LR, Kittleson MD, et al. Bronchomalacia in dogs with myxomatous mitral valve degeneration. J Vet Intern Med 2012;26:312–9.

24. Bauer NB, Schneider MA, Neiger R, et al. Liver disease in dogs with tracheal collapse. J Vet Intern Med 2006;20:845–9.

25. Montgomery JE, Mathews KG, Marcellin-Little DJ, et al. Comparison of radiography and computed tomography for determining tracheal diameter and length in dogs. Vet Surg 2015;44:114–8.

26. Johnson LR, Singh MK, Pollard RE. Agreement among radiographs, fluoroscopy, and bronchoscopy in documentation of airway collapse in dogs. J Vet Intern Med 2015;29(6):1619–26.

27. Heyer CM, Nuesslein TG, Jung D, et al. Tracheobronchial anomalies and stenoses: detection with low-dose multidetector CT with virtual tracheobronchoscopy–comparison with flexible tracheobronchoscopy. Radiology 2007;242:542–9.

28. Leonard HC. Collapse of the larynx and associated structures in the dog. J Am Vet Med Assoc 1960;137:360–3.

29. Amis TC, McKiernan BM. Systemic identification of endobronchial anatomy during bronchoscopy in the dog. Am J Ves Res 1986;47:2649–57.

30. Tangner CH, Hobson HP. A retrospective study of 20 surgically managed cases of collapsed trachea. Vet Surg 1982;11:146–9.

31. Buback JL, Boothe HW, Hobson HP. Surgical treatment of tracheal collapse in dogs; 90 cases (1983-1993). J Am Vet Med Assoc 1996;208(3):380–4.

32. White RN. Unilateral arytenoid lateralization and extraluminal polypropylene ring prosthesis for correction of tracheal collapse in the dog. J Small Anim Pract 1995; 36:151–8.

33. Kirby BM, Bjorling DE, Rankin JH, et al. The effects of surgical isolation and application of polypropylene spiral prostheses on tracheal blood flow. Vet Surg 1992; 20:49–54.

34. Coyne BE, Fingland RB, Kennedy GA, et al. Clinical and pathologic effects of a modified technique for application of spiral prostheses to the cervical trachea of dogs. Vet Surg 1993;22:269–75.

35. Violette NP, Weisse C, Berent AC, et al. Correlations among tracheal dimensions, tracheal stent dimensions, and major complication after endoluminal stenting of tracheal collapse syndrome in dogs. J Vet Intern Med 2019;33(5):2209–16.

36. Sura PA, Krahwinkel DJ. Self-expanding nitinol stents for the treatment of tracheal collapse in dogs: 12 cases (2001-20 04). J Am Vet Med Assoc 2008;232:228–36.

Update on Canine Idiopathic Pulmonary Fibrosis in West Highland White Terriers

Henna P. Laurila, DVM, PhD*, Minna M. Rajamäki, DVM, PhD

KEYWORDS

- Dog • Interstitial lung disease • Idiopathic interstitial pneumonia
- Arterial blood gas analysis • HRCT • Bronchoalveolar lavage • Biomarker

KEY POINTS

- Canine idiopathic pulmonary fibrosis (CIPF) is a chronic, progressive, interstitial lung disease of unknown etiology affecting mainly middle-aged and old West Highland white terriers.
- Typical findings are cough, exercise intolerance, Velcro crackles, abdominal breathing pattern, and hypoxemia.
- Diagnosis is often requires either high-resolution computed tomography (HRCT) or histopathology of the lung tissue, which is seldom performed on live dogs.
- CIPF shares several clinical findings with human idiopathic pulmonary fibrosis, but in HRCT and histopathology, CIPF has features of human idiopathic pulmonary fibrosis as well as nonspecific interstitial pneumonia.
- No curative treatment exists, and clinical treatment trials are lacking in dogs. Symptomatic treatment with corticosteroids and theophylline may alleviate clinical signs.

INTRODUCTION

Idiopathic pulmonary fibrosis (IPF) is a devastating interstitial lung disease (ILD) with no known cure. It is chronic, is inevitably progressive, and leads to death. IPF is recognized in humans and in their animal companions, cats and dogs.[1–3] The term, *canine IPF (CIPF)*, is used to separate the human and canine diseases.

CIPF affects mainly the West Highland white terrier (WHWT). Corcoran and colleagues[3] published the first case series describing the clinical features of this disease in WHWTs. More reports of CIPF in a WHWT and other dog breeds were described around the same time.[4–6] CIPF was found to carry striking similarities to human IPF. The key feature of both diseases is the abnormal accumulation of collagen in the

Discipline of Small Animal Internal Medicine, Department of Equine and Small Animal Medicine, Faculty of Veterinary Medicine, University of Helsinki, PO Box 57 (Viikintie 49), Helsinki 00014, Finland
* Corresponding author.
E-mail address: henna.laurila@helsinki.fi

Vet Clin Small Anim 50 (2020) 431–446
https://doi.org/10.1016/j.cvsm.2019.11.004
vetsmall.theclinics.com
0195-5616/20/© 2019 The Authors. Published by Elsevier Inc. This is an open access article under the CC BY license (http://creativecommons.org/licenses/by/4.0/).

lung parenchyma for no known reason.[7,8] This hampers gas exchange causing cough, exercise intolerance, and, finally, respiratory failure. In humans, IPF diagnosis signifies a worse prognosis than most cancers. During the past 2 decades, CIPF has been the subject of several studies.[9] The possibility that dogs could serve as a spontaneous animal model for human IPF has increased interest in CIPF.

Currently, CIPF is the best-described ILD affecting dogs. Studies on CIPF have focused on detailed clinicopathologic findings, histopathologic features, concomitant pulmonary hypertension (PH), high-resolution computed tomography (HRCT) findings, and outcome and prognostic factors.[8,10–18] Potential blood and bronchoalveolar lavage fluid (BALF) biomarkers of CIPF have been targeted, namely procollagen type III amino-terminal propeptide (PIIINP), endothelin-1 (ET-1), serotonin, vascular endothelial growth factor, serum Krebs von den Lungen-6, and matrix metalloproteinases (MMPs).[9,19–22] New insight has been brought to the pathogenesis and etiology by investigating surfactant protein C, BALF proteome, transforming growth factor ß (TGF-ß) signaling pathway, gene expression profiles, chemokine concentrations, respiratory microbiota, presence of reflux aspiration, association with herpesvirus infection, and potential fungal etiology and by surveying the environment and care of WHWTs with and without CIPF.[9,22–31]

The potential role of dogs in modeling of human respiratory disease has been considered in meetings and reviews of comparative medicine.[32,33] The correlation between CIPF and human IPF is only partially understood at present. Even though CIPF is not identical to human IPF, as a disease model, it is likely superior to models of induced fibrosis in the mouse used today.[33] Several aspects of the disease remain, however, unanswered. The incidence and prevalence of CIPF are not known. A better understanding of the etiology and pathogenesis could help find new therapeutic agents. Finally, the role of genetics in this disorder is still poorly understood but is under active research.

DEFINITION

CIPF and IPF belong to a heterogenous group of ILDs, which consist of several noninfectious and nonmalignant pulmonary diseases with overlapping clinicopathologic and radiographic features. A majority of the ILDs have an unknown etiology. More than 200 ILDs are recognized in humans, but many fewer are reported in dogs.[34] Because diagnosing ILD requires a thorough clinical work-up, histopathologic examination of lung tissue, and a multidisciplinary approach, it is likely that cases are undiagnosed.[34] A classification scheme modified from human medicine was proposed for canine and feline ILDs recently. It divides ILDs into (1) idiopathic interstitial pneumonias (IIPs), (2) ILDs of known cause, and (3) miscellaneous ILDs.[34] CIPF belongs to IIPs. In humans, the IIPs are a group of non-neoplastic disorders that result from damage to the lung parenchyma with varying patterns of inflammation and fibrosis.[35] Canine and feline IIPs are further classified into sporadic and familial fibrotic ILD, nonspecific interstitial pneumonia (NSIP) and lymphocytic interstitial pneumonitis, acute interstitial pneumonia, cryptogenic organizing pneumonia, and other IIPs.[34] CIPF in WHWTs is a familial fibrotic ILD. For the details of the proposed classification and the description of the other IIPs and ILDs affecting dogs and cats, readers are referred to reviews.[34,36]

CIPF is not the only term that has been used to describe this disease affecting WHWTs. Other names include IPF, chronic IPF, canine pulmonary fibrosis, chronic pulmonary disease in WHWTs, and ILD in WHWTs.[3,6,10,13,15,23] By CIPF, the authors refer to a chronic, progressive, familial fibrotic ILD of unknown cause, limited to the lungs, and occurring mainly in older WHWTs.

HISTOPATHOLOGICAL FEATURES

CIPF is characterized histopathologically by 2 different patterns of interstitial fibrosis. All affected dogs have diffuse and mature uniform fibrosis of the alveolar wall.[8,10] This varies from mild to moderate in severity and is distributed throughout the lung (**Fig. 1**A, B).[8] Most affected WHWTs also have multifocal areas of more severe, more cellular, and less mature fibrosis.[3,8,23] These areas of fibrosis occur with pronounced alveolar epithelial and luminal changes, interstitial smooth muscle hyperplasia, proliferating myofibroblasts, and occasional honeycombing (**Fig. 1**C, D).[8] Fibrosis appears accentuated either adjacent to the bronchioli or under the pleura. Only mild to moderate interstitial lymphoplasmacytic inflammation is present.[8]

When compared with human diseases, CIPF in WHWTs shares features of both human usual interstitial pneumonia (UIP), the histopathologic pattern of human IPF, and

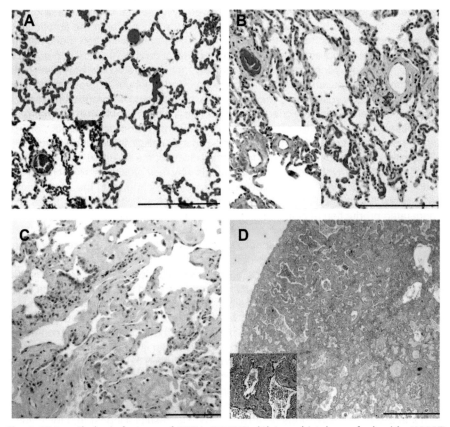

Fig. 1. Histopathologic features of CIPF in WHWTs. (*A*) Lung histology of a healthy WHWT (hematoxylin-eosin [HE]); bar, 200 μm. (*Inset*) Vessel of a healthy WHWT (Masson trichrome). (*B*) Mild diffuse mature interstitial fibrosis (HE); bar 200 μm. (*Inset*) Perivascular concentric fibrosis (Masson trichrome). (*C*) Focus of accentuated disease with severe interstitial fibrosis and type II pneumocyte hyperplasia (HE); bar, 200 μm. (*D*) Subpleural area of honeycombing and severe interstitial fibrosis (HE); bar, 1 mm. (*Inset*) Cystic fibrotic airspace within areas of honeycombing (Masson trichrome). (*From* Laurila HP. Canine idiopathic pulmonary fibrosis - clinical disease, biomarkers and histopathological features. [PhD]. Helsinki, Finland: University of Helsinki; 2015: 3-76; with permission.)

NSIP. The diffuse, mature fibrosis closely resembles the fibrosis pattern of NSIP whereas the accentuation areas are more characteristic of human UIP.[8] Fibroblast foci are a hallmark of human UIP and indicate active, ongoing fibrosis.[1,7] Although not organized in such foci, myofibroblasts likely also participate in fibrogenesis in CIPF.[8]

Whether there are differences in the histopathologic picture between CIPF, the familial fibrotic ILD affecting WHWTs, and a sporadic fibrotic ILD affecting other dog breeds remains to be investigated.

PATHOGENESIS AND ETIOLOGY

As the word idiopathic implies, the etiology of CIPF and IPF is unknown and pathologic processes are incompletely understood. The early idea of IPF as an inflammatory disease has been negated by recent research and the current hypothesis focuses on a repetitive insult to distal lung parenchyma followed by an aberrant wound healing process.[7] The injured alveolar epithelium seems to be the key player in the fibrotic lung response. Increased epithelial cell death, abnormal re-epithelialization, pneumocyte type II hyperplasia, and activation of alveolar epithelial cells participate in creating a profibrotic microenvironment.[7] The abnormally activated alveolar epithelial cells secrete growth factors, such as TGF-ß, cytokines, and other chemotactic mediators, inducing fibroblast proliferation, migration, and recruitment of fibroblast progenitor cells. After epithelial injury, the coagulation cascade is activated, which in turn has profibrotic effects. Exposure to different stimuli, including TGF-ß and wound clotting, transforms epithelial cells into fibroblasts in a process called epithelial mesenchymal cell transition. In humans, fibroblasts form small clusters, the so-called fibroblast foci, and differentiate to myofibroblasts.[7] The reasons why they organize into such foci are unknown. In WHWTs with CIPF, myofibroblasts appear scattered in the interstitium.[8] The final result is an abnormal accumulation of fibroblasts and myofibroblasts and exaggerated production of collagen and other extracellular matrix components, leading to architectural distortion characteristic of IPF lung.

The trigger for this fibrosis cascade is not known. In human IPF, research has revealed several potential epidemiologic risk factors that might contribute to the epithelial injury and apoptosis, such as cigarette smoking, exposure to environmental and occupational agents, gastroesophageal reflux leading to microaspiration, and chronic viral infections, in particular, herpesviruses.[7,37] In dogs, no association between CIPF and herpesvirus infection was found in a recent study.[30] Considering the histopathologic aspect of CIPF, the proximity of the fibrosis accentuation areas to bronchioli could indicate that an inhaled etiologic factor is involved in the pathogenesis of CIPF.[8] An epidemiologic survey for owners of WHWTs with CIPF revealed that living in an old house, lack of ventilation system, and frequent grooming in dedicated grooming facilities were associated with increased risk for CIPF.[9] Määttä and colleagues[31] detected bile acids in BALF of WHWTs with CIPF and healthy WHWTs but not in BALF of healthy dogs of other breeds. The results suggest that microaspiration due to gastroesophageal reflux could be a predisposing factor for CIPF in WHWTs.[31]

Although a majority of human IPF cases are sporadic, several genetic mutations are known to increase the risk for IPF; however, none of these has consistently been associated with IPF.[1,7] In dogs, accumulation of diseased individuals within one breed suggests that CIPF is hereditary in WHWTs. Genetic relationship to another WHWT with CIPF was associated with CIPF in the recent epidemiologic survey.[9] Despite ongoing studies, a unifying genetic factor has not yet been discovered and the strong breed predisposition of WHWTs to CIPF requires further research. One factor predisposing WHWTs to CIPF could be an increase in serum TGF-ß concentration detected both in diseased and healthy WHWTs.[26] TGF-ß is a key mediator of fibrosis and is involved in pathogenesis of CIPF.[26,27]

The diffuse mature, uniform fibrosis detected in the CIPF lung is characteristic of human NSIP. In addition to being an idiopathic disease in humans, NSIP occurs in conjunction with other conditions, such as systemic connective tissue diseases.[35] Such a disease, however, has not been reported in WHWTs to date.

It is likely that CIPF is the result of a complex puzzle of environmental insults, a specific genetic background, and other host factors contributing to the development of the disease.

SIGNALMENT AND CLINICAL SIGNS

CIPF affects mainly WHWTs. Dogs of other breeds, mainly terriers, occasionally can be affected; however, it is unclear whether the fibrotic ILD in these dogs is similar to that of WHWTs. WHWTs tend to be middle-aged or old when they first display signs. The median age at the time of clinical diagnosis varies between 8 years and 13 years in different studies,[3,11,14,16,17] although affected WHWTs as young as 3 years of age have been reported.[11,12] Human IPF typically manifests in the sixth and seventh decades and diagnosis in patients less than 50 years is rare.[1] IPF affects male humans more often than female humans, but there is no sex predisposition in dogs.[1,37]

Commonly, dogs already suffer from advanced disease when they are presented to the veterinarian. The clinical signs develop slowly and at first the affected dogs probably appear normal. The duration of clinical signs varies but usually is between 8 months and 13 months prior to diagnosis.[37] The most common clinical sign is the combination of cough and exercise intolerance, but not all the dogs cough. Other described clinical signs are respiratory difficulty, cyanosis, tachypnea, orthopnea, and collapse.[37] Some dogs develop CIPF-related complications, such as PH. In humans, an association exists between IPF and pulmonary carcinomas,[7] and the authors are aware of some cases of pulmonary carcinoma in WHWTs with CIPF.

DIAGNOSIS AND CLINICAL EXAMINATIONS

Diagnosis of CIPF is based on signalment, anamnestic information, findings in clinical examination, and HRCT as well as exclusion of other respiratory diseases. The typical signalment of a middle-aged to older WHWT improves diagnostic confidence. A definitive diagnosis is provided only by histopathologic examination of lung tissue, but lung biopsies are seldom obtained due to the invasiveness of the procedure; therefore, diagnosis often is confirmed at necropsy. Diagnosing a fibrotic ILD without histopathology in a non-WHWT breed is challenging.

Dogs with CIPF usually are bright and alert due to adaptation to slowly developing respiratory impairment. Some severely affected dogs can be cyanotic and in distress, and an abdominal breathing pattern commonly is present. Lung auscultation reveals bilateral, inspiratory Velcro crackles and sometimes also wheezes.[37] A Velcro crackle is a distinctive pathologic lung sound that mimics the sound heard when separating 2 strips of Velcro.[38] Velcro crackles are hypothesized to result from sudden opening or closing of distorted distal airspaces. In humans, Velcro crackles can be the first sign of IPF.[38] If a WHWT with CIPF is breathing very shallowly, Velcro crackles might not be audible even in advanced CIPF, although in some dogs, crackles can be heard without a stethoscope when the dog is breathing with an open mouth.[14] The authors pay special attention to lung auscultation in older WHWTs even if they do not have clinical signs indicating respiratory disease to provide early detection of potential disease. A soft right-sided murmur is heard in some dogs with tricuspid regurgitation due to PH. CIPF does not cause weight loss.[15]

CIPF is not associated with changes in serum biochemistry or hematology, but these analyses are performed to rule out other reasons for exercise intolerance.[3,14] The lack of polycythemia in CIPF is interesting and, in humans, polycythemia is not linked to IPF as it is to other chronic hypoxemic diseases. The reason for this is not known.[39] CIPF does not cause an elevation in serum C-reactive protein.[40] Fecal examinations, including the flotation and Baermann sedimentation methods, are performed to rule out pulmonary parasites.

ARTERIAL OXYGENATION

Arterial blood gas (ABG) analysis is used to estimate lung function objectively and to determine the severity of CIPF. Repeated ABG analyses also are an easy tool for evaluating disease progression in dogs.[15] Estimates of oxygenation obtained by pulse oximetry can be misleading in unanesthetized WHWTs and, therefore, are not recommended by the authors.[15]

Hypoxemia is a key clinical consequence of CIPF. An ABG analysis can reveal a surprisingly low Pao_2 and high alveolar-arterial oxygen gradient (PAo_2 - Pao_2) in a WHWT with CIPF (**Table 1**). Despite this, most dogs are not in respiratory distress, indicating adaptation to a chronic, slowly progressing disease. Elevation of $Paco_2$ is not a feature of CIPF.[14,16,18] ABG findings of CIPF are in line with those of human IPF.[39,41]

6-MINUTE WALK TEST

A 6-minute walk test is a submaximal exercise test that measures the distance an individual is capable of walking over 6 minutes. It is used to evaluate exercise capacity in human IPF and can be used in CIPF as well without any special equipment or training.[15,16] It is not a diagnostic tool, instead, repeated $P(A-a)o_2$ measurements of the distance walked in 6 minutes can be used to monitor the changes in exercise tolerance of WHWTs with CIPF and, therefore, the progression of the disease. The median distance walked was significantly lower in WHWTs with CIPF (398 m, range 273 m–519 m) compared with healthy aged WHWTs (492 m, range 420 m–568 m).[15]

Table 1 Arterial blood gas analysis in older West Highland white terriers with canine idiopathic pulmonary fibrosis (40 dogs) and healthy West Highland white terriers (32 dogs, all >7 y)		
	West Highland White Terriers with Canine Idiopathic Pulmonary Fibrosis	**Healthy West Highland White Terriers**
Pao_2	60.1 ± 10.2 (33.5–87.4) mm Hg	97.1 ± 6.7 (86.1–113.0) mm Hg
(PAo_2 - Pao_2)	55.0 ± 12.2 (28.0–84.7) mm Hg	18.7 ± 5.3 (9.8–29.9) mm Hg
$Paco_2$	29.2 ± 3.6 (21.2–35.7) mm Hg	29.2 ± 4.3 (19.9–36.8) mm Hg

In CIPF dogs, ABG analysis was performed at the time of diagnosis. CIPF was confirmed by HRCT and/or histopathology. Healthy WHWTs had no clinical signs or HRCT findings indicating respiratory disease. Dogs participated in research projects at the Veterinary Teaching Hospital of the University of Helsinki, Finland. Results are given as mean ± SD and range.

PULMONARY HYPERTENSION

PH develops in many WHWTs with CIPF. Different studies have documented echocardiographic findings indicating PH in approximately 20% to 60% of diseased WHWTs.[12,14,16,17] Similarly, PH is estimated to affect 32% to 50% of human IPF patients and is related to increased mortality.[42] The clinical signs of PH (exercise intolerance and syncope) do not differ from the signs of CIPF.[43] Therefore, Doppler echocardiography is required to search for PH, especially if the dog has a soft right-sided murmur or if thoracic radiographs raise suspicion of right-sided cardiac enlargement. PH is thought to result from an imbalance between pulmonary arterial vasoconstriction and vasodilatation, vascular remodeling due to an advanced lung disease, and chronic hypoxemia. Nevertheless, the pathogenesis of PH is likely much more complex than this and is not yet thoroughly understood.[42]

THORACIC RADIOGRAPHY

Thoracic radiographs of WHWTs with CIPF commonly show a bronchointerstitial pattern, which is already moderate to severe when the animal is presented to the veterinarian.[37] In addition to interstitial infiltrates, predominantly bronchial and patchy alveolar patterns also are reported.[9] Changes in thoracic radiographs are neither sensitive nor specific for CIPF, and the main reason for taking them is to rule out other lung diseases, such as neoplasia.[37]

Identifying early radiographic changes of CIPF is problematic, because healthy older WHWTs also can have mild bronchial or bronchointerstitial patterns in thoracic radiographs.[14] Additionally, the thick skin typical for WHWTs can make the interpretation of subtle changes difficult. Thoracic radiography is not helpful in evaluating the progression of CIPF, because the changes vary independently of clinical signs (**Fig. 2**).[15] Cardiac and pulmonary arterial enlargement can be present in thoracic radiographs, caused mainly by PH.

HIGH-RESOLUTION COMPUTED TOMOGRAPHY

HRCT provides superior evaluation of the lung compared with conventional radiographs. If HRCT findings are characteristic, lung biopsy is not necessary to confirm IPF in humans.[1] HRCT also is useful in diagnosing CIPF. The HRCT features of WHWTs with CIPF have been assessed by several studies.[11,13,14,16–18] The most frequent finding is ground-glass opacity (GGO) described as a hazy increased opacity of the lungs, with preservation of bronchial and vascular margins. Mosaic attenuation pattern also is frequently observed[16,17] and may indicate a more advanced disease.[17] Linear and reticular opacities are common, whereas traction bronchiectasis and honeycombing are detected more rarely. Consolidation can occur, and, in some dogs, bronchial wall thickening or nodules have been described (**Fig. 3**).

In humans, extensive GGO points toward an alternative diagnosis, such as NSIP, whereas honeycombing, traction bronchiectasis, coarse reticulation, and architectural distortion are characteristic of IPF.[44] Therefore, the HRCT features of CIPF share characteristics of both human IPF and NSIP.[9]

When lung tissue attenuation is evaluated quantitatively by measuring computed tomography values, values are significantly higher in WHWTs with CIPF than in healthy WHWTs.[14,17,18]

To avoid the risks of general anesthesia, the authors use a modified VetMouseTrap positioning device (Universal Medical Systems Inc., Solon, OH) (**Fig. 4**). It limits the dog's motion and enables HR CT imaging with no or only minimal sedation. The

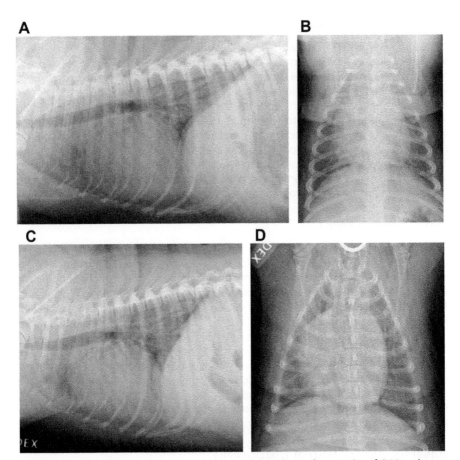

Fig. 2. Thoracic radiography is not a sensitive tool to evaluate the severity of CIPF as demonstrated by these images. Right lateral and ventrodorsal radiographs from a 12-year-old WHWT with moderate CIPF (Pao$_2$ 82 mm Hg) (*A, B*) and from another 12-year-old WHWT with more severe CIPF (Pao$_2$ 64 mm Hg) (*C, D*). The images show moderate (*B*) to severe (*A, C, D*) generalized bronchointerstitial lung patterns and a large cardiac shadow. Extreme skin folds increase the overall opacity of the lungs. ([*A, B*] *From* Laurila HP. Canine idiopathic pulmonary fibrosis - clinical disease, biomarkers and histopathological features. [PhD]. Helsinki, Finland: University of Helsinki; 2015: 3-76; with permission; and [*C, D*] *Courtesy of* Anu K. Lappalainen, DVM, PhD, University of Helsinki, Finland.)

method was found feasible in discriminating healthy from diseased WHWTs.[18] When HR CT images obtained under sedation were compared with those obtained under anesthesia, both underestimation and overestimation of GGO and mosaic attenuation patterns were observed.[16]

BRONCHOSCOPY AND BRONCHOALVEOLAR LAVAGE

Bronchoscopy and BALF provide useful information about the lung and airways, but the findings are not specific for CIPF. Many dogs with CIPF have some degree of bronchial involvement (**Fig. 5**). It is not known whether this is an individual phenomenon, related to underlying CIPF, or connected to cough. The presence of bronchoscopic

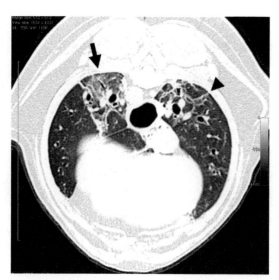

Fig. 3. A transverse HRCT image at the level of caudal lung lobes in an 11-year-old WHWT with CIPF and a Pao₂ of 57 mm Hg. Areas of GGO (*arrow*) and traction bronchiectasis (*arrowhead*) are seen dorsally. The images were obtained under general anesthesia. (*Courtesy of* Anu K. Lappalainen, DVM, PhD, University of Helsinki, Finland.)

changes cannot be used to differentiate CIPF from CB. Bronchial changes, however, such as hyperemia, mucus accumulation, and mucosal irregularities, usually are more profound in CB than in CIPF.[37] Bronchoscopy requires general anesthesia. The decision to perform bronchoscopy must be considered from the perspective of benefits versus risks. Bronchoscopy should be pursued, especially when there is discrepancy between clinical data and HRCT findings or suspicion of infection or other disease process or if CIPF is suspected in a young WHWT or in a dog of a non-WHWT breed. The general condition and the severity of hypoxemia determine whether a dog is fit for the procedure. In the authors' experience, careful planning of anesthesia with

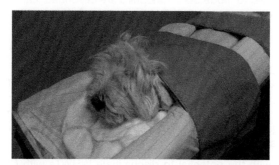

Fig. 4. Photograph illustrating use of the modified VetMouseTrap™ (Universal Medical Systems Inc., Solon, OH.) The device is used without the lid, and padding is added inside the device. (From Holopainen S, Rautala E, Lilja-Maula L, et al. Thoracic high resolution CT using the modified VetMousetrap™ device is a feasible method for diagnosing canine idiopathic pulmonary fibrosis in awake West Highland white terriers. Vet Radiol Ultrasound. 2019; 60(5):525-532; with permission.)

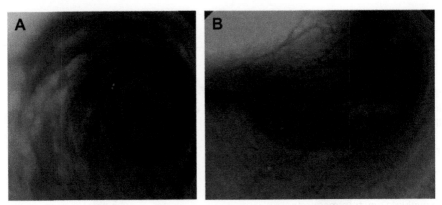

Fig. 5. Bronchoscopic images from WHWTs with CIPF. (*A*) Moderate bronchial mucosal irregularity in a 12-year-old WHWT with CIPF. (*B*) Grade II tracheal collapse viewed at the level of carina in a 12-year-old WHWT with CIPF. (*From* Laurila HP. Canine idiopathic pulmonary fibrosis - clinical disease, biomarkers and histopathological features. [PhD]. Helsinki, Finland: University of Helsinki; 2015: 3-76; with permission.)

supplemental oxygen before, during, and after bronchoscopy make scoping possible even in severely hypoxemic WHWTs with CIPF.

Bronchoscopic changes reported in CIPF are bronchial mucosal irregularity, mild to moderate increases in bronchial mucus, bronchomalacia, dynamic airway collapse, and bronchiectasis.[3,14,16] Additionally, tracheal collapse, usually mild to moderate, seems to be common in WHWTs with CIPF.[3,14,16] The significance of this finding and its possible relationship to the underlying ILD is unclear, and the authors have also detected tracheal collapse in clinically healthy old WHWTs.[14] Bronchial mucosal irregularity can be explained at least partly by age-related changes.[14,45]

BALF analysis of WHWTs with CIPF usually shows an increase in the total cell count due to increased numbers of macrophages, neutrophils, and mast cells. Bacterial growth is uncommon.[9,14] BALF analysis is not routinely recommended in the diagnostic evaluation of human IPF, but it can be useful in excluding other ILDs or evaluating infection or malignancy.[1] In human IPF, increased total cell count, BALF neutrophilia, and mild to moderate eosinophilia are described. Lack of lymphocytosis supports the IPF diagnosis. In NSIP, BALF lymphocytosis is typical.[46,47]

BIOMARKERS

Reaching CIPF diagnosis can require HRCT, which is expensive and not always applicable, or histologic investigation of lung tissue. The lack of CIPF-specific therapy, however, questions the benefits of surgical lung biopsy. Therefore, identification of a noninvasive fibrosis biomarker could be helpful. Both screening and targeted investigational approaches have been used in the biomarker search with promising results.[9]

- Biomarkers with the potential to discriminate WHWTs with CIPF from healthy WHWTs are serum and BALF ET-1, serum and BALF chemokine (C-C) ligand 2, BALF interleukin-8, BALF PIIINP, and BALF MMP-9.[19–21,29]
- Biomarkers with the potential to differentiate WHWTs with CIPF from dogs with chronic bronchitis (CB) are serum and BALF ET-1, BALF PIIINP, BALF MMP-9, and BALF MMP-2.[19–21]

- Biomarkers that might be related to the predisposition of WHWT breed for CIPF are serum TGF-ß, serum interleukin-8, and possibly serum Krebs von den Lungen-6. The concentrations of these markers were higher in serum of WHWTs compared with other breeds.[9,22,26]

Further studies are necessary to confirm these findings, to find novel biomarkers, and to investigate combinations of these that have the highest predictive values. Ideally, a biomarker that differentiates WHWTs that will develop CIPF from those that will not would be available to select WHWTs for breeding.

TREATMENT

Currently, there are no effective treatments for CIPF. No treatment trials have been performed on dogs with CIPF, and the studies published on CIPF have not been designed to evaluate any treatment effect.[37] Pharmacologic treatment options for human IPF are scarce as well. No known treatment can stop the progression or reverse the fibrotic changes. IPF is the leading indication for lung transplantation in humans worldwide.[48]

Knowledge about IPF pathogenesis has shifted treatment targets from inflammation toward the aberrant wound healing process. What used to be a standard-of-care combination therapy with prednisone, azathioprine, and N-acetylcysteine was revealed to be harmful in human IPF. At present, human IPF-specific therapy is based on 2 novel antifibrotics, pirfenidone and nintedanib. Both can slow the decline in lung function but do not result in cure.[49]

Pirfenidone has well-established antifibrotic, antioxidant, and anti-inflammatory effects.[49] It might be considered for treatment of CIPF. Although the pharmacokinetics of pirfenidone have been studied in dogs, the safety is not known and there are no clinical reports of its use in dogs.[37] Currently, pirfenidone is expensive: treating a WHWT would cost 12€ to 17€ ($13–$20) per day (July 2019) if the pirfenidone dose is extrapolated from humans.

Nintedanib is an intracellular inhibitor of multiple tyrosine kinases with potent antifibrotic and anti-inflammatory effects in animal models.[49] A recent study suggested that nintedanib extends life expectancy in human patients with IPF.[50] Unfortunately, in toxicology studies of nintedanib, dogs suffered from severe gastrointestinal adverse effects even with low doses of the drug.[51]

In CIPF, treatment is used mainly to reduce clinical signs on an individual basis and to alleviate complications.[37] Many WHWTs with CIPF receive corticosteroids. Corcoran and colleagues[3] reported that some dogs with CIPF seem to respond to corticosteroid treatment. Based on the authors' experience, corticosteroids reduce cough in many dogs; however, the authors have not observed any clear long-term improvement in arterial oxygenation.[15] In human IPF, corticosteroids are not recommended as disease-modifying therapy due to adverse effects and lack of efficacy.[52] In NSIP, however, oral corticosteroids form the basis of the treatment alone or in combination with other immunosuppressive agents. Human patients with a less common, cellular NSIP respond well whereas patients with a more common, fibrosing NSIP do far worse but still survive longer than patients with IPF.[53] If corticosteroids are chosen as an empirical therapy for CIPF, it is up to the veterinarian to decide whether to give it orally or via inhalation. No studies exist to support either use. Given the potential benefit of corticosteroids in human NSIP, an oral route might be elected. On the other hand, considering the lack of efficacy in human IPF, concurrent bronchial changes could be targeted instead of the interstation, and, therefore, inhaled steroids might be a better option, especially in old WHWTs with concomitant diseases.

Combination therapy with corticosteroids and theophylline has been recommended for treatment of CIPF and is also the authors' choice.[3] Theophylline causes mild bronchodilatation, enhances mucociliary clearance, and increases contractibility of the diaphragmatic muscle.[54]

WHWTs with CIPF might benefit from use of proton pump inhibitors or histamine H_2 receptor blockers. This is supported by the finding of microaspiration in WHWTs with CIPF.[31] Gastroesophageal reflux with microaspiration is common in human IPF and predisposes to lung injury. Antiacid therapy is recommended for the treatment of all human patients with IPF[1] because it could slow disease progression and reduce the risk of acute worsening of IPF in humans.[55] Because it is a low-cost treatment and unlikely harmful, it can be used in WHWTs with CIPF as well.

Treatment of PH usually focuses first on management of the underlying disease; however, because no effective treatment exists for CIPF, treatment of concurrent PH is directly targeted to reduce pulmonary arterial pressure. A recent meta-analysis in human medicine did not support the theoretic concern that hypoxemia could worsen with PH treatment because of deterioration in ventilation-perfusion mismatch.[56] Data on the use of sildenafil in human IPF-related PH are conflicting and the authors of the official management guidelines of human IPF do not take a stand for or against its use.[49] Although no study has evaluated the benefits and adverse effects of sildenafil in CIPF-related PH, sildenafil therapy has been investigated in dogs with PH in general and has been reported to improve clinical signs and quality of life. The authors prescribe sildenafil to WHWTs with CIPF that have echocardiographic measurements suggesting PH.

WHWTs with CIPF can experience acute worsening of respiratory function during the disease course. The cause for such worsening, for example, a bacterial pneumonia, should be treated appropriately. If no cause is found, the dog could be suffering from an acute exacerbation (AE) of CIPF, histopathologically characterized by diffuse alveolar damage.[15,28] The etiology of AE in human IPF is unknown, but it is likely triggered by an acute insult, for example, microaspiration, infection, or stress due to bronchoscopy or surgery, which then leads to severe acute lung injury. Despite empirical treatment with a high dose of corticosteroids and broad-spectrum antibiotics, the short-term mortality of AE of IPF in humans is very high.[57] Likewise, the expected outcome for a WHWT having AE of CIPF is poor.

Pulmonary rehabilitation and long-term oxygen therapy are recommended for humans with IPF.[1] The authors encourage the owners of WHWTs with CIPF to continue routine daily walks with their dogs, unless the dog shows signs of exhaustion. Long-term oxygen therapy is not feasible in dogs, although intermittent treatment might be possible in some dogs.

CLINICAL COURSE AND SURVIVAL

Although diseased WHWTs usually are already old at the time of disease recognition, CIPF has a negative impact on survival. Median survival was reported to be 32 months (range 2–51 months) from the onset of clinical signs and 11 months (range 0–40 months) from diagnosis (**Fig. 6**).[15] In humans, the median survival after diagnosis is 2 years to 3 years in IPF and 6 years to 13.5 years in fibrotic NSIP.[1,53] Predicting the disease course for an individual WHWT is difficult, because of the lack of prognostic markers. Only high-serum chemokine (C-C) ligand 2 at the time of diagnosis and the severity of CT findings were found to be negatively associated with survival.[9] As in human IPF, CIPF in WHWTs can have either a slow or rapid disease progression. When diseased WHWTs were followed over time, 5 of 15 WHWTs with CIPF needed to

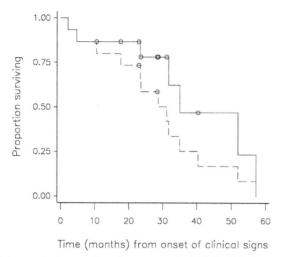

Fig. 6. Kaplan-Meier survival curves for all-cause survival (*dashed line*) and CIPF-specific survival (*solid line*) of WHWTs with CIPF from onset of clinical signs. Circles indicate censored animals (all-cause survival: WHWTs alive at study endpoint; CIPF-specific survival: WHWTs alive and those who died of non–CIPF-related causes). (*From* Lilja-Maula LIO, Laurila HP, Syrjä P, et al. Long-term outcome and use of 6-minute walk test in West Highland white terriers with idiopathic pulmonary fibrosis. J Vet Intern Med 2014;28:379-85; with permission.)

be euthanized because of AE.[15] Further research into the etiopathogenesis and genetics of CIPF is needed, along with searches for viable biomarkers for disease as well as disease progression.

DISCLOSURE

The authors have nothing to disclose.

ACKNOWLEDGMENTS

The authors thank the funding sources: Orion-Farmos Research Foundation, Finnish Veterinary Association, Finnish Veterinary Research Foundation, and the Finnish West Highland White Terrier Breeding Club.

REFERENCES

1. Raghu G, Collard HR, Egan JJ, et al. An official ATS/ERS/JRS/ALAT statement: idiopathic pulmonary fibrosis: evidence-based guidelines for diagnosis and management. Am J Respir Crit Care Med 2011;183:788–824.
2. Cohn LA, Norris CR, Hawkins EC, et al. Identification and characterization of an idiopathic pulmonary fibrosis-like condition in cats. J Vet Intern Med 2004;18: 632–41.
3. Corcoran BM, Cobb M, Martin MW, et al. Chronic pulmonary disease in West Highland white terriers. Vet Rec 1999;144:611–6.
4. Corcoran BM, Dukes-McEwan J, Rhind S, et al. Idiopathic pulmonary fibrosis in a Staffordshire bull terrier with hypothyroidism. J Small Anim Pract 1999;40:185–8.
5. Lobetti RG, Milner R, Lane E. Chronic idiopathic pulmonary fibrosis in five dogs. J Am Anim Hosp Assoc 2001;37:119–27.

6. Webb JA, Armstrong J. Chronic idiopathic pulmonary fibrosis in a West Highland white terrier. Can Vet J 2002;43:703–5.

7. King TE Jr, Pardo A, Selman M. Idiopathic pulmonary fibrosis. Lancet 2011;378: 1949–61.

8. Syrjä P, Heikkilä H, Lilja-Maula L, et al. The histopathology of idiopathic pulmonary fibrosis in West Highland white terriers shares features of both nonspecific interstitial pneumonia and usual interstitial pneumonia in man. J Comp Pathol 2013;149:303–13.

9. Clercx C, Fastrès A, Roels E. Idiopathic pulmonary fibrosis in West Highland white terriers: an update. Vet J 2018;242:53–8.

10. Norris AJ, Naydan DK, Wilson DW. Interstitial lung disease in West Highland White Terriers. Vet Pathol 2005;42:35–41.

11. Johnson VS, Corcoran BM, Wotton PR, et al. Thoracic high-resolution computed tomographic findings in dogs with canine idiopathic pulmonary fibrosis. J Small Anim Pract 2005;46:381–8.

12. Schober KE, Baade H. Doppler echocardiographic prediction of pulmonary hypertension in West Highland white terriers with chronic pulmonary disease. J Vet Intern Med 2006;20:912–20.

13. Corcoran BM, King LG, Schwarz T, et al. Further characterisation of the clinical features of chronic pulmonary disease in West Highland white terriers. Vet Rec 2011;168:355.

14. Heikkilä HP, Lappalainen AK, Day MJ, et al. Clinical, bronchoscopic, histopathologic, diagnostic imaging, and arterial oxygenation findings in West Highland white terriers with idiopathic pulmonary fibrosis. J Vet Intern Med 2011;25:433–9.

15. Lilja-Maula LIO, Laurila HP, Syrjä P, et al. Long-term outcome and use of 6-minute walk test in West Highland white terriers with idiopathic pulmonary fibrosis. J Vet Intern Med 2014;28:379–85.

16. Roels E, Couvreur T, Farnir F, et al. Comparison between sedation and general anesthesia for high resolution computed tomographic characterization of canine idiopathic pulmonary fibrosis in West Highland white terriers. Vet Radiol Ultrasound 2017;58:284–94.

17. Thierry F, Handel I, Hammond G, et al. Further characterization of computed tomographic and clinical features for staging and prognosis of idiopathic pulmonary fibrosis in West Highland white terriers. Vet Radiol Ultrasound 2017;58: 381–8.

18. Holopainen S, Rautala E, Lilja-Maula L, et al. Thoracic high resolution CT using the modified VetMousetrap™ device is a feasible method for diagnosing canine idiopathic pulmonary fibrosis in awake West Highland White Terriers [published online ahead of print, June 7, 2019]. Vet Radiol Ultrasound 2019. https://doi.org/10.1111/vru.12779.

19. Heikkilä HP, Krafft E, de Lorenzi D, et al. Matrix metalloproteinase -2 and -9 in bronchoalveolar lavage fluid of dogs with idiopathic pulmonary fibrosis and chronic bronchitis. Proceedings of the 21st ECVIM-CA Congress. Seville, Spain, September 8-10, 2011. p. 213.

20. Krafft E, Heikkilä H, Jespers P, et al. Serum and bronchoalveolar lavage fluid endothelin-1 concentrations as diagnostic biomarkers of canine idiopathic pulmonary fibrosis. J Vet Intern Med 2011;25:990–6.

21. Heikkilä HP, Krafft E, Jespers P, et al. Procollagen type III amino terminal propeptide concentrations in dogs with idiopathic pulmonary fibrosis compared with chronic bronchitis and eosinophilic bronchopneumopathy. Vet J 2013;196:52–6.

22. Roels E, Krafft E, Antoine N, et al. Evaluation of chemokines CXCL8 and CCL2, serotonin, and vascular endothelial growth factor serum concentrations in healthy dogs from seven breeds with variable predisposition for canine idiopathic pulmonary fibrosis. Res Vet Sci 2015;101:57–62.
23. Erikson M, von Euler H, Ekman E, et al. Surfactant protein C in canine pulmonary fibrosis. J Vet Intern Med 2009;23:1170–4.
24. Lilja-Maula LIO, Palviainen MJ, Heikkilä HP, et al. Proteomic analysis of bronchoalveolar lavage fluid samples obtained from West Highland White Terriers with idiopathic pulmonary fibrosis, dogs with chronic bronchitis, and healthy dogs. Am J Vet Res 2013;74:148–54.
25. Krafft E, Laurila HP, Peters IR, et al. Analysis of gene expression in canine idiopathic pulmonary fibrosis. Vet J 2013;198:479–86.
26. Krafft E, Lybaert P, Roels E, et al. Transforming growth factor beta 1 activation, storage, and signaling pathways in idiopathic pulmonary fibrosis in dogs. J Vet Intern Med 2014;28:1666–75.
27. Lilja-Maula L, Syrjä P, Laurila HP, et al. Comparative study of transforming growth factor-β signaling and regulatory molecules in human and canine idiopathic pulmonary fibrosis. J Comp Pathol 2014;150:399–407.
28. Lilja-Maula L, Syrjä P, Laurila HP, et al. Upregulation of alveolar levels of activin B, but not activin A, in lungs of West Highland white terriers with idiopathic pulmonary fibrosis and diffuse alveolar damage. J Comp Pathol 2015;152:192–200.
29. Roels E, Krafft E, Farnir F, et al. Assessment of CCL2 and CXCL8 chemokines in serum, bronchoalveolar lavage fluid and lung tissue samples from dogs affected with canine idiopathic pulmonary fibrosis. Vet J 2015;206:75–82.
30. Roels E, Dourcy M, Holopainen S, et al. No evidence of Herpesvirus infection in West Highland White Terriers with canine idiopathic pulmonary fibrosis. Vet Pathol 2016;53:1210–2.
31. Määttä OLM, Laurila HP, Holopainen S, et al. Reflux aspiration in lungs of dogs with respiratory disease and in healthy West Highland White Terriers. J Vet Intern Med 2018;32:2074–81.
32. Williams K, Roman J. Studying human respiratory disease in animals–role of induced and naturally occurring models. J Pathol 2016;238:220–32.
33. Barnes T, Brown KK, Corcoran B, et al. Research in pulmonary fibrosis across species: unleashing discovery through comparative biology. Am J Med Sci 2019;357:399–404.
34. Reinero C. Interstitial lung diseases in dogs and cats part I: the idiopathic interstitial pneumonias. Vet J 2019;243:48–54.
35. Travis WD, Costabel U, Hansell DM, et al. An official American Thoracic Society/European Respiratory Society statement: update of the international multidisciplinary classification of the idiopathic interstitial pneumonias. Am J Respir Crit Care Med 2013;188:733–48.
36. Reinero C. Interstitial lung diseases in dogs and cats part II: known cause and other discrete forms. Vet J 2019;243:55–64.
37. Heikkilä-Laurila HP, Rajamäki MM. Idiopathic pulmonary fibrosis in West Highland white terriers. Vet Clin North Am Small Anim Pract 2014;44:129–42.
38. Sgalla G, Walsh SLF, Sverzellati N, et al. "Velcro-type" crackles predict specific radiologic features of fibrotic interstitial lung disease. BMC Pulm Med 2018;18:103.
39. Crystal RG, Fulmer JD, Roberts WC, et al. Idiopathic pulmonary fibrosis: clinical, histologic, radiographic, physiologic, scintigraphic, cytologic, and biochemical aspects. Ann Intern Med 1976;85:769–88.

40. Viitanen SJ, Laurila HP, Lilja-Maula LI, et al. Serum C-reactive protein as a diagnostic biomarker in dogs with bacterial respiratory diseases. J Vet Intern Med 2014;28:84–91.

41. Nava S, Rubini F. Lung and chest wall mechanics in ventilated patients with end stage idiopathic pulmonary fibrosis. Thorax 1999;54:390–5.

42. Collum SD, Amione-Guerra J, Cruz-Solbes AS, et al. Pulmonary hypertension associated with idiopathic pulmonary fibrosis: current and future perspectives. Can Respir J 2017;2017:1430350.

43. Kellihan HB, Waller KR, Pinkos A, et al. Acute resolution of pulmonary alveolar infiltrates in 10 dogs with pulmonary hypertension treated with sildenafil citrate: 2005–2014. J Vet Cardiol 2015;17:182–91.

44. Gotway MB, Freemer MM, King TE Jr. Challenges in pulmonary fibrosis. 1: use of high resolution CT scanning of the lung for the evaluation of patients with idiopathic interstitial pneumonias. Thorax 2007;62:546–53.

45. Mercier E, Bolognin M, Hoffmann AC, et al. Influence of age on bronchoscopic findings in healthy beagle dogs. Vet J 2011;187:225–8.

46. Domagala-Kulawik J, Skirecki T, Chazan R. Diagnostic value of total cell count in bronchoalveolar lavage fluid from patients with interstitial lung diseases. Eur Respir J Suppl 2009;34:107.

47. Meyer KC, Raghu G, Baughman RP, et al. An official American Thoracic Society clinical practice guideline: the clinical utility of bronchoalveolar lavage cellular analysis in interstitial lung disease. Am J Respir Crit Care Med 2012;185:1004–14.

48. George PM, Patterson CM, Reed AK, et al. Lung transplantation for idiopathic pulmonary fibrosis. Lancet Respir Med 2019;7:271–82.

49. Raghu G, Rochwerg B, Zhang Y, et al. An official ATS/ERS/JRS/ALAT clinical practice guideline: treatment of idiopathic pulmonary fibrosis. an update of the 2011 clinical practice guideline. Am J Respir Crit Care Med 2015;192:e3–19.

50. Lancaster L, Crestani B, Hernandez P, et al. Safety and survival data in patients with idiopathic pulmonary fibrosis treated with nintedanib: pooled data from six clinical trials. BMJ Open Respir Res 2019;6:e000397.

51. Ofev. Available at: https://www.ema.europa.eu/en/documents/assessment-report/ofev-epar-public-assessment-report_en.pdf. Accessed July 10, 2019.

52. Sköld CM, Bendstrup E, Myllärniemi M, et al. Treatment of idiopathic pulmonary fibrosis: a position paper from a Nordic expert group. J Intern Med 2016;281:149–66.

53. Kim DS, Collard HR, King TE Jr. Classification and natural history of the idiopathic interstitial pneumonias. Proc Am Thorac Soc 2006;3:285–92.

54. Plumb DC. Plumb's veterinary drug handbook. 7th edition. Ames (IA): Wiley-Blackwell; 2011.

55. Lee JS, Collard HR, Anstrom KJ, et al. Anti-acid treatment and disease progression in idiopathic pulmonary fibrosis: an analysis of data from three randomised controlled trials. Lancet Respir Med 2013;1:369–76.

56. Prins KW, Duval S, Markowitz J, et al. Chronic use of PAH-specific therapy in World Health Organization Group III Pulmonary Hypertension: a systematic review and meta-analysis. Pulm Circ 2017;7:145–55.

57. Collard HR, Ryerson CJ, Corte TJ, et al. Acute exacerbation of idiopathic pulmonary fibrosis. An international working group report. Am J Respir Crit Care Med 2016;194:265–75.

Bacterial Pneumonia in Dogs and Cats: An Update

Jonathan D. Dear, MAS, DVM

KEYWORDS

- Bacterial pneumonia • Lower respiratory tract infection • Canine • Feline
- Lower airway disease

KEY POINTS

- Clinically, bacterial pneumonia is diagnosed much more commonly in dogs than in cats, although it is likely under-recognized in cats.
- Viral infection followed by bacterial invasion is common in young dogs, whereas aspiration pneumonia and foreign body pneumonia seem to be more common in older dogs.
- Clinical signs can be acute or chronic and do not always reflect the underlying respiratory condition.
- Definitive diagnosis requires detection of intracellular bacteria in airway cytology or clinically significant bacterial growth from an airway sample, although relevant clinical findings can also support a clinical diagnosis.
- Treatment requires identification and management of underlying diseases associated with pneumonia, appropriate antimicrobial therapy, and control of airway secretions.

INTRODUCTION

Bacterial pneumonia remains one of the most common clinical diagnoses in dogs with acute or chronic respiratory disease. Research suggests a complex relationship between viral respiratory diseases, environmental factors, and development of bacterial and mycoplasmal respiratory infection in dogs. In cats, bacterial pneumonia is less commonly identified than is inflammatory feline bronchial disease, although it might be overlooked because of similarities in clinical presentation and diagnostic findings.

CLASSIFICATION OF BACTERIAL PNEUMONIA
Aspiration

Aspiration pneumonia results from the inadvertent inhalation of gastric acid, oropharyngeal secretions, and/or ingesta and remains a common cause of bacterial

Department of Medicine and Epidemiology, University of California, Davis, One Shields Avenue, Davis, CA 95616, USA
E-mail address: jddear@ucdavis.edu
Twitter: @jddear (J.D.D.)

Vet Clin Small Anim 50 (2020) 447–465
https://doi.org/10.1016/j.cvsm.2019.10.007
0195-5616/20/© 2019 Elsevier Inc. All rights reserved.
vetsmall.theclinics.com

pneumonia, accounting for roughly 23% of clinical diagnoses in a study of human patients admitted to the intensive care unit.[1] Although the true incidence of aspiration pneumonia related to all causes is not well described in veterinary medicine, the incidence of postanesthesia or sedation aspiration pneumonia was reported to be 0.17% in 1 large multi-institution study.[2] Other than anesthesia, various conditions predispose to this disease. Risk factors that have been identified for the development of aspiration pneumonia include esophageal disease, refractory vomiting, seizures, and laryngeal dysfunction[3] (**Table 1**).

In healthy animals, physiologic and anatomic features reduce the chance of aspiration. During a normal swallow, fluid and food are propelled caudally into the oropharynx and through the upper esophageal sphincter by contraction of the oral cavity, pharynx, and tongue. Concurrently, the epiglottis retracts to cover the laryngeal aditus and protect the trachea from particulate inhalation. In addition, adduction of the arytenoid cartilages contributes to further occlusion of the upper airways. Any process impeding these primary defenses or inhibiting normal swallowing reflexes greatly enhances the likelihood of aspiration.

Aspiration injury results from inhalation of either sterile, acidic gastric contents (resulting from vomiting or gastric regurgitation) or of septic material from either gastric or oral secretions. Irritation induced by acid inhalation promotes a local environment in which bacterial colonization can develop and lead to bacterial pneumonia.[4] The severity of disease varies depending on the quantity and nature of the material aspirated as well as the length of time between the event and diagnosis. Conscious animals with intact airway reflexes tend to cough and prevent massive aspiration injury. Animals under anesthesia or with reduced airway reflexes caused by neurologic disorders are less likely to cough in response to the aspiration event and are, therefore, more likely to develop diffuse pulmonary infiltrates and serious lung injury. In many instances, aspiration injuries occur under general anesthesia and it should be noted that the presence of a cuffed endotracheal tube does not prevent inadvertent aspiration.

Table 1
Factors associated with aspiration pneumonia

• Gastrointestinal disease o Refractory vomiting caused by systemic or metabolic disease o Pancreatitis o Intussusception o Foreign body obstruction o Ileus	• Anesthesia o Prolonged anesthesia o Postprocedural upper airway obstruction
• Esophageal disease o Megaesophagus o Esophageal motility disorder o Hiatal hernia o Esophageal stricture o Esophagitis	• Neurologic disease o Polyneuropathy o Myasthenia gravis o Seizure o Conditions leading to prolonged recumbency
• Cricopharyngeal dyssynchrony • Muscular dystrophy • Oropharyngeal dysphagia • Laryngeal disease • Tracheostomy	• Breed o Brachycephalic breeds o Golden retriever o Cocker spaniel o English springer spaniel o Irish wolfhound

Data from Refs.[18,33–35]

Studies have shown that concurrent use of cisapride with a proton-pump inhibitor reduces the incidence of gastroesophageal reflux under anesthesia[5,6] and therefore might reduce the likelihood of aspiration pneumonia.

Canine Infectious Pneumonia

Infectious, or community-acquired, pneumonias in dogs often begin with viral colonization and infection of the upper respiratory tract with canine respiratory coronavirus, adenovirus, herpesvirus, pneumovirus, parainfluenza virus, or others.[7] Often, such diseases are acute and self-limiting, but, in a subset of dogs, inflammation associated with these organisms immobilizes the host's immune defenses and predisposes to infection with other (often bacterial) respiratory pathogens.[8] Many bacteria have been implicated in canine infectious respiratory disease, although special focus has been directed toward *Streptococcus* (specifically *Streptococcus equi* subsp *zooepidemicus* and *Streptococcus canis*), *Mycoplasma cynos*, and *Bordetella bronchiseptica*.[9]

Canine infectious respiratory disease (CIRD) is especially prevalent in dogs naïve to the pathogens and exposed in overcrowded, stressful environments such as animal shelters, boarding kennels, and treatment facilities, although it is important to remember that all dogs remain susceptible to these pathogens in any environment. The pathophysiology associated with infectious respiratory disease in dogs and cats is discussed later in this article (**Boxes 1** and **2**).

Foreign Body

Inhaled foreign bodies carry mixed bacterial and fungal organisms into the lung and are associated with focal or lobar pneumonias that are often initially responsive to

---

Box 1
Canine infectious respiratory disease complex: changing the face of kennel cough

CIRD complex (formerly known as kennel cough) is a syndrome in which multiple pathogens, both viral and bacterial, coinfect either naïve, immunocompromised dogs or previously vaccinated dogs. This complex is multifactorial and it seems likely that both host and environmental factors play a role in the development of illness.[40] Organisms associated with this disease are ubiquitous, especially in overcrowded housing facilities such as animal shelters and training facilities. It is likely that stress induced by the new environment and exposure to novel pathogens both play a role in development of disease.

In most cases, respiratory signs are present for days to weeks and most animals show mild to moderate clinical signs. Typically, viral infections cause either a bronchopneumonia or bronchointerstitial pneumonia because of their propensity to infect and damage type I pneumocytes.[41] As the condition progresses, desquamation of the respiratory epithelium and aggregation of inflammatory cells further reduce the lungs' natural defenses, increasing the potential for secondary bacterial colonization and infection.

Previous studies have implicated viral organisms such as canine adenovirus or canine parainfluenza[42] as major participants in CIRD, although recent studies have proposed novel respiratory pathogens such as canine respiratory coronavirus,[7,43–45] canine influenza virus,[43] and canine herpesvirus[46] as additional important pathogens associated with CIRD. *B bronchiseptica*,[9,47] *S canis*, *S equi* subsp *zooepidemicus*,[42] and *M cynos*[7,48] have been implicated as secondary bacterial infections associated with CIRD. *S equi* subsp *zooepidemicus* infections, in particular, have been associated with a rapidly progressive and often fatal hemorrhagic pneumonia.[40,49] Of note, some strains identified in outbreaks of this pathogen have been identified as resistant to tetracycline antibiotics, often the drug of choice prescribed for other bacterial pathogens associated with this complex.

Box 2
Feline lower respiratory tract infections

Organisms that have been reported as lower respiratory pathogens of cats include *Pasteurella* spp, *Escherichia coli*, *Staphylococcus* spp, *Streptococcus* spp, *Pseudomonas* spp, *B bronchiseptica*, and *Mycoplasma* spp,[50] and specific attention has been paid to *Mycoplasma* spp because of a possible association with the induction and exacerbation of asthma in adult and pediatric human patients.[51] However, the association between lower respiratory infection and chronic inflammatory lower airway disease in cats is unclear and a topic of ongoing interest.

Mycoplasma spp are considered normal flora in the upper respiratory tract and their role is controversial in lower respiratory tract infection. Because they are rarely identified cytologically and specific culture or polymerase chain reaction is needed to document the presence of these organisms, the role of *Mycoplasma* in cats (as well as in dogs) remains difficult to define.

---

antimicrobial medications but relapse shortly after discontinuation of therapy.[10,11] Foreign bodies reported in the veterinary literature include grass awns and plant or plastic materials.[11] Organisms associated with grass awn inhalation include *Pasteurella*, *Streptococcus*, *Nocardia*, *Actinomyces*, and anaerobic bacteria.[10–12] Most often, foreign material remains at the carina or enters caudodorsal principal bronchi (accessory, right and left caudal lobar bronchi).

Features associated with pulmonary foreign bodies include:

- Young, sporting breeds
- Environmental exposure to grass awns
- Focal, recurrent radiographic alveolar pattern
- History of other cutaneous or visceral foreign bodies
- Spontaneous pneumothorax or pyothorax

Importantly, normal thoracic radiographs do not rule out the possibility of an airway foreign body and even computed tomography (CT) can fail to identify an affected bronchus.[12] Chronic pulmonary foreign bodies are associated with marked inflammation that can lead to massive airway remodeling and bronchiectasis, which, when seen on radiographs, should raise the degree of suspicion for foreign body.[10]

Nosocomial

Ventilator-associated pneumonia (VAP) is a common cause of hospital-acquired pneumonia in people, although there are few reports in the veterinary literature. Colonization of the oropharynx by pathogenic and multidrug-resistant bacteria occurs and the endotracheal tube acts as a conduit to transmit pathogens into the airways, which leads to tracheobronchitis and potentially pneumonia. In addition, any animal with a compromised respiratory tract or serious systemic disease is particularly prone to development of infectious airway disease while hospitalized.

The use of mechanical ventilation in human patients increases the risk of nosocomial infection by 6-fold to 20-fold.[13] No published studies assess the risk in ventilated veterinary patients, although a study investigating the difference in bacterial sensitivity between ventilated and nonventilated animals suggested that dogs requiring mechanical ventilation were more likely to be infected with bacteria resistant to the antimicrobials most commonly used empirically to treat pneumonia in veterinary practice.[14] This suggestion parallels the increase in incidence of multidrug-resistant VAP in human medicine.[13] In a recent outbreak of *Acinetobacter calcoaceticus–Acinetobacter baumannii* complex infections in a teaching hospital, 9 of 11 animals were suspected of developing pneumonia caused by use of contaminated equipment during general anesthesia.[15]

Immune Dysfunction

Both the innate and adaptive immune systems protect against the development of infectious airway disease, and a breakdown in either increases the likelihood of opportunistic infection (**Table 2**). Congenital immunodeficiencies have been recognized that make animals particularly sensitive to infectious organisms. Young animals are especially prone to the development of bacterial pneumonia because of their naive immune systems, and when coupled with alterations to the innate immune system, such as primary ciliary dyskinesia (PCD), complement deficiency, or bronchiectasis (congenital or acquired), the risk of life-threatening infection increases tremendously (see Veterinary Clinics of North America September 2007, Vol 37 (5): pp 845–860 for a comprehensive review of respiratory defenses in health and disease).

Any cause of systemic immunocompromise increases the risk for bacterial pneumonia, and any additional alterations to the body's natural defense mechanisms dramatically increase the risk. Specifically, medications such as chemotherapy, immunosuppressive therapy, or antitussive therapy increase the likelihood of bacterial pneumonia. Underlying respiratory viruses or systemic viruses such as feline leukemia virus (FeLV) and feline immunodeficiency virus (FIV) have the potential to enhance the severity of respiratory illness.

CLINICAL SIGNS

Clinical signs of bacterial pneumonia vary depending on its cause, severity, and chronicity. They can be acute or peracute in onset or can show an insidious onset, resulting in chronic illness, particularly in animals with preexisting chronic airway disease. Early in disease, mild signs such as an intermittent, soft cough might be the only evidence of disease. As infection spreads, clinical signs worsen and often include a refractory, productive cough; exercise intolerance; anorexia; and severe lethargy. Owners might note a change in the respiratory pattern, with increased panting or rapid breathing and, in cases of severe infection, cyanosis and orthopnea can be observed. In general, these systemic signs are more often recognized in dogs than in cats.

Cats with pneumonia can show similar clinical signs to dogs, although the cough can be misinterpreted as a retch or vomit by owners. Clinical signs and radiographic

Table 2		
Conditions leading to impaired immune function and resulting in increased risk of pneumonia		
	Congenital	**Acquired**
Innate	Primary ciliary dyskinesia Complement deficiency Leukocyte adhesion deficiency	Bronchiectasis Secondary ciliary dyskinesia

Adaptive	Immunoglobulin deficiency
	Severe combined
	  immunodeficiency
		Retrovirus infection (eg, feline
		  immunodeficiency virus, feline
		  leukemia virus)
		Endocrine or metabolic disease (eg,
		  diabetes mellitus or hyperadrenocorticism)
		Chemotherapy and other
		  immunosuppressive therapy
		Splenectomy

Data from Refs.[36–38]

findings (eg, right middle lobar consolidation or collapse) can also be considered suggestive of inflammatory airway disease rather than pneumonia.[16] As disease worsens, cats can become tachypneic with short, shallow breaths and nasal flaring.[17] Rarely do cat owners notice exercise intolerance associated with bacterial pneumonia.

PHYSICAL EXAMINATION

As with the history and clinical signs of bacterial pneumonia, physical examination findings vary greatly with the state and severity of disease. Dogs or cats with mild disease might have no abnormalities detected on physical examination. A change in the respiratory pattern, with an increase in rate and effort, can be an early clue to the diagnosis. Clinicians must pay close attention to thoracic auscultation because adventitious lung sounds (crackles and wheezes) can be subtle, focal, or intermittent. In many cases, only harsh or increased lung sounds are detected rather than crackles.[18] Physical examination should assess for evidence of upper airway signs (eg, nasal congestion or discharge) that can result from lower airway infection, either as an extension of epithelial infection or from nasopharyngeal regurgitation of lower airway secretions. Thorough auscultation of the trachea and upper airway is important for detecting upper airway obstructive disease that could predispose to pneumonia.

Animals with bacterial pneumonia generally present with mixed inspiratory and expiratory signs, similar to those seen with other diseases of the pulmonary parenchyma. Fever is detected in 16% to 50% of cases, so it is not a reliable indicator of disease.[8,16,18–20]

DIAGNOSIS

Bacterial pneumonia implies sepsis of the lower airway and lungs; consequently, the diagnosis is confirmed by the presence of septic suppurative inflammation on airway cytology obtained through bronchoalveolar lavage (BAL) or tracheal wash, along with a positive microbiology culture. In some cases, this is completed easily and yields results consistent with clinical suspicion. However, financial limitations or anesthetic concerns sometimes inhibit the ability to collect the samples needed to confirm a bacterial infection, and in those cases a clinical diagnosis of bacterial pneumonia might be presumed based on available information.

A clinical diagnosis of bacterial pneumonia should be reached after obtaining compelling evidence to suggest a bacterial cause for the animal's clinical signs (after excluding other causes), and is confirmed by resolution of signs following appropriate antimicrobial therapy. Acute bacterial pneumonia is a common diagnosis in the small animal clinic and can often be easily identified; however, early and chronic pneumonias are more challenging to recognize because clinical signs can be subtle.

Hematology

The complete blood count is a useful diagnostic test in animals with respiratory signs. Bacterial pneumonias are often associated with an inflammatory leukogram, characterized primarily by a neutrophilia, with or without a left shift and variable evidence of toxic changes,[12,21] although the absence of inflammatory change does not exclude the possibility of pneumonia.[8,18] Furthermore, the leukogram and differential can provide clues that suggest bacterial pneumonia is less likely. For example, eosinophilia in an animal with respiratory signs would be more suggestive of eosinophilic bronchopneumopathy, granulomas, or parasitic lung diseases as an underlying cause than a bacterial cause. The erythrogram and platelet evaluation are generally not helpful in determining a bacterial cause of respiratory disease.

A biochemistry panel and urinalysis do not always contribute to the diagnosis of bacterial pneumonia but can provide clues to the presence of metabolic or endocrine diseases that could make the development of bacterial pneumonia more likely. Similarly, fecal flotation, sedimentation, and Baermann or heartworm test do not provide evidence for bacterial pneumonia but can be helpful in excluding parasitic pneumonia in areas where these organisms are endemic. Cats with respiratory conditions should be screened for FeLV and FIV to detect systemic causes of immunosuppression.

Pulmonary Function Testing

Arterial blood gas analysis is a useful test to measure the lung's ability to oxygenate. Ideally, for animals with significant respiratory compromise, arterial blood samples should be collected and analyzed to determine the severity of pulmonary disease. Furthermore, trends in arterial oxygen partial pressure can be used to track progression or resolution of disease. In many cases, blood gas analysis is not available or patient factors preclude the acquisition of samples. Pulse oximetry is a quick, noninvasive evaluation of oxygen delivery to body tissues that measures percentage of hemoglobin saturation with oxygen. It provides only a crude assessment of oxygenation and is subject to variability; however, trends in hemoglobin saturation can provide additional clinical support to progression or resolution of disease. In addition, pulse oximetry provides a practical measure of oxygen desaturation during anesthesia for airway lavage and should be monitored closely during this procedure.

Thoracic Radiography

Thoracic radiographs are crucial diagnostic tests in the evaluation of lower airway and pulmonary parenchymal disease. Radiographic evidence of bacterial pneumonia can appear as a focal, multifocal, or diffuse alveolar pattern, although early in the disease process infiltrates can be primarily interstitial (**Figs. 1** and **2**).[16,22] Ventral lung lobes are most commonly affected in aspiration pneumonia, and a caudodorsal pattern would be expected with inhaled foreign bodies or hematogenous bacterial spread. A lobar sign is often seen in cases of aspiration pneumonia in which the right middle lung lobe is affected (**Table 3**).

Three-view thoracic radiographs (left lateral, right lateral, and either dorsoventral or ventrodorsal views) should be obtained when screening for pneumonia because

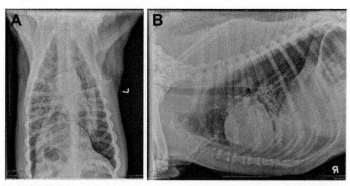

Fig. 1. Dorsoventral (*A*) and right lateral (*B*) thoracic radiographs from a dog with an alveolar pattern in the cranioventral lung lobes, suggestive of aspiration. Note that in many cases the right middle lung lobe is most affected, which is best seen on a left lateral orthogonal view.

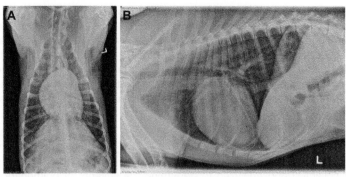

Fig. 2. Dorsoventral (*A*) and right lateral (*B*) thoracic radiographs of a dog with a focal, patchy interstitial to alveolar pattern in the left cranial lung lobe. This dog was diagnosed with a foxtail foreign body, which was removed thoracoscopically via lung lobectomy. (*From* Dear JD. Bacterial pneumonia in dogs and cats. Vet Clin North Am Small Anim Pract. 2014; 44(1): 143-159; with permission.)

differential aeration associated with positional atelectasis can either mask or highlight pulmonary changes. For example, a radiograph taken in left lateral recumbency is preferred when aspiration is suspected because it increases aeration of the right middle lung lobe, the most commonly affected lobe.

Diffuse radiographic involvement would be expected to suggest more severe disease, although radiographic changes lag behind clinical disease. Consequently, bacterial pneumonia cannot be ruled out in animals with acute onset of clinical signs and unremarkable radiographs.[12]

Advanced Imaging

Advanced imaging is rarely necessary in the diagnosis of uncomplicated bacterial pneumonia, although it can be helpful in more complicated cases. Thoracic ultrasonography can be used to characterize peripheral areas of consolidation and to obtain fine-needle aspirates for cytology. Cytology is often helpful in distinguishing

Table 3	
Differential diagnoses for specific radiographic patterns	
Lobar alveolar consolidation	Focal alveolar consolidation
Aspiration pneumonia (cranioventral, right middle)	Airway foreign body
	Granuloma
Lung lobe torsion (cranial)	Primary pulmonary neoplasia (caudal lobes)
Atelectasis secondary to mucus plugging (right middle most commonly)	Metastatic neoplasia
	Noncardiogenic pulmonary edema
Diffuse alveolar pattern	Diffuse or focal interstitial pattern
Acute respiratory distress syndrome	Early bacterial pneumonia
Congestive heart failure (perihilar in dogs)	Imminent congestive heart failure
Fluid overload	*Pneumocystis canis* infection
Eosinophilic bronchopneumopathy	Inhalant toxicity (eg, paraquat)
Coagulopathy	Viral pneumonia
Metastatic neoplasia	
Fungal pneumonia	

Modified from Dear JD. Bacterial pneumonia in dogs and cats. Vet Clin North Am Small Anim Pract. 2014; 44(1): 143-159; with permission.

inflammation from neoplastic or fungal disease. In addition, sonographic evaluation can be useful in the detection of superficial foxtail foreign bodies when they remain in the periphery of the lobe (**Figs. 3** and **4**).[12]

CT provides greater detail and resolution of lesions within the pulmonary parenchyma and gives clinicians better spatial information regarding the severity and extent of pulmonary involvement. In particular, CT is much better at identifying the presence and extent of bronchiectasis compared with thoracic radiography. In some cases, CT can be useful to identify migration tracts associated with inhaled foreign bodies.[12] However, in most cases general anesthesia is required for CT acquisition, and prolonged recumbency can lead to atelectasis, which is difficult to differentiate radiographically from infiltrates. Repeating the CT in a different position after providing several maximal inspirations can alleviate atelectasis. Nuclear scintigraphy can be useful for the evaluation of ciliary dyskinesia, although secondary causes of mucociliary stasis (eg, infection with *Mycoplasma* or *Bordetella*, exposure to smoke) must be excluded before assuming the diagnosis of PCD. Because of the time necessary for image acquisition, MRI is not commonly used for the diagnosis of most respiratory diseases. PET has not been evaluated for use in bacterial pneumonia, although it might be useful in evaluating patients with atypical infiltrates or mass lesions when a definitive diagnosis is not forthcoming.

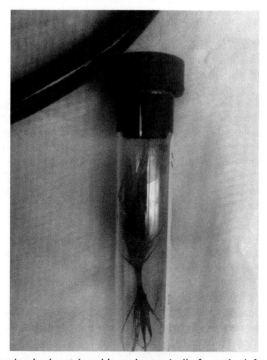

Fig. 3. A foxtail foreign body retrieved bronchoscopically from the left principle bronchus of a dog with chronic respiratory signs. Foxtails are endemic to the Western and Midwestern United States as well as some parts of Europe and are associated with mixed aerobic and anaerobic infections. Fungal infections seem to occur rarely as a consequence of bronchopulmonary foreign bodies. (*From* Dear JD. Bacterial pneumonia in dogs and cats. Vet Clin North Am Small Anim Pract. 2014; 44(1): 143-159; with permission.)

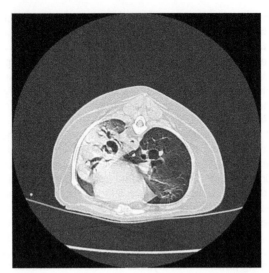

Fig. 4. CT image of a dog with severe, diffuse pneumonia resulting from a chronic foxtail foreign body (see **Fig. 3**). The foreign body was not visible on thoracic radiographs, but is clearly evident in the left principal bronchus on this image. (*From* Dear JD. Bacterial pneumonia in dogs and cats. Vet Clin North Am Small Anim Pract. 2014; 44(1): 143-159; with permission.)

Bronchoscopic Evaluation

Examination of the trachea and bronchial tree should be performed systematically. Endoscopists should note the color and character of the mucosa and any airway sections, making sure to evaluate all branches of the lower airways for evidence of foreign bodies, bronchiectasis, or collapse (diffuse or focal changes). Airway mucosa in normal animals should be pale pink with visible mucosal and pulmonary vessels. Airway bifurcations should appear as narrow, crisp mucosal margins.

Animals with pneumonia can have hyperemia of the epithelium, prominent mucosal vessels, and evidence of airway inflammation, appearing as rounded, thickened airway bifurcations and airway nodules. Airway secretions are usually opaque, therefore viscous and discolored (brown, yellow-green, or red-tinged) secretions can indicate inflammation or pneumonia.

Airway Sampling

When available, BAL is preferred for collection of lower airway samples rather than tracheal wash because the trachea and carina are not sterile, even in healthy dogs.[23] In addition, the sensitivity for detecting cytologic features of sepsis is greater with BAL than with tracheal wash.[19] However, when only a tracheal wash specimen can be obtained, because of the lack of equipment for BAL or because of patient instability, collection of a lower airway sample is desirable to identify infecting bacteria and to determine appropriate antimicrobial therapy through susceptibility testing. Oropharyngeal swabs are not suitable substitutes for making a diagnosis of pneumonia.

BAL cell counts in animals with bacterial pneumonia are markedly higher than in dogs with chronic bronchitis or other respiratory disease.[21] Septic, suppurative inflammation is a reliable indicator of bacterial pneumonia in dogs[21] and is likely to indicate bacterial pneumonia in cats. In cases that lack evidence of airway sepsis (intracellular bacteria), BAL cytology generally reveals suppurative or mixed inflammation.[20] Note that animals with mycoplasma pneumonia can have positive culture in the absence of cytologic evidence of sepsis.

In animals with suspected or confirmed foreign bodies, a BAL sample should always be obtained from the affected airway as well as an additional site, with both submitted individually for cytologic analysis. Airway bacteria are more likely to be seen in the cytologic sample from the site of the foreign body than from an alternate site.[11] Furthermore, cytology of BAL samples obtained from multiple lobes can reveal different findings, even in cases of sterile inflammatory diseases such as feline bronchial disease, thus reliance on single-segment BAL cytology could lessen the chance of yielding diagnostic results.[24]

Microbiology

Diagnosis of bacterial pneumonia relies on identification of septic inflammation in conjunction with a positive bacterial culture. Typically, aerobic and *Mycoplasma* culture and sensitivity are requested, and, in cases with markedly purulent secretions or a history of known aspiration or foreign bodies, anaerobic cultures should also be requested. Samples should be refrigerated in sterile containers until submitted. If multiple alveolar segments are sampled during BAL, these are usually pooled for culture submission. When anaerobic cultures are desired, BAL fluid should be inoculated into the appropriate transport media and kept at room temperature until submission.

Cultures should be performed whenever possible in order to guide appropriate antimicrobial therapy. With overly liberal use of antibiotics, increasing populations of resistant microbes are being identified, particularly in animals with hospital-acquired pneumonia.[25,26] However, airway samples cannot be collected in all animals, and, in those instances, recommendations regarding antimicrobial stewardship should be followed.[27]

Bacteria commonly isolated from lung washes of cats or dogs with bacterial pneumonia include enteric organisms (*Escherichia coli*, *Klebsiella* spp), *Pasteurella* spp, coagulase-positive *Staphylococcus* spp, beta-hemolytic *Streptococcus* spp, *Mycoplasma* spp, and *B bronchiseptica* (**Table 4**).[20,22]

TREATMENT

Treatment of bacterial pneumonia varies depending on the severity of disease, and appropriate antimicrobial therapy is essential. The International Society for

Table 4	
Bacteria commonly isolated from airway samples of canine patients with pneumonia	
Organism	**Isolates (%)**
B bronchiseptica	22–71
E coli	11–51
Klebsiella pneumoniae	2–25
Pasteurella spp	3–21
Mycoplasma spp	30–70
Streptococcus spp	6–21
Staphylococcus spp	7–20
Anaerobes	5–17
Enterococcus spp	4–11

Data from Refs.[8,20,28,39]

Companion Animal Infectious Disease (ISCAID) has published guidelines for treatment of dogs and cats with respiratory infections and these should be consulted for further details about recommendations.[27] For stable animals with mild disease, outpatient therapy consisting of administration of a single, oral antibiotic is often all that is necessary (**Table 5**). Ideally, antimicrobial choices should be based on culture and sensitivity results from airway lavage samples because resistance to antimicrobials selected empirically has been reported in up to 26% of cases.[28] For critically ill animals in which airways samples cannot be obtained, blood cultures might be considered, although there is a lack of data on sensitivity in veterinary patients. Regardless, in cases of severe pneumonia, initial empiric therapy should be instituted while awaiting culture results. Traditionally, antimicrobials have been administered for 3 to 6 weeks, and at least 1 to 2 weeks beyond the resolution of clinical and/or radiographic signs of disease, although there is no evidence to support this practice. ISCAID recommendations suggest that shorter durations might be appropriate, but there are few data to support this suggestion. One observational study found similar radiographic and clinical cures in dogs treated with a short course of antibiotic (<14 days) compared with those that received a longer duration of treatment.[29] Regardless of the intended duration of therapy, reevaluation within 10 to 14 days of starting treatment is important to determine response and to define optimal length of treatment.

Animals with more advanced disease require more intensive care, including hospitalization with intravenous fluids to maintain hydration. Adequate hydration is essential to facilitate clearance of respiratory exudates. Nebulization to create liquid particles that enter the lower airways (<5 μm) can also enhance clearance of secretions.

Table 5
Empiric antibiotic choice for patients with pneumonia

Stable patient, mild clinical signs	Monotherapy:
	  Doxycycline 5 mg/kg PO every 12 h
	  Amoxicillin-clavulanic acid 13.75 mg/kg PO every 12 h (dog)
	  62.5 mg PO every 12 h (cat)

Moderate clinical signs	Monotherapy:
	  As above
	Dual therapy:
	  Amoxicillin 22 mg/kg PO every 12 h
	  Ampicillin 22–30 mg/kg IV every 8 h
	  Clindamycin 10 mg/kg PO/SQ every 12 h (dog)
	  10–15 mg/kg PO/SQ every 12 h (cat)
	  And
	  Enrofloxacin 10 mg/kg PO/IV every 24 h (dog)
	  5 mg/kg PO/IV every 24 h (cat)
	  Pradofloxacin 7.5 mg/kg PO every 24 h (cat)
	  Amikacin 15 mg/kg SQ every 24 h

Critical patient, severe clinical signs	Dual therapy
	  As above
	Monotherapy:
	  Piperacillin-tazobactam 50 mg/kg IV every 6 h
	  Meropenem 24 mg/kg IV every 24 h
	  Imipenem 10 mg/kg IV every 8 h

Abbreviations: IV, intravenous; PO, by mouth; SQ, subcutaneous.
   Data from Lappin MR, Blondeau J, Boothe D, et al. Antimicrobial use Guidelines for Treatment of Respiratory Tract Disease in Dogs and Cats: Antimicrobial Guidelines Working Group of the International Society for Companion Animal Infectious Diseases. *J Vet Intern Med.* 2017;31(2):279-294.

Nebulizer types include ultrasonic devices, compressed air nebulizers, and mesh nebulizers. Nebulization with sterile saline can be achieved by directing the hosing from the nebulizer into a cage or animal carrier covered in plastic. Depending on how viscous secretions are, therapy can be provided for 15 to 20 minutes 2 to 4 times daily. In many cases, nebulization coupled with coupage can help the animal expectorate airway secretions, although no specific studies in veterinary medicine have evaluated this technique. Coupage is performed by cupping the hands and gently, rhythmically pounding on both lateral thoracic walls in a dorsal to ventral and caudal to cranial direction. Coupage should not be performed in animals with regurgitation because any increase in intrathoracic pressure could exacerbate regurgitation and subsequent reaspiration.

Supplemental oxygen is necessary for animals with moderate to marked hypoxemia (documented by a Pao_2 <80 mm Hg or SpO_2 <94% on room air) in conjunction with increased respiratory effort. Oxygen supplementation at 40% to 60% is provided until respiratory difficulty lessens and the animal can be weaned to room air. Animals with refractory pneumonia that fail to improve on supplemental oxygen can succumb to ventilatory fatigue and need to be referred to an intensive care facility for mechanical ventilation.

Clinically, it seems that administration of an oral mucolytic agent such as N-acetylcysteine can be useful for animals with retention of thick respiratory secretions. In particular, this can be helpful in dogs with moderate to severe bronchiectasis that are prone to chronic or recurrent pneumonia. Decreasing the viscosity of airway secretions might improve expectoration of fluid and debris that accumulates in dependent airways, although no published information is available on the use of mucolytics in animals. N-acetylcysteine is typically not used via nebulization because of risks of bronchoconstriction and epithelial toxicity. Under no circumstances is it appropriate to use cough suppressants (eg, butorphanol or hydrocodone) in the management of bacterial pneumonia, particularly when it is complicated by bronchiectasis. By decreasing the cough reflex, these drugs perpetuate retention of mucus, debris, and other material in the airways and therefore hinder clearance of infection. Also, furosemide should not be used because drying of secretions traps material in the lower airway and perpetuates infection.

In cases in which aspiration pneumonia is suspected, strategies should be used to reduce the chance of reaspirating through appropriate treatment of the underlying condition. With disorders of esophageal motility, upright feedings of either slurry or meatballs can enhance esophageal transit. Furthermore, diets low in fat can increase gastric emptying. In patients with refractory vomiting, antiemetic and prokinetic agents can be used to reduce the episodes of vomiting. Drugs such as maropitant (Cerenia; 1 mg/kg intravenously or subcutaneously once daily) or ondansetron (Zofran; 0.3–1 mg/kg intravenously or subcutaneously once to twice daily) act peripherally or centrally to decrease the urge to vomit and are safe to use in both cats and dogs.

The role of antacids in management of aspiration pneumonia remains controversial. By neutralizing the pH of gastric secretions, animals with refractory vomiting or regurgitation are less likely to succumb to chemical injury related to aspiration. However, in cases treated with acid suppression, the aspirant could be more likely to contain a greater concentration of bacteria that can colonize the airways and lead to bacterial pneumonia. Although treatment with proton pump inhibitors has been shown to reduce the incidence of acid reflux events in both dogs and cats undergoing anesthesia,[5,30] no controlled studies have assessed the severity of aspiration pneumonia or relative risk of using antacid therapy in dogs or cats as a preventive measure.

Because radiographic findings lag behind clinical disease, recheck radiographs are not helpful early in the disease process, although they are useful to document resolution of disease and should be obtained either before or within a week of discontinuation of antimicrobial therapy. In cases of refractory pneumonia, recheck radiographs midway through therapy can assess resolution or progression of disease and help to guide further diagnostics and therapy.

Serum biomarkers such as acute phase proteins are associated with inflammatory disease. Being nonspecific, these biomarkers are not clinically useful for diagnosis but might be helpful in determining treatment response, facilitating better antimicrobial stewardship by suggesting resolution of disease more rapidly than thoracic radiographs.[31] Further studies are required to establish their utility in management of pneumonia.

In animals suspected of having contagious or multidrug-resistant pathogens, appropriate contact precautions should be used. Isolation gowns, examination gloves, and good hand washing technique along with appropriate quarantine facilities are essential to prevent transmission of disease to other animals or members of the health care team.

Prognosis

Prognosis for animals with bacterial pneumonia varies depending on the severity of disease, the animal's immunocompetence, and the virulence of the infectious agent. In general, between 77% and 94% of patients diagnosed with pneumonia are discharged from the hospital.[8,28,32] No large, long-term studies have assessed the overall prognosis of animals with multidrug-resistant bacteria or recurrent pneumonia. Presumably, the outcome associated with these cases will be worse. In a recent case series of presumed nosocomial multidrug resistant *A calcoaceticus–A baumannii* complex infections, 8 out of 11 animals with pneumonia died or were euthanized as a consequence of their disease.[15]

CASE STUDIES
Case Study 1

A 7-year-old male castrated bichon frise presented for a chronic cough.

History

Six-year history of progressive cough since adoption. The cough is described as nonproductive, worse in the morning, and exacerbated by aerosols and heavy fragrances. Previous treatment with theophylline and doxycycline have not lessened the severity of cough.

Physical Examination

Temperature (38.9°C [101.9°F]), pulse (72 beats/min), and respiratory rate (32 breaths/min) were normal. No heart murmur but soft crackles were auscultated on inspiration. A cough was elicited on tracheal palpation.

Diagnostic Evaluation

Chronic cough in a small-breed dog is often associated with airway collapse or chronic bronchitis; however, infectious and neoplastic disease must remain on the differential list. Congestive heart failure is unlikely in this case given the lack of a heart murmur and normal heart rate.

A white blood cell count was normal (6650 cells/μL) with 4722 neutrophils. Thoracic radiographs revealed dynamic lower airway narrowing between lateral projections and

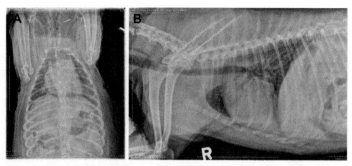

Fig. 5. Dorsoventral (*A*) and right lateral (*B*) thoracic radiographs revealing bronchiectasis and a diffuse prominent bronchointerstitial pattern, most prominent in the caudal thorax (case study 1).

a diffuse prominent bronchointerstitial pattern, most prominent in the caudal thorax (**Fig. 5**). The larynx seemed to have normal function at anesthetic induction. Bronchoscopy revealed mild to moderate dynamic lower airway collapse and bronchiectasis of caudodorsal bronchi along with airway exudate. BAL samples were hypercellular on cytology (2500 cells/μL) and revealed septic suppurative inflammation (55%, normal 5%–8%) with degenerate neutrophils. Bacterial cultures were positive for *Pasteurella dagmatis* and *Fusobacterium* sp. In this case, chronic inflammatory airway disease likely contributed to the dog's bronchiectasis, which then predisposed to bronchopneumonia.

Case Study 2

A 5-year-old MC domestic medium hair was presented for evaluation of acute respiratory distress.

History

Lethargy and anorexia had been noted 3 days before the onset of respiratory signs.

Physical Examination

Temperature (38.7°C [101.6°F]) and pulse (210 beats/min) were normal. Tachypnea was noted (respiratory rate 60 breaths/min) along with increased respiratory effort on inspiration and expiration. Diffuse expiratory wheezes were auscultated.

Diagnostic Evaluation

Acute onset of respiratory difficulty in a cat is most commonly related to inflammatory airway disease. The physical examination is consistent with this diagnosis, although it is uncommon for affected cats to show lethargy and anorexia. Infectious and neoplastic diseases were also on the differential diagnosis list, along with aspiration and foreign body pneumonia.

Thoracic radiographs showed a focal opacity in the left caudal lung lobe and a diffuse bronchial pattern (**Fig. 6**). Complete blood count revealed a normal white blood cell count (8500 cells/μL) with a left shift (6800 neutrophils, 1000 bands). Bronchoscopy with lavage was performed. A moderate amount of airway hyperemia and edema was noted along with purulent material obstructing several airways. BAL cytology had increased cellularity (1500 cells/μL, normal 500 cells/μL) with neutrophilic inflammation (84%, normal 5%–8%). Neutrophils contained dark blue granular debris,

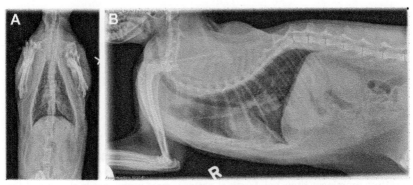

Fig. 6. Dorsoventral (*A*) and right lateral (*B*) thoracic radiographs revealing a focal opacity in the left caudal lung lobe and a diffuse bronchial pattern (case study 2).

suspicious for sepsis. Aerobic and anaerobic cultures were negative, but a pure culture of *Mycoplasma* was isolated on special media. A diagnosis of mycoplasma bronchopneumonia was made.

DISCLOSURE

The author has nothing to disclose.

REFERENCES

1. Leroy O, Vandenbussche C, Coffinier C, et al. Community-acquired aspiration pneumonia in intensive care units. Epidemiological and prognosis data. Am J Respir Crit Care Med 1997;156(6):1922–9.

2. Ovbey DH, Wilson DV, Bednarski RM, et al. Prevalence and risk factors for canine post-anesthetic aspiration pneumonia (1999-2009): a multicenter study. Vet Anaesth Analg 2014;41(2):127–36.

3. Tart KM, Babski DM, Lee JA. Potential risks, prognostic indicators, and diagnostic and treatment modalities affecting survival in dogs with presumptive aspiration pneumonia: 125 cases (2005-2008). J Vet Emerg Crit Care (San Antonio) 2010;20(3):319–29.

4. Mitsushima H, Oishi K, Nagao T, et al. Acid aspiration induces bacterial pneumonia by enhanced bacterial adherence in mice. Microb Pathog 2002;33(5):203–10.

5. Zacuto AC, Marks SL, Osborn J, et al. The influence of esomeprazole and cisapride on gastroesophageal reflux during anesthesia in dogs. J Vet Intern Med 2012;26(3):518–25.

6. Ogden J, Ovbey D, Saile K. Effects of preoperative cisapride on postoperative aspiration pneumonia in dogs with laryngeal paralysis. J Small Anim Pract 2019;60(3):183–90.

7. Brownlie J, Mitchell J, Walker CA, et al. Mycoplasmas and novel viral pathogens in canine infectious respiratory disease. J Vet Intern Med (Seattle) 2013.

8. Radhakrishnan A, Drobatz KJ, Culp WTN, et al. Community-acquired infectious pneumonia in puppies: 65 cases (1993-2002). J Am Vet Med Assoc 2007;230(10):1493–7.

9. Taha-Abdelaziz K, Bassel LL, Harness ML, et al. Cilia-associated bacteria in fatal Bordetella bronchiseptica pneumonia of dogs and cats. J Vet Diagn Invest 2016; 28(4):369–76.

10. Workman HC, Bailiff NL, Jang SS, et al. Capnocytophaga cynodegmi in a rottweiler dog with severe bronchitis and foreign-body pneumonia. J Clin Microbiol 2008;46(12):4099–103.

11. Tenwolde AC, Johnson LR, Hunt GB, et al. The role of bronchoscopy in foreign body removal in dogs and cats: 37 cases (2000-2008). J Vet Intern Med 2010; 24(5):1063–8.

12. Schultz RM, Zwingenberger A. Radiographic, computed tomographic, and ultrasonographic findings with migrating intrathoracic grass awns in dogs and cats. Vet Radiol Ultrasound 2008;49(3):249–55.

13. Craven DE, Hjalmarson KI. Ventilator-associated tracheobronchitis and pneumonia: thinking outside the box. Clin Infect Dis 2010;51(Suppl 1):S59–66.

14. Epstein SE, Mellema MS, Hopper K. Airway microbial culture and susceptibility patterns in dogs and cats with respiratory disease of varying severity. J Vet Emerg Crit Care (San Antonio) 2010;20(6):587–94.

15. Kuzi S, Blum SE, Kahane N, et al. Multi-drug-resistant Acinetobacter calcoaceticus-Acinetobacter baumannii complex infection outbreak in dogs and cats in a veterinary hospital. J Small Anim Pract 2016;57(11):617–25.

16. Levy N, Ballegeer E, Koenigshof A. Clinical and radiographic findings in cats with aspiration pneumonia: retrospective evaluation of 28 cases. J Small Anim Pract 2019;60(6):356–60.

17. Egberink H, Addie D, Belak S, et al. Bordetella bronchiseptica infection in cats. ABCD guidelines on prevention and management. J Feline Med Surg 2009; 11(7):610–4.

18. Kogan DA, Johnson LR, Jandrey KE, et al. Clinical, clinicopathologic, and radiographic findings in dogs with aspiration pneumonia: 88 cases (2004-2006). J Am Vet Med Assoc 2008;233(11):1742–7.

19. Hawkins EC, DeNicola DB, Plier ML. Cytological analysis of bronchoalveolar lavage fluid in the diagnosis of spontaneous respiratory tract disease in dogs: a retrospective study. J Vet Intern Med 1995;9(6):386–92.

20. Johnson LR, Queen EV, Vernau W, et al. Microbiologic and cytologic assessment of bronchoalveolar lavage fluid from dogs with lower respiratory tract infection: 105 cases (2001-2011). J Vet Intern Med 2013;27(2):259–67.

21. Peeters DE, McKiernan BC, Weisiger RM, et al. Quantitative bacterial cultures and cytological examination of bronchoalveolar lavage specimens in dogs. J Vet Intern Med 2000;14(5):534–41.

22. Cohn LA. Pulmonary parenchymal disease. In: Ettinger SJ, Feldman EC, editors. Textbook of veterinary internal medicine: diseases of the dog and the cat, vol. 2, 7th edition. St Louis (MO): Saunders, Elsevier; 2010.

23. McKiernan BC, Smith AR, Kissil M. Bacterial isolates from the lower trachea of clinically healthy dogs. J Am Anim Hosp Assoc 1984;20:139–42.

24. Ybarra WL, Johnson LR, Drazenovich TL, et al. Interpretation of multisegment bronchoalveolar lavage in cats (1/2001-1/2011). J Vet Intern Med 2012;26(6): 1281–7.

25. Chalker VJ, Waller A, Webb K, et al. Genetic diversity of Streptococcus equi subsp. zooepidemicus and doxycycline resistance in kennelled dogs. J Clin Microbiol 2012;50(6):2134–6.

26. Foley JE, Rand C, Bannasch MJ, et al. Molecular epidemiology of feline bordetellosis in two animal shelters in California, USA. Prev Vet Med 2002;54(2):141–56.

27. Lappin MR, Blondeau J, Boothe D, et al. Antimicrobial use guidelines for treatment of respiratory tract disease in dogs and cats: antimicrobial guidelines Working Group of the International Society for Companion Animal Infectious Diseases. J Vet Intern Med 2017;31(2):279–94.

28. Proulx A, Hume DZ, Drobatz KJ, et al. In vitro bacterial isolate susceptibility to empirically selected antimicrobials in 111 dogs with bacterial pneumonia. J Vet Emerg Crit Care (San Antonio) 2014;24(2):194–200.

29. Wayne A, Davis M, Sinnott VB, et al. Outcomes in dogs with uncomplicated, presumptive bacterial pneumonia treated with short or long course antibiotics. Can Vet J 2017;58(6):610–3.

30. Garcia RS, Belafsky PC, Della Maggiore A, et al. Prevalence of gastroesophageal reflux in cats during anesthesia and effect of omeprazole on gastric pH. J Vet Intern Med 2017;31(3):734–42.

31. Viitanen SJ, Lappalainen AK, Christensen MB, et al. The utility of acute-phase proteins in the assessment of treatment response in dogs with bacterial pneumonia. J Vet Intern Med 2017;31(1):124–33.

32. Kogan DA, Johnson LR, Sturges BK, et al. Etiology and clinical outcome in dogs with aspiration pneumonia: 88 cases (2004-2006). J Am Vet Med Assoc 2008; 233(11):1748–55.

33. Viitanen SJ, Lappalainen AK, Koho NM, et al. Recurrent bacterial pneumonia in Irish Wolfhounds: clinical findings and etiological studies. J Vet Intern Med 2019;33(2):846–55.

34. McBrearty A, Ramsey I, Courcier E, et al. Clinical factors associated with death before discharge and overall survival time in dogs with generalized megaesophagus. J Am Vet Med Assoc 2011;238(12):1622–8.

35. Bedu AS, Labruyere JJ, Thibaud JL, et al. Age-related thoracic radiographic changes in golden and labrador retriever muscular dystrophy. Vet Radiol Ultrasound 2012;53(5):492–500.

36. Watson PJ, Herrtage ME, Peacock MA, et al. Primary ciliary dyskinesia in Newfoundland dogs. Vet Rec 1999;144(26):718–25.

37. Watson PJ, Wotton P, Eastwood J, et al. Immunoglobulin deficiency in Cavalier King Charles spaniels with pneumocystis pneumonia. J Vet Intern Med 2006; 20(3):523–7.

38. Jezyk PF, Felsburg PJ, Haskins ME, et al. X-linked severe combined immunodeficiency in the dog. Clin Immunol Immunopathol 1989;52(2):173–89.

39. Foster SF, Martin P, Braddock JA, et al. A retrospective analysis of feline bronchoalveolar lavage cytology and microbiology (1995-2000). J Feline Med Surg 2004;6(3):189–98.

40. Pesavento PA, Hurley KF, Bannasch MJ, et al. A clonal outbreak of acute fatal hemorrhagic pneumonia in intensively housed (shelter) dogs caused by Streptococcus equi subsp. zooepidemicus. Vet Pathol 2008;45(1):51–3.

41. Mellema M. Viral pneumonia. In: King LG, editor. Textbook of respiratory disease in dogs and cats, vol. 1. St Louis (MO): Saunders; 2004. p. 431–45.

42. Chalker VJ, Brooks HW, Brownlie J. The association of Streptococcus equi subsp. zooepidemicus with canine infectious respiratory disease. Vet Microbiol 2003; 95(1–2):149–56.

43. An DJ, Jeoung HY, Jeong W, et al. A serological survey of canine respiratory coronavirus and canine influenza virus in Korean dogs. J Vet Med Sci 2010;72(9): 1217–9.

44. Knesl O, Allan FJ, Shields S. The seroprevalence of canine respiratory coronavirus and canine influenza virus in dogs in New Zealand. N Z Vet J 2009;57(5): 295–8.

45. Mitchell JA, Brooks HW, Szladovits B, et al. Tropism and pathological findings associated with canine respiratory coronavirus (CRCoV). Vet Microbiol 2013; 162(2–4):582–94.

46. Kawakami K, Ogawa H, Maeda K, et al. Nosocomial outbreak of serious canine infectious tracheobronchitis (kennel cough) caused by canine herpesvirus infection. J Clin Microbiol 2010;48(4):1176–81.

47. Keil DJ, Fenwick B. Canine respiratory bordetellosis: keeping up with an evolving pathogen. In: Carmichael LE, editor. Recent advances in canine infectious disease. Ithaca (NY): International Veterinary Information Service; 2000. Available at: http://www.ivis.org/advances/Infect_Dis_Carmichael/keil/chapter.asp?LA=1. Accessed November 23, 2019.

48. Chalker VJ, Owen WM, Paterson C, et al. Mycoplasmas associated with canine infectious respiratory disease. Microbiology 2004;150(Pt 10):3491–7.

49. Priestnall S, Erles K. Streptococcus zooepidemicus: an emerging canine pathogen. Vet J 2011;188(2):142–8.

50. Foster SF, Martin P, Allan GS, et al. Lower respiratory tract infections in cats: 21 cases (1995-2000). J Feline Med Surg 2004;6(3):167–80.

51. Wood PR, Hill VL, Burks ML, et al. Mycoplasma pneumoniae in children with acute and refractory asthma. Ann Allergy Asthma Immunol 2013;110(5): 328–334 e321.

Canine and Feline Exudative Pleural Diseases

Steven E. Epstein, DVM*, Ingrid M. Balsa, DVM

KEYWORDS

- Pyothorax • Chylothorax • Bilothorax • Hemothorax

KEY POINTS

- Exudative pleural effusions have high total protein and high nucleated cell counts.
- Hemothorax is most frequently caused by trauma or a coagulopathy, with neoplasia, infectious causes, or lung lobe torsion implicated less commonly.
- Pyothorax in dogs and cats can be successfully managed medically or surgically. Surgical indications include migrating foreign bodies or pulmonary abscessation.
- Chylothorax is a rare disease, and idiopathic effusion is the most common diagnosis. Surgical intervention is typically needed for resolution and involves thoracic duct ligation with pericardectomy or cisterna chyli ablation for optimal chances of success and can be performed with minimally invasive techniques.

ANATOMY AND DEVELOPMENT OF PLEURAL EFFUSIONS

The pleural cavity is a potential space formed by the visceral and parietal pleura. There is a right and left pleural cavity separated by the mediastinum. There is controversy in the anatomy of dogs and cats as to whether the right and left pleural cavities communicate or are isolated structures representing a barrier to movement of fluid from 1 side of the pleural cavity to the other.[1] Anatomists have described the mediastinum to be complete in the dog, whereas clinical experience suggests this might not be accurate. Infusion of saline into 1 side of the pleural cavity in dogs has resulted in bilateral distribution,[2] whereas infusion of air has remained localized unilaterally in some experimental dogs.[3] Clinical experience suggests pleural effusion that is initially unilateral can become bilateral or stay unilateral. The presence of bilateral effusions likely indicates that some dogs and cats have a communication between the left and right pleural space, whereas in other animals it does not communicate, or that communications can be sealed because of disease.

Department of Veterinary Surgical and Radiological Sciences, School of Veterinary Medicine, University of California–Davis, 1 Shields Avenue, 2112 Tupper Hall, Davis, CA 95616, USA
* Corresponding author.
E-mail address: seepstein@ucdavis.edu

Vet Clin Small Anim 50 (2020) 467–487
https://doi.org/10.1016/j.cvsm.2019.10.008
0195-5616/20/Published by Elsevier Inc.

vetsmall.theclinics.com

In health, a small volume of fluid is present in the pleural space to minimize friction during movement of the lungs throughout respiration. The amount of fluid in normal dogs and cats is approximately 0.1 and 0.3 mL/kg body weight, respectively.[4,5] The amount of fluid present is related to production through Starling forces and removal by pleural lymphatic drainage. Starling forces that promote development of pleural effusion include an increase in capillary hydrostatic pressure, a decrease in capillary colloid osmotic pressure, and an increase in permeability of the capillary wall. Alterations in the first 2 tend to lead to a transudate or modified transudate (**Table 1**).

Exudative effusions usually result from an inflammatory process within the pleural cavity that causes elaboration of cytokines or other vasoactive mediators. These substances cause an increase in capillary permeability (filtration coefficient), allowing protein-rich fluid to enter the pleural space along with a variety of inflammatory cells. This initial inflammatory response can be related to endogenous insults (eg, chyle, bile, neoplastic cells) or exogenous stimuli (eg, bacteria, virus, or fungus). The lymphatic system is responsible for draining fluid formed within the pleural space. Obstruction, disruption, or decreased efficacy of the lymphatic drainage system can also result in exudative effusions.

CLASSIFICATION AND TYPES OF EFFUSIONS

Sampling of pleural effusion via diagnostic or therapeutic thoracocentesis is indicated to classify the fluid as either a pure transudate, a modified transudate, or an exudate, as outlined in **Table 1**. The main causes of exudative pleural effusions are listed in **Box 1**.

HEMOTHORAX
Diagnosis

There is no standardized definition of hemothorax in veterinary medicine, because the hematocrit in the effusion will depend on the peripheral circulating hematocrit. Hemothorax can be defined as a pleural space effusion with a hematocrit that is at least 25% of the peripheral blood.[6] Iatrogenic hemorrhage caused by thoracocentesis can be differentiated from an existing hemorrhagic effusion by the presence of platelets in the fluid and the lack of erythrophagocytosis.

Cause

There is a multitude of causes of hemothorax in cats and dogs. The first cause to consider is blunt, sharp, or iatrogenic trauma. The history of the patient can be used to determine if the patient was hit by a car or suffered some other trauma, although sometimes this can be difficult to discern. It is usually obvious if the animal has had

Table 1 Fluid type and characteristics			
Type of Effusion	**Transudate**	**Modified Transudate**	**Exudate**
Total protein, g/dL	<2.5	2.5–7.5	>3.0
Total nucleated cell count, cells/μL	<1500	1000–7000	>7000

Data from Rizzi TE, Cowell RL, Tyler RD, et al. Effusions: abdominal, thoracic and pericardial. In: Cowell RL, Tyler RD, Menkoth JH, et al editors. Diagnostic cytology and hematology of the dog and cat. 3rd ed. St. Louis: Mosby; 2008:235-255.

Box 1
Exudative pleural effusions

Hemorrhage (dog and cat)

Bile (dog and cat)

Chyle (dog and cat)

Infectious
    Bacterial (pyothorax) (dog and cat)
    Fungal (rare)

Immune mediated
    Feline infectious peritonitis (cat)

Neoplasia (dog and cat, can also be modified transudate)

Modified from Epstein SE. Exudative pleural diseases in small animals. Vet Clin North Am Small Anim Pract. 2014; 44(1):161-180; with permission.

---

recent thoracic surgery, thoracocentesis, intrathoracic fine needle aspirate, venipuncture, or jugular catheter placement. When there is no history of trauma, coagulopathies, neoplasia, lung lobe torsion, or infectious causes can be considered.

Disorders of either primary or secondary hemostasis can lead to hemothorax, with anticoagulant rodenticide intoxication (inhibiting secondary hemostasis) being the most frequent coagulation disturbance encountered in clinical practice that results in pleural effusion. In a study of noncoagulopathic spontaneous hemothorax in dogs, the most common cause was neoplasia (14/16 dogs).[7] Identified malignancies included hemangiosarcoma, mesothelioma, metastatic carcinoma, osteosarcoma, and pulmonary carcinoma.

Other causes of hemothorax are less common and include lung lobe torsion, pancreatitis, and infectious or parasitic causes, including *Streptococcus equi* subspecies *zooepidemicus*, *Angiostrongylus vasorum*, *Spirocerca lupi*, or *Dirofilaria immitis*.[8–10] Lung lobe torsion as a cause of hemothorax has been reported in both the dog and the cat.[11] Afghan hounds and pugs are overrepresented,[12,13] and the finding of hemothorax in these breeds warrants investigation of lung lobe torsion as the underlying cause.

Treatment

Treatment of hemothorax is based on correcting the underlying cause if possible. For most traumatic cases, no specific treatment is indicated. If cardiovascular shock is present, it should be treated immediately with fluid resuscitation. Respiratory distress should be alleviated with thoracocentesis. Only sufficient blood should be removed to maintain patient comfort because the remainder of red blood cells will be reabsorbed over time. If intrathoracic neoplasia is diagnosed in a location amenable to surgical removal, resection should be considered because it can improve survival.[14]

Secondary coagulopathies should be treated with fresh frozen plasma to normalize hemostasis. As above, limited thoracocentesis is recommended initially because blood will continue to effuse until the coagulopathy is corrected. Red blood cell transfusions are sometimes needed to maintain an appropriate level of oxygen delivery. Specific treatment of an infectious disease is indicated when diagnosed. Animals with lung lobe torsion required lung lobectomy to resolve clinical signs. The prognosis for hemothorax ranges from poor to excellent depending on the underlying cause.

BILOTHORAX

Bilothorax is a rare condition in both human and veterinary medicine. It has been reported in the literature in just 5 dogs and 3 cats, although additional cases have likely been diagnosed. In dogs, 2 cases were associated with gunshot injuries, resulting in diaphragmatic tears; 1 case was due to traumatic bile duct rupture with an intact diaphragm, and the fourth case occurred after cholecystectomy in a dog with an intact diaphragm.[15–18] In cats, bilothorax was identified after thoracostomy tube placement and subsequent pleurobiliary fistula in 1 case; after suspected bite wounds over the thorax in a second cat; and after gunshot injury and diaphragmatic tear in the other.[19–21]

Diagnosis of bilothorax is based on detection of a pleural fluid-to-serum bilirubin ratio greater than 1:1. Development of bilothorax appears to occur through formation of a pleurobiliary fistula formation or in association with bile leakage into the abdomen. Bile can traverse the intact diaphragm in the lymphatics, with subsequent leakage into the pleural space.

Medical treatment of bilothorax includes placing a thoracostomy tube to allow frequent drainage of the fluid in order to minimize the degree of pleuritis resulting from bile-induced inflammation. Lavage of the pleural space with warm saline can be considered. If medical therapy fails or if a pleurobiliary fistula is identified, exploratory surgery is indicated. In veterinary medicine, bilothorax is apparently associated with an excellent prognosis, as all case reports were successfully treated.

PYOTHORAX
Cause: Dogs

Potential causes of pyothorax include migrating foreign material, penetrating bite wounds, hematogenous spread, esophageal perforation, parasitic migration, previous thoracocentesis or thoracic surgery, progression of discospondylitis, and thoracic neoplasia with abscessation. The cause of pyothorax may or may not be identified, and in 2 large retrospective series, the cause in dogs was determined in only 2% to 19% of cases.[22,23] When an underlying cause can be documented, the most common cause is a migrating grass awn or plant material. In a large-scale study of grass awn migration, approximately 3% of patients had intraabdominal or intrathoracic migration.[24] The most common cause of pyothorax is likely to be regionally dependent (eg, migrating grass awns are common in California), breed dependent (eg, prevalence of working dog breeds), and time dependent (grass awns are more often found in July to December).[25]

When a grass awn enters the mouth and migrates down the respiratory tree, it can carry oral microbiological organisms into the lower respiratory tract, resulting in infection. The shape of the grass awn favors forward migration because of barbing of the awn, and they often penetrate into the pleural space. The grass awn can then stay in the pleural space, causing pyothorax, or migrate elsewhere (eg, retroperitoneal space or out the thoracic wall into the subcutis)[26] (**Fig. 1**).

Cause: Cats

Reported causes of pyothorax in cats include parapneumonic spread, foreign body migration, hematogenous spread, or penetrating thoracic wounds. The predominant cause of feline pyothorax is not clear at this time. There is a common belief that the primary route of infection is due to bite wounds from other cats. Support for this is based on data indicating that organisms isolated from feline pyothorax are similar to those found in bite wound abscesses. In addition, affected cats are 3.8 times more

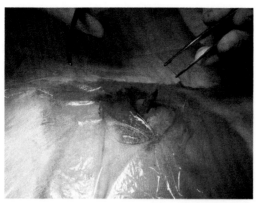

Fig. 1. Migrating plant awn removed from subcutaneous swelling in a dog with pyothorax. (*Courtesy of* Guillaume Hoareau, DVM, PhD, DACVECC, DECVECC, Salt Lake City, UT.)

likely to live in a multicat than in a single-cat household,[27] and a seasonal association has been found, with higher incidence in late summer or fall, when enhanced outdoor activity would be expected. Recent history of wounds was also documented in 14.5% to 40% of cases in 2 studies,[27,28] and a review article reported evidence supporting bite wounds as the cause in 20 out of 128 cases (15.6%).[29]

An alternate hypothesis was suggested in a retrospective study from Australia, which suggested that 15/27 (56%) cats had parapneumonic spread of infection as the likely mechanism associated with pyothorax.[30] A case series describing pneumonectomy for parapneumonic spread in 4 cats supported this cause.[31] In 2 historical studies of pleural effusion, cats with pyothorax and an identified cause of effusion had pneumonia or a focal pulmonary abscess in 7/15 (47%) cats.[32,33] At this time, the most likely cause of pyothorax has not been established, and there is evidence to support multiple causes in cats.

Diagnosis

Diagnosis of pyothorax is made based on cytologic examination of pleural fluid in combination with aerobic and anaerobic bacterial cultures. Gross characteristics of the fluid that supports the diagnosis of pyothorax include a turbid to opaque appearance and the presence of flocculent material. If anaerobic infection is present, there is often a malodorous smell. In a retrospective study of pleural and mediastinal effusions in dogs, pyothorax was the diagnosis in 13/81 (16%) cases.[34]

Analysis of fluid typically reveals an exudate, and bacteria are often identified on microscopic evaluation (**Fig. 2**). In fact, bacteria were cytologically apparent in pleural fluid of 68% of dogs and 91% of cats in 1 study.[35] Mixed populations of bacteria are commonly seen. Identification of long filamentous bacteria is suggestive of involvement with *Actinomyces* or *Nocardia* species, which are often associated with grass awn migration and can be difficult to culture.[24] Bacteria may not be identified on cytology if antimicrobials have already been administered or if nonstaining infectious organism (eg, *Mycoplasma*) is the causative agent. Nematode eggs have rarely been reported in pleural exudates of dogs.[36]

Microbiology

Multiple bacterial organisms have been cultured from dogs and cats with pyothorax. Aerobic, anaerobic, and mixed infections are documented most commonly.[22,35]

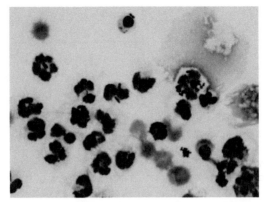

Fig. 2. Cytology of a dog with pyothorax showing both intracellular and extracellular bacteria. (*From* Epstein SE. Exudative pleural diseases in small animals. Vet Clin North Am Small Anim Pract. 2014; 44(1):161-180; with permission.)

Pasteurella spp are reported most commonly in cats, whereas in dogs, *Pasteurella* spp, the family Enterobacteriaceae, anaerobes, and *Actinomyces/Nocardia* spp, are the most common organisms isolated. **Box 2** lists other commonly identified bacteria. The fungal organisms *Cryptococcus*, *Candida*, and *Blastomyces* have been reported, but are considered rare.[30,37,38]

Signalment

Cats and dogs with pyothorax tend to be younger, with an average age of 3 to 5 years; however, it has been noted in a 1-month-old kitten[40] and even in a neonatal boxer.[41] Males of both species are overrepresented in multiple studies. Hunting dogs are overrepresented; however, no clear breed disposition compared with a general hospital population has been identified. No breed dispositions have been reported in cats, with domestic shorthairs and domestic longhairs representing the most frequently affected breeds.

Box 2
Bacteria commonly associated with pyothorax in dogs and cats

Aerobes: *Pasteurella* spp
  Escherichia coli
  Actinomyces spp
  Streptococcus canis
  Staphylococcus spp
  Corynebacterium spp (dog only)

Anaerobes: *Peptostreptococcus anaerobius*
  Bacteriodes spp
  Fusobacterium spp
  Porphyromonas spp
  Prevotella spp

Mycoplasma spp (cat only)

Data from Refs.[22,23,27,28,35,39]

Clinical Features

Animals with pyothorax have clinical signs related to pleural effusion and abscess formation. These signs can be either acute or chronic in duration. A restrictive breathing pattern can be noted in some animals, with tachypnea expected most commonly. Other common but nonspecific clinical signs include fever, anorexia, coughing, and lethargy, and these can predominate over respiratory signs. Fifty percent or less of cats with pyothorax will present with fever, showing that lack of an increase in body temperature should not exclude pyothorax from the differential list.[23,27,30]

Sepsis in cats is a common sequelae to pyothorax, and in 29 cats with severe sepsis, pyothorax was the most common underlying disease.[42] Also, in a separate retrospective study of cats diagnosed with pyothorax, greater than 50% had a concurrent clinical diagnosis of sepsis.[27] The proportion of dogs with sepsis owing to pyothorax is unknown at this time.

Clinicopathologic Findings

Abnormalities in serum biochemical analysis are common in dogs and cats with pyothorax. Elevations in liver enzyme activities, electrolyte disturbances, hypoproteinemia, and hypoglycemia or hyperglycemia are often documented. In a retrospective study, lower cholesterol concentration was a prognostic marker for survival in cats, although both groups had mean cholesterol concentrations within the reference interval, making this finding of questionable value.[27] No biochemical abnormalities detected in dogs have been associated with survival.

Hematologic abnormalities of anemia and leukocytosis with neutrophilia are common in dogs and cats. In cats with pyothorax, lower leukocyte counts were observed in cats that died compared with those that survived, but this was nonsignificant when neutrophil counts were compared.[27] Dogs showed no association of survival with leukocyte count or band neutrophil count.[43]

Diagnostic Imaging

Thoracic ultrasonography is a frequently used technique to document moderate to large volumes of pleural effusion at the cage allowing for the diagnosis of pleural effusion without moving a patient with respiratory compromise. With pyothorax, fluid is often echogenic, and fibrinous strands can be visualized between the pleural margins. Pulmonary foreign bodies can sometimes be detected,[26] and abscessation might also be detected. In 1 study, ultrasonography was a valuable tool in locating grass awns in the pleural space of 13/43 dogs, and in the pulmonary parenchyma of 10/43 dogs with suspected intrathoracic grass awn migration.[44]

Thoracic radiographs are indicated to diagnose pleural effusion when ultrasonography is not available. However, if the respiratory distress is severe, therapeutic thoracocentesis should be considered before taking radiographs, or only a dorsoventral projection should be obtained to confirm the diagnosis of pleural effusion without overly stressing the animals. However, it is important to remember that in cases of small-volume effusion, the ventrodorsal radiographic view has an increased ability to detect fluid.

If imaging is performed before thoracocentesis, radiographs will demonstrate the classic signs of pleural effusion (retraction of lung borders from thoracic wall, interlobar fissure lines, loss of ventral cardiac silhouette, and so forth). Although most cases of pyothorax show bilateral effusion, unilateral effusion is not uncommon and is easily visualized on a dorsoventral radiograph (**Fig. 3**). If radiographs are taken before pleural

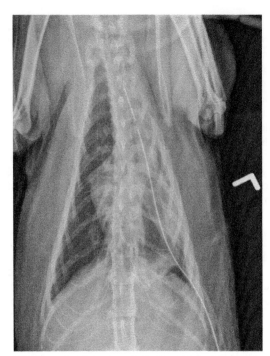

Fig. 3. Dorsoventral radiograph of a cat with unilateral pleural effusion secondary to pyothorax. A chest tube is appropriately placed in the left hemithorax to the level of the second rib. (*From* Epstein SE. Exudative pleural diseases in small animals. Vet Clin North Am Small Anim Pract. 2014; 44(1):161-180; with permission.)

drainage, they should be repeated after drainage to look for specific causes of pyothorax, such as a mass lesion, focal pulmonary opacity, or foreign body.

Computed tomography (CT) is commonly used in veterinary medicine for assessment of intrathoracic disease, including pyothorax. A study of dogs and cats analyzing results of radiographs, CT, and ultrasonography in dogs and cats with migrating intrathoracic grass awns found a significant association between radiographic and CT localization with the gross site of lesions. Importantly, CT was able to detect more sites of abnormalities and trace the path of the foreign body more accurately than radiographs.[26] In a group of 8 dogs with pyothorax, CT localization of lesions was also highly correlated to surgical findings.[45] Although 1 study suggests grass seeds were visible within the bronchus more commonly on CT than in radiographs,[25] other studies[26,39] have pointed out the weakness of CT in identifying the actual plant awn. CT is useful to determine animals in which surgical therapy is indicated due to extrapulmonary abnormalities, pulmonary abscessation, or possibly a migrating foreign body (**Fig. 4**). At the authors' institution (an area endemic for grass awns), CT is routinely used to determine extent of disease in cases where migrating grass awns are suspected as the underlying cause of the pyothorax; however, bronchoscopy is also performed as a means for confirming the presence and location of awns and potentially extracting awns in order to preserve lung lobes that are deemed salvageable.[39]

Treatment

Treatment of pyothorax can be divided into medical or surgical management. Medical management involves thoracocentesis or thoracostomy tube placement. Surgical

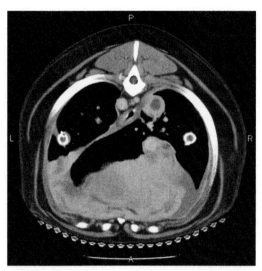

Fig. 4. CT of a dog with a pulmonary abscess secondary to a migrating plant awn. (*From* Epstein SE. Exudative pleural diseases in small animals. Vet Clin North Am Small Anim Pract. 2014; 44(1):161-180; with permission.)

intervention usually refers to exploratory thoracotomy (median sternotomy or lateral thoracotomy), although video-assisted thoracic surgery (VATS) and thoracoscopic lung lobectomy have been reported.[39,46,47] The mainstays of treatment revolve around drainage of the purulent material, removal of the underlying cause, supportive care, and systemic antimicrobial therapy.

Depending on the cause of pyothorax and thus on geographic location, drainage alone by thoracocentesis or thoracostomy tube placement can result in a good success rate in dogs[48] (**Table 2**). It should be noted however that studies with high success of medical therapy alone in dogs were performed in areas with low levels of migrating grass awns.[48] In contrast, Rooney and Monnet[43] found that treatment

Table 2		
Summary of outcome in canine pyothorax with various methods of treatment		
Study, y	Procedure (n)	Survival to Discharge, n (%)
Piek & Robben,[49] 2000	Thoracostomy tube (9) No evidence of migrating foreign body	9 (100)
Demetriou et al,[23] 2002	Thoracostomy tube (29) Surgical exploration (7)	25 (86) 6 (86)
Rooney & Monnet,[43] 2002	Thoracostomy tube (7) Thoracostomy tube followed by surgery (12) Surgical exploration (7)	5 (71) 16 (84)
Johnson & Martin,[48] 2007	Thoracocentesis (16) No evidence pulmonary mass or consolidation	15 (94)
Boothe et al,[22] 2010	Thoracocentesis (7) Thoracostomy tube (26) Surgical exploration (13)	2 (29) 20 (77) 12 (92)

Data from Refs.[22,23,43,48,49]

was 5.4 times as likely to fail in dogs treated medically as in dogs treated surgically, and 14/26 dogs (54%) had evidence of mediastinal or pulmonary lesions that necessitated surgical intervention. A more recent study by Boothe and colleagues,[22] however, failed to support that a better long-term outcome was achieved with surgical intervention. At present, there is no consensus on the ideal therapy for all cases of canine pyothorax. Most clinicians would agree that if thoracic radiography or CT suggests pulmonary abscessation or migrating foreign material, surgical exploration of the thorax is warranted. However, successful treatment with thoracostomy tube and supportive care could still be attempted when the owner is unable to pursue surgery.

Cats with pyothorax also have improved outcomes with either thoracostomy tube placement or surgical exploration over thoracocentesis alone (**Table 3**). Although there are reports of successful outcomes with single or repeated thoracocentesis, the largest retrospective study does not support this as a routine recommendation. Use of thoracostomy tubes for drainage is indicated in cats unless, similar to dogs, pulmonary abscessation or migrating foreign material is suspected, which would necessitate surgery.

If thoracostomy tubes are chosen as the drainage technique of choice, the decision to place unilateral or bilateral tubes should be made on a case-by-case basis. The authors typically will place 1 thoracostomy tube and drain the pleural space. Thoracic radiographs will be obtained, and if effective drainage with 1 tube can be accomplished leaving minimal residual effusion, only 1 tube is used. If a significant effusion is present in the hemithorax contralateral to the tube, a second thoracostomy tube can be placed. If the pyothorax is initially bilateral, then the likelihood that bilateral thoracostomy tubes will be needed is greater, and some investigators recommend routine bilateral placement. Drainage from the thoracostomy tube can be accomplished by intermittent manual drainage, or continuous suction, although this has not been shown to provide an advantage over intermittent fluid removal.

There are 2 main methods for placement of a thoracostomy tube. A small-bore wire-guided chest drain can be placed via a modified Seldinger technique, or a larger-gauge thoracostomy tube can be inserted in dogs or cats. One advantage to the small-bore (typically 14 gauge) thoracostomy tube is that it can be placed under sedation alone. Placement of this type of thoracostomy tube has been shown to be

Table 3		
Summary of outcome in feline pyothorax with various methods of treatment		
Study, y	**Procedure (n)**	**Survival to Discharge, n (%)**
Demetriou et al,[23] 2002	Thoracostomy tube (11)	10 (91)
	Surgical exploration (3)	3 (100)
Waddell et al,[27] 2002	Thoracocentesis (39)	3 (8)
	Thoracostomy tube (48)	35 (73)
	Surgical exploration (5)	5 (100)
Barrs et al,[30] 2005[a]	Thoracocentesis (2) Small volume only	2 (100)
	Thoracostomy tube (19)	18 (95)
	Surgical exploration (1)	1 (100)
Crawford et al,[31] 2011	Surgery/pneumonectomy (4)	4 (100)

[a] Five cats died or were euthanized before initiation of therapy.
Data from Refs.[23,27,30,31]

effective in 1 study involving a small group of dogs and cats with pyothorax.[50] Currently, at the authors' institution, the majority of pyothorax in dogs and cats are being treated with small-bore chest tubes.

Thoracic Lavage

Many investigators recommend thoracic lavage via a thoracostomy tube to facilitate evacuation of viscous pleural fluid. To date, no large-scale study in cats or dogs has compared outcome of lavage versus no lavage, and no information is available on optimal dwell time. In theory, the benefits of lavage include minimizing bacteria and inflammatory mediators in the pleural space as well as increased removal of thick exudate that can plug the tube. Boothe and colleagues[22] showed improved outcome when pleural lavage was performed compared with thoracocentesis only or thoracostomy tube without pleural lavage, but only 4 patients with thoracostomy tubes did not receive pleural lavage, making it difficult to interpret the results.

The addition of heparin to lavage fluid to assist with fibrin breakdown was evaluated in 1 canine study. Dogs with heparin (10 U/mL) added to their lavage fluid had improved short-term survival but no difference in long-term survival.[22] Because of this short-term survival benefit, addition of heparin is not routinely recommended for pleural lavage in pyothorax cases. Addition of fibrinolytics, such as tissue plasminogen activator or urokinase, to lavage fluid is not regularly used in human medicine for thoracic empyema and cannot be recommended for veterinary patients. More recently, the investigation of the combination of tissue plasminogen activator and deoxyribonuclease in thoracic lavage was evaluated in humans. Multiple studies have shown a benefit to this combination in the form of improved prognosis or reduced need for surgery.[51,52] No investigations of this technique have been reported in dogs or cats to date.

If pleural lavage is chosen, warmed sterile isotonic saline is used at a dose of 10 to 20 mL/kg and is infused slowly into the thoracostomy tube and left in the pleural space for 10 to 15 minutes before withdrawal. Typically, less fluid is removed than is infused. Accurate record keeping of volume in and volume out should be performed to avoid fluid overload in the patient. Hypokalemia was documented in 1 cat undergoing pleural lavage.[30]

Indwelling thoracostomy tubes are generally removed when fluid production has decreased to 3 to 5 mL/kg/d and improvement is noted clinically, radiographically, and clinicopathologically. Either ultrasonography or thoracic radiographs should be performed confirming minimal effusion in the pleural space before withdrawal of the tube. Cytologic analysis of the fluid should demonstrate no evidence of infectious organisms, and neutrophils will be nondegenerate. Generally, the neutrophil count will decline markedly with successful treatment. However, this is not always a definitive indicator of resolution of disease because the tube will generate some degree of inflammation, and when fluid production is minimal, there can be an artificial elevation of cellular concentration. Median duration of an indwelling thoracostomy tube has been reported as 5 to 8 days in patients medically managed.[22,27]

Antimicrobial Therapy

Initial antimicrobial therapy is broad spectrum and is often administered intravenously. Given the variety of pathogens reported, final therapy should be based on culture and susceptibility results; however, initially, a ß-lactam with ß-lactamase inhibitor (amoxicillin/sulbactam) antimicrobial combination is chosen because of efficacy against *Actinomyces* spp as well as anaerobes. Therapy with enrofloxacin is often added for improved gram-negative coverage pending culture results.

Antimicrobial treatment is often long term, although there is little evidence to support this. It seems likely that animals treated medically would require longer therapy than those treated surgically; however, this has also not been evaluated. One clinical approach is to have the patient return at 2-week intervals for clinical assessment and thoracic radiographs and to treat with antimicrobials for an additional 2 weeks beyond resolution of radiographic signs. Mean duration of antimicrobial therapy in 2 studies on cats with pyothorax was 5 to 7 weeks.[23,30] The British Thoracic Society recommends treatment with oral antimicrobials for at least 3 weeks for humans with pleural empyema, with the ultimate duration based on clinical, biochemical, and radiological response.[53] The International Society for Companion Animal Infectious Diseases currently recommends treatment for a minimum of 3 weeks and ideally 4 to 6 weeks[54]; however, recognizing additional research is needed to determine if shorter course may be appropriate.

Infusion of intrapleural antimicrobials has not been evaluated in veterinary pyothorax; however, it is not used in human medicine and is unlikely to be beneficial in veterinary patients. Systemic delivery results in adequate pleural concentrations for effective therapy.

Indications for Surgery

The main indications for exploratory thoracotomy are failure to respond to medical therapy or diagnostic imaging findings supportive of mediastinal or pulmonary abscessation or migrating foreign material. Failure of medical therapy would include persistence of effusion despite thoracostomy drainage, persistence of infectious organisms despite appropriate antimicrobial therapy and thoracostomy drainage, or failure of clinical improvement in the first 72 hours. The presence of Actinomyces could be considered an indication for a thoracotomy because of the association of migrating grass awns with that bacterium, although in a recent study only 20% to 30% of dogs with intrathoracic migrating plant awn cultured Actinomyces spp.[39] Clinically, it is important to note that this bacterium can be difficult to isolate, and a presumptive diagnosis of Actinomyces is often made on cytology alone; therefore, if a migrating plant awn is suspected, surgery should not be withheld because of the lack of isolation of Actinomyces on culture.

Goals at the time of surgery are to remove inciting causes that can be discovered (eg, pulmonary abscess or migrating plant awn), to debride necrotic material, such as mediastinal or pulmonary tissue, and to break down any adhesions causing pocketing of fluid that cannot be drained by a thoracostomy tube.

Bronchoscopy

The role of bronchoscopy in pyothorax secondary to grass awn migration has been investigated in veterinary medicine.[39,46] Used as an adjunctive to CT, bronchoscopy is both a diagnostic and a minimally invasive therapeutic modality to remove intrabronchial migrating plant awns.[26,39] Bronchoscopy has been shown to be successful in removal of foreign bodies in up to 76% of animals[39,55]; therefore, bronchoscopy should be considered before exploratory thoracotomy when a migrating grass awn is the suspected cause of pyothorax.

Prognosis

The prognosis for canine and feline pyothorax with appropriate treatment can be good. Ultimately, it depends on the severity of clinical signs, and animals with severe sepsis have a worse prognosis than clinically healthy animals. **Tables 2** and **3** summarize survival data from the literature since 2000 and provide an overall survival of 83% in dogs and 62% in cats using various treatment options.

CHYLOTHORAX

Chylothorax is an accumulation of chyle (lymph) within the pleural cavity resulting from impaired or obstructed lymphatic drainage. The primary lymphatic vessel within the thorax is the thoracic duct. The thoracic duct is the cranial continuation of the cisterna chyli, which returns chyle from the intestines, liver, and caudal half of the body. The thoracic duct typically converges with the venous system at the point where the internal and external jugular veins meet the cranial vena cava.

Cause

Chylothorax can result from abnormalities of the lymphatic vessels, increased venous hydrostatic pressure at the level of the right heart, abnormal organ positioning, neoplasia, or idiopathic causes. Trauma to the thoracic duct is also reported to cause chylothorax; however, in experimental models of laceration and transection of the thoracic duct in dogs, sustained chylothorax was not observed.[56] Clinically, animals with thoracic duct rupture are unlikely to develop significant pleural effusion, and such cases are not commonly recognized. Other causes of thoracic duct abnormalities include fungal granulomas, congenital abnormalities of the thoracic duct,[57] or transmural leakage across an intact but dilated vessel (lymphangiectasia). Finally, mediastinal neoplasia (lymphoma or thymoma) can result in chylothorax because of physical obstruction of the thoracic duct as it enters the jugular vein or cranial vena cava.

Increased venous pressures can be due to cardiac disease, cranial vena cava obstruction, pericardial effusion, heartworm disease, congenital cardiac abnormalities (tetralogy of Fallot, tricuspid dysplasia, double right ventricular outflow tract, or cor triatriatum dexter), or associated with primary portal venous hypoplasia.[58-61] Abnormal organ positioning from peritoneal-pericardial diaphragmatic hernia or lung lobe torsion has also been associated with chylothorax in the dog and cat.[12,62] However, the most common diagnosis in veterinary medicine appears to be idiopathic chylothorax.[63,64]

Diagnosis

Diagnosis of chylothorax is made on gross, cytologic, and biochemical examination of pleural fluid. Typically, fluid has a milky white appearance, and lymphocytes are the predominant cell, although with chronicity, the number of nondegenerate neutrophils tends to increase. Small numbers of macrophages may also be noted. A Sudan stain can be used to verify lipid content in the sample. Cytologic evaluation is also important for investigating neoplasia as a potential cause. Definitive diagnosis of chylothorax is based on detection of a triglyceride level in fluid that is higher than serum with paired sample analysis.[65] If progressive disease and anorexia result in transudation of fewer lipids into the fluid, the effusion can lose its milky white appearance and appear more similar to serum. Therefore, in an anorectic patient with pleural effusion, chylothorax should remain on the differential list until triglycerides are measured or another disease is diagnosed.

Once chylothorax has been diagnosed, further diagnostic testing, such as heartworm testing, echocardiography, thoracic ultrasound, and radiography or CT, should be performed to identify a potential cause. Abdominal imaging and assessment of gastrointestinal function can be used to investigate systemic lymphatic abnormalities. Owners should be questioned for any potential trauma in the history. If no identifiable cause is present, a diagnosis of idiopathic chylothorax is made.

Signalment

Chylothorax can occur in any breed of dog or cat; however, the Afghan hound is over-represented among dog breeds because of the association of chylothorax with lung lobe torsion.[12,66] In cats, Siamese are reported to be affected more commonly than other breeds.[67] Older cats develop chylothorax more often than younger ones, likely associated with the increased occurrence of cardiac disease and neoplasia in older cats.

Clinical Findings

Clinical signs of chylothorax are related to the development of pleural effusion. Animals can present with either acute or chronic disease. Abnormalities, such as cardiac murmurs, can be present depending on the underlying cause of the chylothorax. There are no consistent clinicopathologic abnormalities found on routine blood work associated with chylothorax.

Medical Treatment

The cornerstone of medical management of chylothorax is control of the underlying condition; however, because most cases are idiopathic, specific therapy is rarely possible. Initial therapy involves removal of pleural effusion when respiratory distress is present. Removal of the effusion alone is very unlikely to resolve the animal's condition, although there are rare reports of spontaneous resolution of chylothorax.[68] Nonetheless, surgical options are generally not pursued immediately because of the chance for spontaneous resolution or for the possibility that medical therapy will control clinical signs.

Given the lack of specific medical management possible in most cases, alternate therapies can be used on a trial basis. Rutin is a nutraceutical purported to increase uptake of edema fluid by lymphatic vessels. Rutin has been evaluated in 3 reports with 5 of 6 cats showing some degree of improvement.[69–71] The efficacy of rutin for idiopathic chylothorax in dogs has not been reported at this time. Octreotide is a somatostatin analogue that has been used in dogs and cats for management of chylothorax; however, given its low success rate, expense, and parental route of delivery, it is not widely used.

Surgical Treatment

Because of the inflammatory nature of chyle and the risks for the development of pleuritis and pericarditis, surgical intervention is recommended if chylothorax persists longer than 4 weeks despite medical therapy. Both minimally invasive and open surgical procedures to treat chylothorax are described in the veterinary literature. There are several combinations of procedures: thoracic duct ligation (TDL), cisterna chyli ablation, and pericardiectomy used in veterinary medicine to stop the accumulation of chyle in the thorax with a varying success rates reported.

Given the variation in branching of canine and feline thoracic duct anatomy, imaging of the duct before surgery and during surgery is essential to provide the surgeon with a roadmap of the branches and to allow ligation at an area of minimal branching and of all the branches to stop the flow of chyle into the thoracic cavity. Thoracic duct imaging requires injection of a contrast agent into a lymph node or tissue caudal to the thorax followed by preoperative radiographs or CT lymphangiogram (CTLA) and direct intraoperative visualization of the thoracic duct.

Currently, minimally invasive or percutaneous ultrasound-guided techniques are commonly being used for both preoperative and intraoperative imaging. The ideal preoperative technique for visualization of the thoracic duct appears to be CT because of increased identification of thoracic duct branches through CTLA versus radiography using popliteal lymphangiography.[72] Ultrasound-guided injection into mesenteric lymph node and direct injection into the popliteal lymph node and perianal region have been evaluated in dogs and cats.[72–79] In addition, intrahepatic injections have been successfully evaluated for thoracic duct visualization in normal cats.[78] CTLA appears to be adequate for the visualization of the thoracic ducts and to determine if there is cessation of flow in the thoracic following TDL (**Fig. 5**).

Intraoperative injection of methylene blue or indocyanine green (ICG) into the popliteal, mesenteric lymph nodes and diaphragmatic crus has also been reported. The purpose of this procedure is to colorize the thoracic duct in either white light (methylene blue) or near-infrared light (ICG) in order to make it easier to identify at the time of surgery. Based on a small study of normal dogs, it appears that injection into the diaphragmatic crus is less reliable than injection into a mesenteric lymph node to create coloration of the thoracic duct.[80] Thoracic duct coloration is most often identified within 10 minutes of injection with either dye.[81,82]

TDL is the most common procedure used for surgical treatment of idiopathic chylothorax in dogs and cats. The thoracic duct can be directly visualized and ligated along with each branch, or an en bloc ligation can be performed by clipping all of the structures in the caudal mediastinum dorsal to the aorta but ventral to the sympathetic ganglion.[83] This en bloc technique was evaluated in cadaveric dogs and was 93% successful in encircling all branches of the thoracic duct.[84] In clinical patients with chylothorax, ligation of the thoracic duct alone yielded a success rate of 50% to 59% in dogs and 14% to 53% in cats.[83]

Because of the relatively low success rate when performing TDL alone, it is usually combined with pericardectomy and/or cisterna chyli ablation. Previous studies have shown similar success rates for open surgical TDL combined with pericardectomy compared with TDL with cisterna chyli ablation. TDL combined with pericardectomy resolved idiopathic chylothorax in 43/55 (78%) animals.[85–88] TDL combined with cisterna chyli ablation resolved idiopathic chylothorax in 23/27 (85%) patients.[88–91]

VATS has also been used for TDL, pericardectomy, and cisterna chyli ablation in dogs and cats as a less invasive technique.[91–94] With recent advances in both preoperative and intraoperative imaging and surgery, 95% resolution of chylothorax has been reported for dogs undergoing preoperative CTLA followed by VATS TDL and

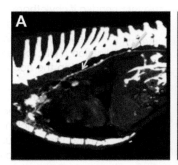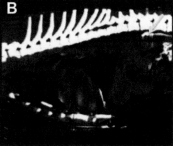

Fig. 5. (*A*) Reconstructed CT image of a dog after ultrasound-guided mesenteric lymphangiography documenting cranial mediastinal lymphangiectasia with leakage of contrast medium from the lymphatics into the cranial mediastinum. Yellow arrows highlight the thoracic duct. (*B*) Reconstructed CT image of the same dog following VATS TDL.

pericardiectomy.[95] An alternative minimally invasive approach involving catheterization of the cisterna chyli and embolization of the thoracic duct has reported success experimentally and in clinical patients with recurrent chylous effusion.[96,97]

As mentioned above, prognosis following surgical treatment of chylothorax in the veterinary literature ranges from good to excellent. It is difficult to draw a definitive conclusion as to the optimal surgical procedures to treat canine chylothorax owing to low case numbers and the variety of interventions investigated. In addition, it should be noted that several late recurrences of chylothorax in dogs have been noted in the literature.[96,97] The complication of fibrosing pleuritis as a sequela to long-term chylous effusion can also reduce surgical success rates.

If surgical intervention does not resolve chylothorax or if it recurs, pleurodesis can be considered to create adhesions between the parietal and visceral pleura; however, experimentally, it has been challenging to achieve complete adhesions that resolve chylous effusion. An alternative to pleurodesis is placement of a pleural-peritoneal shunt to allow active or passive movement of chyle into the peritoneal space for resorption. A PleuralPort (Norfolk Vet Products, Skokie, IL, USA) can also be placed. A PleuralPort is a thoracostomy tube attached to a titanium access port that is surgically placed into the subcutaneous space. Pleural effusion can then be aspirated directly by insertion of a Huber needle into the silicon port septum. Complications include blockage of the port and infection.

SUMMARY

Successful management of an exudative pleural effusion requires an accurate diagnosis of the type of effusion present and identification of the underlying condition responsible for fluid accumulation. Prognosis can be favorable; however, expensive and invasive techniques are often required for resolution.

DISCLOSURE

None.

REFERENCES

1. Evans HE. The respiratory system. In: Evans HE, editor. Miller's anatomy of the dog. Philadelphia: WB Saunders; 1993. p. 463–93.
2. Von Recum AF. The mediastinum and hemothorax, pyothorax and pneumothorax in the dog. J Am Vet Med Assoc 1977;171(6):531–3.
3. Moran JF, Jones RH, Wolfe WG. Regional pulmonary function during experimental unilateral pneumothorax in the awake state. J Thorac Cardiovasc Surg 1977;74(3):396–402.
4. Miserocchi G, Negrini D, Mortola JP. Comparative features of Starling-lymphatic interaction at the pleural level in mammals. J Appl Physiol Respir Environ Exerc Physiol 1984;54:1151–6.
5. Lai-fook SJ. Pleural mechanics and fluid exchange. Physiol Rev 2004;84:385–410.
6. Prittie J, Barton L. Hemothorax and sanguinous effusions. In: King LG, editor. Textbook of respiratory diseases in dogs and cats. St Louis (MO): Saunders; 2004. p. 610–6.
7. Nakamura RK, Rozanski EA, Rush JE. Non-coagulopathic spontaneous hemothorax in dogs. J Vet Emerg Crit Care 2008;18(3):292–7.

8. Sasanelli M, Paradies P, Otranto D, et al. Haemothorax associated with Angiostrongylus vasorum infection in a dog. J Small Anim Pract 2008;49(8):417–20.

9. Chikweto A, Bhaiyat MI, Tiwari KP, et al. Spirocercosis in owned and stray dogs in Grenada. Vet Parasitol 2012;190(3–4):613–6.

10. Byun JW, Yoon SS, Woo GH, et al. An outbreak of fatal hemorrhagic pneumonia caused by Streptococcus equi subsp. zooepidemicus in shelter dogs. J Vet Sci 2009;10(3):269–71.

11. Schultz RM, Peters J, Zwingenbuerger A. Radiography, computed tomography and virtual bronchoscopy in four dogs and two cats with lung lobe torsion. J Small Anim Pract 2009;50:360–3.

12. Neath PJ Brockman DJ, King LG. Lung lobe torsion in dogs: 22 cases (1981-1999). J Am Vet Med Assoc 2000;217(7):1041–4.

13. Murphy KA, Brisson BA. Evaluation of lung lobe torsion in pugs: 7 cases 1991-2004. J Am Vet Med Assoc 2006;228:86–90.

14. Rutherford L, Stell A, Smith K, et al. Hemothorax in three dogs with intrathoracic extracardiac hemangiosarcoma. J Am Anim Hosp Assoc 2016;52:325–9.

15. Guillaumin J, Chanoit G, Decosne-Junot C, et al. Bilothorax following cholecystectomy in a dog. J Small Anim Pract 2006;47:733–6.

16. Barnhart MD, Rasmussen LM. Pleural effusion as a complication of extrahepatic biliary tract rupture in a dog. J Am Anim Hosp Assoc 1996;32:409–12.

17. Bellenger CR, Trim C, Summer-Smith G. Bile pleuritis in a dog. J Small Anim Pract 1975;16:575–7.

18. Davis KM, Spaulding KA. Imaging diagnosis: biliopleural fistula in a dog. Vet Radiol Ultrasound 2004;45:70–2.

19. Wustefeld-Janssens BG, Loureiro JF, Dukes-McEwan J, et al. Bilothorax in a Siamese cat. J Feline Med Surg 2011;13:984–7.

20. Murgia D. A case of combined bilothorax and bile peritonitis secondary to gunshot wounds in a cat. J Feline Med Surg 2012;15(6):513–6.

21. Mullins RA, Barandun MA, Gallagher B, et al. Non-iatrogenic traumatic isolated bilothorax in a cat. JFMS Open Rep 2017;3(1). 2055116917714871.

22. Boothe HW, Howe LM, Boothe DM, et al. Evaluation of outcomes in dogs treated for pyothorax: 46 cases (1983-2001). J Am Vet Med Assoc 2010;236(6):657–63.

23. Demetriou JL, Foale RD, Ladlow J, et al. Canine and feline pyothorax: a retrospective study of 50 cases in the UK and Ireland. J Small Anim Pract 2002;43:388–94.

24. Brennan KE, Ihrke PJ. Grass awn migration in dogs and cats: a retrospective study of 182 cases. J Am Vet Med Assoc 1983;182:1201–4.

25. Vansteenkiste DP, Lee KCL, Lamb CR. Computed tomographic findings in 44 dogs and 10 cats with grass seed foreign bodies. J Small Anim Pract 2014;55(11):579–84.

26. Schultz RM, Zwingenberger A. Radiographic, computed tomographic, and ultrasonographic findings with migrating intrathoracic grass awns in dogs and cats. Vet Radiol Ultrasound 2008;49(3):249–55.

27. Waddell LS, Brady CA, Drobatz KJ. Risk factors, prognostic indicators, and outcome of pyothorax in cats: 80 cases (1986-1999). J Am Vet Med Assoc 2002;221(6):819–24.

28. Jonas LD. Feline pyothorax: a retrospective study of twenty cases. J Am Anim Hosp Assoc 1983;19:865–71.

29. Stillion JR, Letendre JA. A clinical review of the pathophysiology, diagnosis, and treatment of pyothorax in dogs and cats. J Vet Emerg Crit Care 2015;25(1):113–29.

30. Barrs VR, Allan GS, Martin P, et al. Feline pyothorax: a retrospective study of 27 cases in Australia. J Feline Med Surg 2005;7:211–22.

31. Crawford AH, Halfacree ZJ, Lee KCL, et al. Clinical outcome following pneumonectomy for management of chronic pyothorax in four cats. J Feline Med Surg 2011;13:762–7.

32. Davies C, Forrester SD. Pleural effusion in cats: 82 cases (1987-1995). J Small Anim Pract 1996;37:217–24.

33. Hayward AHS. Thoracic effusions in the cat. J Small Anim Pract 1968;9:75–82.

34. Mellanby RJ, Villiers E, Herrtage ME. Canine pleural and mediastinal effusions: a retrospective study of 81 cases. J Small Anim Pract 2002;43:447–51.

35. Walker AL, Jang SS, Hirsh DC. Bacteria associated with pyothorax of dogs and cats: 98 cases (1989-1998). J Am Vet Med Assoc 2000;216(3):359–63.

36. Klainbart S, Mazaki-Tovi M, Auerbach N, et al. Spirocercosis-associated pyothorax in dogs. Vet J 2007;173:209–14.

37. Barrs VR, Beatty JA. Feline pyothorax–new insights into an old problem: part 1. Aetiopathogenesis and diagnostic investigation. Vet J 2009;179(2):163–70.

38. McCaw D, Franklin R, Fales W, et al. Pyothorax caused by Candida albicans in a cat. J Am Vet Med Assoc 1984;85(3):311–2.

39. Gibson EA, Balsa IM, Mayhew PD, et al. Utility of bronchoscopy combined with surgery in the treatment and outcomes of dogs with intrathoracic disease secondary to plant awn migration. Vet Surg 2019. https://doi.org/10.1111/vsu.13287.

40. Gulbahar M, Gurturk K. Pyothorax associated with Mycoplasma spp and Arcanobacterium pyogenes in a kitten. Aust Vet J 2002;80(6):344–5.

41. Schoeffler GL, Rozanski EA, Rush JE. Pyothorax in a neonatal boxer. J Vet Emerg Crit Care 2001;11(2):147–52.

42. Brady CA, Otto CM, Van Winkle TJ, et al. Severe sepsis in cats: 29 cases (1986-1998). J Am Vet Med Assoc 2000;217(4):531–5.

43. Rooney MB, Monnet E. Medical and surgical treatment of pyothorax in dogs: 26 cases (1991-2001). J Am Vet Med Assoc 2002;221(1):86–92.

44. Caivano D, Birettoni F, Rishniw M, et al. Ultrasonographic findings and outcomes of dogs with suspected migrating intrathoracic grass awns: 43 cases (2010-2013). J Am Vet Med Assoc 2016;248:413–21.

45. Swinbourne F, Baines EA, Baines SJ, et al. Computed tomographic findings in canine pyothorax and correlation with findings at exploratory thoracotomy. J Small Anim Pract 2011;52:203–8.

46. Shamir S, Mayhew PD, Zwingenberger A, et al. Treatment of intrathoracic grass awn migration with video-assisted thoracic surgery in two dogs. J Am Vet Med Assoc 2016;249:214–20.

47. Pelaez MJ, Jolliffe C. Thoracoscopic foreign body removal and right middle lung lobectomy to treat pyothorax in a dog. J Small Anim Pract 2012;53(4):240–4.

48. Johnson MS, Martin MWS. Successful medical treatment of 15 dogs with pyothorax. J Small Anim Pract 2007;48:912–6.

49. Piek CJ, Robben JH. Pyothorax in nine dogs. Vet Q 2000;22(2):107–11.

50. Valtolina C, Adamantos S. Evaluation of small-bore wire-guided chest drains for management of pleural space disease. J Small Anim Pract 2009;50:290–7.

51. Piccolo F, Pitman N, Bhatnagar R, et al. Intrapleural tissue plasminogen activator and deoxyribonuclease for pleural infection. An effective and safe alternative to surgery. Ann Am Thorac Soc 2014;11(9):1419–25.

52. Piccolo F, Popowicz N, Wong D, et al. Intrapleural tissue plasminogen activator and deoxyribonuclease therapy for pleural infection. J Thorac Dis 2015;7(6): 999–1008.

53. Davies HE, Davies RJO, Davies CWH. Management of pleural infection in adults: British Thoracic Society pleural disease guideline 2010. Thorax 2010;65(suppl 2): ii41–53.

54. Lappin MR, Blondeau J, Boothe D, et al. Antimicrobial use guidelines for the treatment of respiratory tract disease in dogs and cats: antimicrobial guidelines working group of the International Society for Companion Animal Infectious Diseases. J Vet Intern Med 2017;31:279–94.

55. Tenwolde AC, Johnson LR, Hunt GB, et al. The role of bronchoscopy in foreign body removal in dogs and cats: 37 cases (2000-2008). J Vet Intern Med 2010; 24:1063–8.

56. Hodges CC, Fossum TW, Evering W. Evaluation of thoracic duct healing after experimental laceration and transection. Vet Surg 1993;22(6):431–5.

57. Schuller S, Le Garreres A, Remy I, et al. Idiopathic chylothorax and lymphedema in 2 whippet littermates. Can Vet J 2011;52:1243–5.

58. Fossum TW, Miller MW, Rogers KS, et al. Chylothorax associated with right-sided heart failure in five cats. J Am Vet Med Assoc 1994;204(1):84–9.

59. Dixon-Jimenez A, Margiocco ML. Infectious endocarditis and chylothorax in a cat. J Am Anim Hosp Assoc 2011;47(6):e121–6.

60. Singh A, Brisson BA. Chylothorax associated with thrombosis of the cranial vena cava. Can Vet J 2010;51:847–52.

61. Konstantinidis AO, Pardali D, Batra MM, et al. Chylothorax in a dog with primary hypoplasia of the portal vein. Vet Rec Case Rep 2015;3:e000210.

62. Mclane MJ, Buote NJ. Lung lobe torsion associated with chylothorax in a cat. J Feline Med Surg 2011;13:135–8.

63. Ludwig LL, Simpson AM, Han E. Pleural and extrapleural diseases. In: Ettinger SJ, Feldman EC, editors. Textbook of veterinary internal medicine. St Louis (MO): WB Saunders; 2010. p. 1131–335.

64. Singh A, Brisson B, Nykamp S. Idiopathic chylothorax: pathophysiology, diagnosis, and thoracic duct imaging. Compend Contin Educ Vet 2012;34(8):E1–8.

65. Fossum TW, Jacobs RM, Birchard SJ. Evaluation of cholesterol and triglyceride concentrations in differentiating chylous and nonchylous pleural effusions in dogs and cats. J Am Vet Med Assoc 1986;188(1):49–51.

66. Fossum TW, Brichard SJ, Jacobs RM. Chylothorax in 34 dogs. J Am Vet Med Assoc 1986;188(11):1315–8.

67. Fossum TW, Forrester SD, Swenson CL, et al. Chylothorax in cats: 37 cases (1969-1989). J Am Vet Med Assoc 1991;198(4):672–8.

68. Greenberg MJ, Weisse CW. Spontaneous resolution of iatrogenic chylothorax in a cat. J Am Vet Med Assoc 2005;226(10):1667–9.

69. Gould L. The medical management of idiopathic chylothorax in a domestic long-haired cat. Can Vet J 2004;45(1):51–4.

70. Kopko SH. The use of rutin in a cat with idiopathic chylothorax. Can Vet J 2005; 46(8):729–31.

71. Thompson MS, Cohn LA, Jordan RC. Use of rutin for medical management of idiopathic chylothorax in four cats. J Am Vet Med Assoc 1999;215(3):345–8.

72. Singh A, Brisson BA, Nykamp S, et al. Comparison of computed tomographic and radiographic popliteal lymphangiography in normal dogs. Vet Surg 2011; 40:762–7.

73. Kim M, Lee H, Lee N, et al. Ultrasound-guided mesenteric lymph node iohexol injection for thoracic duct computed tomographic lymphography in cats. Vet Radiol Ultrasound 2011;52(3):302–5.

74. Johnson EG, Wisner ER, Kyles A, et al. Computed tomographic lymphography of the thoracic duct by mesenteric lymph node injection. Vet Surg 2009;38:361–7.

75. Naganobu K, Ohigashi Y, Akiyoshi T, et al. Lymphography of the thoracic duct by percutaneous injection of iohexol into the popliteal lymph node of dogs: experimental study and clinical application. Vet Surg 2006;35:377–81.

76. Lee N, Won S, Choi M, et al. CT thoracic duct lymphography in cats by popliteal lymph node iohexol injection. Vet Radiol Ultrasound 2012;53(2):174–80.

77. Millward IR, Kirberger RM, Thompson PN. Comparative popliteal and mesenteric computed tomography lymphangiography of the canine thoracic duct. Vet Radiol Ultrasound 2011;52(3):295–301.

78. Mitchell JW, Mayhew PD, Johnson EG, et al. Video-assisted thoracoscopic thoracic duct sealing is inconsistent when performed with a bipolar vessel-sealing device in healthy cats. Vet Surg 2018;47(S1):O84–90.

79. Iwanaga T, Tokunaga S, Momoi Y. Thoracic duct lymphography by subcutaneous contrast agent injection in a dog with chylothorax. Open Vet J 2016;6(3):238–41.

80. Bayer BJ, Dujowich M, Krebs AI, et al. Injection of the diaphragmatic crus with methylene blue for coloration of the canine thoracic duct. Vet Surg 2014;43(7):829–33.

81. Enwiller TM, Radlinsky MG, Mason DE, et al. Popliteal and mesenteric lymph node injection with methylene blue for coloration of the thoracic duct in dogs. Vet Surg 2003;32:359–64.

82. Steffey MA, Mayhew PD. Use of direct near-infrared fluorescent lymphography for thoracoscopic thoracic duct identification in 15 dogs with chylothorax. Vet Surg 2018;47(2):267–76.

83. Singh A, Brisson B, Nykamp S. Idiopathic chylothorax in dogs and cats: nonsurgical and surgical management. Compend Contin Educ Vet 2012;34(8):E1–8.

84. MacDonald MH, Noble PJM, Burrow RD. Efficacy of en bloc ligation of the thoracic duct: descriptive study in 14 dogs. Vet Surg 2008;37:696–701.

85. Fossum TW, Merens MM, Miller MW, et al. Thoracic duct libation and pericardectomy for treatment of idiopathic chylothorax. J Vet Intern Med 2004;18:307–10.

86. Carobbi B, White RAS, Romanelli G. Treatment of idiopathic chylothorax in 14 dogs by ligation of the thoracic duct and partial pericardectomy. Vet Rec 2008;163:743–5.

87. Adrega da Silva C, Monnet E. Long-term outcome of dogs treated surgically for idiopathic chylothorax: 11 cases (1995-2009). J Am Vet Med Assoc 2011;239(1):107–13.

88. McAnulty JF. Prospective comparison of cisterna chyli ablation to pericardectomy for the treatment of spontaneously occurring idiopathic chylothorax in the dog. Vet Surg 2011;40:926–34.

89. Hayashi K, Sicard G, Gellash K, et al. Cisterna chyli ablation with thoracic duct ligation for chylothorax: results in eight dogs. Vet Surg 2005;34:519–24.

90. Staiger BA, Stanley BJ, McAnulty JF. Single paracostal approach to thoracic duct and cisternal chyli: experimental study and case series. Vet Surg 2011;40:786–94.

91. Mayhew PD, Culp WTN, Mayhew KN, et al. Minimally invasive treatment of idiopathic chylothroax in dogs by thoracoscopic thoracic duct ligation and subphrenic pericardiectomy: 6 cases (2007-2010). J Am Vet Med Assoc 2012;241(7):904–9.

92. Allman DA, Radlinsky MG, Ralph AG, et al. Thoracoscopic thoracic duct ligation and thoracoscopic pericardectomy for treatment of chylothorax in dogs. Vet Surg 2010;39:21–7.

93. Haimel G, Liehmann L, Dupre G. Thoracoscopic en bloc thoracic duct sealing and partial pericardectomy for the treatment of chylothorax in two cats. J Feline Med Surg 2012;14(12):928–31.
94. Morris KP, Singh A, Hold DE, et al. Hybrid single-port laparoscopic cisterna chyli ablation for the adjunct treatment of chylothorax disease in dogs. Vet Surg 2019; 48(S1):O121–9.
95. Mayhew PD, Steffey MA, Fransson BA, et al. Long-term outcome of video-assisted thoracoscopic thoracic duct ligation and pericardectomy in dogs with chylothorax: a multi-institutional study of 39 cases. Vet Surg 2019;48(S1):O112–20.
96. Singh A, Brisson BA, O'Sullivan ML, et al. Feasibility of percutaneous catheterization and embolization of the thoracic duct in dogs. Am J Vet Res 2011;72(11): 1527–34.
97. Clendaniel DC, Weisse C, Culp WT, et al. Salvage cisterna chyli and thoracic duct glue embolization in 2 dogs with recurrent idiopathic chylothorax. J Vet Intern Med 2014;28(2):672–6.

Moving?

Make sure your subscription moves with you!

To notify us of your new address, find your **Clinics Account Number** (located on your mailing label above your name), and contact customer service at:

Email: journalscustomerservice-usa@elsevier.com

800-654-2452 (subscribers in the U.S. & Canada)
314-447-8871 (subscribers outside of the U.S. & Canada)

Fax number: 314-447-8029

Elsevier Health Sciences Division
Subscription Customer Service
3251 Riverport Lane
Maryland Heights, MO 63043

*To ensure uninterrupted delivery of your subscription, please notify us at least 4 weeks in advance of move.